Workbook to Accompany

DENTAL ASSISTING

A Comprehensive Approach

Fourth Edition

6705 Hanley Dr.
Feb 3 1pm a 5pm

Workbook to Accompany

DENTAL ASSISTING

A Comprehensive Approach

Fourth Edition

Donna J. Phinney, CDA, FADAA, BA, MEd
Professor Spokane Community College

Judy H. Halstead, CDA, BA
Professor Emeritus Spokane Community College

Part II: Practice Management Software
prepared by
Cynthia Lamkin

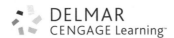
DELMAR
CENGAGE Learning™

Australia • Brazil • Japan • Korea • Mexico • Singapore • Spain • United Kingdom • United States

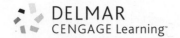
DELMAR
CENGAGE Learning™

Workbook to Accompany Dental Assisting: A Comprehensive Approach Fourth Edition

Donna J. Phinney and Judy H. Halstead

Vice President, Editorial: Dave Garza

Director of Learning Solutions: Matthew Kane

Acquisitions Editor: Tari Broderick

Managing Editor: Marah Bellegarde

Senior Product Manager: Darcy M. Scelsi

Editorial Assistant: Nicole Manikas

Vice President, Marketing: Jennifer Baker

Marketing Manager: Scott Chrysler

Production Director: Wendy Troeger

Production Manager: Andrew Crouth

Senior Content Project Manager: Kenneth McGrath

Senior Art Director: Jack Pendleton

Technology Project Manager: Brandon Dingeman

Production Technology Analyst: Mary Colleen Liburdi

For product information and technology assistance, contact us at
Cengage Learning Customer & Sales Support, 1-800-354-9706
For permission to use material from this text or product,
submit all requests online at **www.cengage.com/permissions**
Further permissions questions can be e-mailed to
permissionrequest@cengage.com

Library of Congress Control Number: 2011943937

ISBN-13: 978-1-1115-4299-3

ISBN-10: 1-1115-4299-6

Delmar
5 Maxwell Drive
Clifton Park, NY 12065-2919
USA

Cengage Learning is a leading provider of customized learning solutions with office locations around the globe, including Singapore, the United Kingdom, Australia, Mexico, Brazil, and Japan. Locate your local office at: **international.cengage.com/region**

Cengage Learning products are represented in Canada by Nelson Education, Ltd.

To learn more about Delmar, visit **www.cengage.com/delmar**

Purchase any of our products at your local college store or at our preferred online store **www.cengagebrain.com**

Notice to the Reader

Publisher does not warrant or guarantee any of the products described herein or perform any independent analysis in connection with any of the product information contained herein. Publisher does not assume, and expressly disclaims, any obligation to obtain and include information other than that provided to it by the manufacturer. The reader is expressly warned to consider and adopt all safety precautions that might be indicated by the activities described herein and to avoid all potential hazards. By following the instructions contained herein, the reader willingly assumes all risks in connection with such instructions. The publisher makes no representations or warranties of any kind, including but not limited to, the warranties of fitness for particular purpose or merchantability, nor are any such representations implied with respect to the material set forth herein, and the publisher takes no responsibility with respect to such material. The publisher shall not be liable for any special, consequential, or exemplary damages resulting, in whole or in part, from the readers' use of, or reliance upon, this material.

Printed in the United States of America
4 5 6 7 8 9 10   20 19 18 17 16

CONTENTS

This workbook is designed to accompany *Dental Assisting: A Comprehensive Approach,* Fourth Edition. The workbook also contains a DENTRIX® Learning Edition CD with introductory content and practice activities. Using the textbook and this Workbook, along with other components of Cengage's complete learning system, will help you become a successful dental assistant. The complete learning system will help reinforce all the essential competencies you will need to enter the field of dental assisting and become a highly skilled professional in today's multiskilled health care environment. In addition, this workbook will challenge you to apply basic skills, use assessment evaluations, and integrate your knowledge effectively.

WORKBOOK ORGANIZATION

The Workbook has been divided into two parts. Part I is a review of the concepts presented in the textbook and correlates to the chapters in the textbook. These Workbook chapters are divided into the following sections: Specific Instructional Objectives, Summary, Exercises and Activities, and Skill Competency Assessments.

Specific Instructional Objectives

The list of objectives reiterates those found at the beginning of each textbook chapter. Reviewing these objectives will reinforce the facts and principles that need to be understood in each chapter.

Summary

The summary provides a brief overview of the chapter content and describes the responsibilities of the dental assistant.

Exercises and Activities

These exercises cover the basic chapter content and terminology, further reinforcing your understanding and mastery of chapter material. Activities include true or false, multiple choice, matching, labeling, critical thinking, and case studies.

Skill Competency Assessments

This workbook provides Skill Competency Assessment checklists that are designed to correlate with specific information and procedures found in *Dental Assisting: A Comprehensive Approach,* Fourth Edition.

The checklists are designed to set criteria or standards that should be observed while a specific procedure is performed. They follow the same procedural steps as listed in the textbook. As you perform each procedure, the evaluation sections of the sheet are used to judge your performance with an opportunity for self-evaluation.

The instructor will also use this sheet to evaluate your competency in performing the specific skill identified in each procedure. The comment portion of the checklist allows for constructive feedback.

The Skill Competency Assessment sheet is organized as follows:

- *Skill*—Describes the procedure.

- *Performance Objective*—Identifies what must be successfully demonstrated by the student.

- *Equipment and Supplies*—Lists the equipment and supplies required to perform the procedure, along with the possible points earned for successfully gathering each piece.

- *Competency Steps*—Lists each step to be described or performed by the student in order to successfully complete the procedure, along with the possible points earned for completing each step.

- *Total Points*—Lists the total points possible for a first or second attempt at performing the procedure along with a space for entering the actual points earned.

The points assigned to each step reflect the importance of that step in meeting the performance objective. An important step is valued with 1 point, an essential step with 2 points, and a critical step with 3 points. Failure results if any of the critical steps are missed or performed incorrectly.

A Skill Tracking Sheet is provided on pages ix–xv to serve as a table of contents for all assessments, as well as a guide to easily view your performance.

Part Two of the Workbook is to be used with the DENTRIX® Learning Edition CD. Information is provided in two sections, Patient Management and Practice Management. An overview of the functions of the various tools within the software is provided along with exercises to use as practice to allow you to become accustomed to working with the software. While DENTRIX® is just one of several different practice management systems you may encounter in your career, the skills you learn using this one will easily allow you to adapt to any other system that may be in use when you begin your work in a dental office.

GENERAL STUDY TIPS

- Feel certain that each procedure and concept that you master is an important step toward preparing you for the workplace. The textbook, CDs, workbook, and instructor materials have all been coordinated to meet the specific instructional objectives. Review the objectives before you begin to study as they are a road map that will take you to your goal.

- Remember that you are the learner, so you can take credit for your success. The instructor is an important guide on this journey, and the textbook, CDs, workbook, and clinical experiences are tools. Whether you use these tools wisely is ultimately up to you.

- Evaluate yourself and your study habits. Take positive action toward improving yourself, and avoid habits that could limit your success. For example, do you let family responsibilities or social opportunities interfere with your study? If so, sit down with your family and plan a schedule for study that they will support and to which you will adhere. Find a special place to study that is free from distraction.

Because regulations vary from state to state regarding which procedures can be performed by a dental assistant, checking specific regulations in your state will be important. A dental assistant should never perform a procedure without being aware of legal responsibilities, correct procedure, and proper authorization. Enjoy your new career in dental assisting!

SKILL COMPETENCY ASSESSMENT TRACKING SHEET

Date Assessment Completed and Competency Achieved

Assessment No. and Title	Workbook Page No.	Self-Evaluation Date/Initials	Student Evaluation Date/Initials	Instructor Evaluation Date/Initials
4-1 Applying Disclosing Agent for Plaque Identification				
4-2 Bass or Modified Bass Brushing Technique				
4-3 Charters Brushing Technique				
4-4 Modified Stillman Brushing Technique				
4-5 Rolling Stroke Brushing Technique				
4-6 Fones Brushing Technique				
4-7 Modified Scrub Brushing Technique				
4-8 Dental Flossing Technique				
4-9 Fluoride Application				
11-1 Handwashing				
11-2 Putting on Personal Protective Equipment				
11-3 Removing Personal Protective Equipment				
11-4 Preparing the Dental Treatment Room				
11-5 Completion of Dental Treatment				
11-6 Final Treatment Room Disinfecting and Cleaning				
11-7 Treatment of Contaminated Tray in the Sterilization Center				
11-8 Dental Radiography Infection Control Protocol				
13-1 Taking an Oral Temperature Using a Digital Thermometer				
13-2 Taking Tympanic Temperature				
13-3 Taking a Radial Pulse and Measuring the Respiration Rate				
13-4 Measuring Blood Pressure				
16-1 Administration of Oxygen				
16-2 CPR for an Adult, One Rescuer				

Assessment No. and Title	Workbook Page No.	Self-Evaluation Date/Initials	Student Evaluation Date/Initials	Instructor Evaluation Date/Initials
16-3 Rescue Breathing for Adults				
16-4 Operating an Automated External Defibrillation (AED) Unit				
16-5 Heimlich Maneuver (Subdiaphragmatic Thrusts) for a Conscious Adult				
16-6 Adult with Airway Obstruction				
16-7 Treatment of a Patient with Syncope				
17-1 Daily Routine to Open the Office				
17-2 Daily Routine to Close the Office				
17-3 Seating the Dental Patient				
17-4 Dismissing the Dental Patient				
19-1 One-Handed Instrument Transfer				
19-2 Specific Tip Placements for Evacuation of Oral Cavity				
20-1 Preparing the Anesthetic Syringe				
20-2 Assisting with the Administration of Topical and Local Anesthetics				
20-3 Administration and Monitoring of Nitrous Oxide Sedation				
22-1 Radiography Infection Control				
22-2 Full-Mouth X-Ray Exposure with Paralleling Technique				
22-3 Exposing Occlusal Radiographs				
22-4 Full-Mouth Pediatric X-Ray Exposure				
22-5 Processing Radiographs Using a Manual Tank				
22-6 Processing Radiographs Using an Automatic Processor				
22-7 Mounting Radiographs				
22-8 Processing Duplicating Technique				
23-1 Exposing Panoramic Radiographs				
23-2 Digital Radiology Techniques				

Assessment No. and Title	Workbook Page No.	Self-Evaluation Date/Initials	Student Evaluation Date/Initials	Instructor Evaluation Date/Initials
24-1 Electronic Pulp Testing				
24-2 Root Canal Treatment				
24-3 Apicoectomy				
25-1 Surgical Scrub				
25-2 Routine or Uncomplicated Extraction				
25-3 Multiple Extractions and Alveoplasty				
25-4 Removal of Impacted Third Molars				
25-5 Biopsy				
25-6 Dental Implant Surgery				
25-7 Treatment for Alveolitis				
25-8 Removal of Simple and Continuous Simple Sutures				
25-9 Removal of Sling and Continuous Sling Sutures				
25-10 Removal of Horizontal and Vertical Mattress Sutures				
27-1 Placement and Removal of Elastic Separators				
27-2 Placement and Removal of Steel Spring Separators				
27-3 Placement and Removal of Brass Wire Separators				
27-4 Cementation of Orthodontic Bands				
27-5 Direct Bonding of Brackets				
27-6 Placement of the Arch Wire and Ligature Ties				
27-7 Completion Appointment				
28-1 T-Band Placement				
28-2 Spot-Welded Matrix Band Placement				
28-3 Pulpotomy				
28-4 Stainless Steel Crown Placement				
28-5 Procedure for Placing Dental Sealants				

Assessment No. and Title	Workbook Page No.	Self-Evaluation Date/Initials	Student Evaluation Date/Initials	Instructor Evaluation Date/Initials
29-1 Occlusal Adjustment				
29-2 Scaling, Curettage, and Polishing				
29-3 Gingivectomy				
29-4 Osseous Surgery				
29-5 Preparation and Placement of Noneugenol Periodontal Dressing				
29-6 Removal of the Periodontal Dressing				
29-7 Polishing with Rubber Cup				
29-8 Using Prophy Brush				
29-9 Polishing with Dental Tape and Floss				
29-10 Coronal Polishing Procedure				
30-1 Porcelain Veneers				
30-2 Preparation for Porcelain-Fused-to-Metal Crown				
30-3 Cementation of Porcelain-Fused-to-Metal Crown				
30-4 Placing and Removing Retraction Cord				
31-1 Nonvital Whitening				
31-2 In-Office Whitening for Vital Teeth				
31-3 Home Whitening				
32-1 Final Impressions for Partial Denture				
32-2 Try-In Appointment for Partial Denture				
32-3 Delivery Appointment for Partial Denture				
32-4 Final Impression Appointment				
32-5 Jaw Relationship Appointment				
32-6 Try-In Appointment				
32-7 Appointment for Delivery of Complete Denture				
32-8 Chairside Denture Relining				
33-1 Mixing Zinc Phosphate Cement				

Assessment No. and Title	Workbook Page No.	Self-Evaluation Date/Initials	Student Evaluation Date/Initials	Instructor Evaluation Date/Initials
33-2 Mixing Zinc Oxide Eugenol Cement—Powder/Liquid Form				
33-3 Mixing Zinc Oxide Eugenol Cement—Two-Paste System				
33-4 Mixing Polycarboxylate Cement				
33-5 Mixing Glass Ionomer Cement				
33-6 Mixing of Calcium Hydroxide Cement—Two-Paste System				
33-7 Preparing Cavity Varnish				
33-8 Placing Resin Cement—Dual-Curing Technique				
33-9 Placing Etchant				
33-10 Placing Bonding Agent				
33-11 Placing Cavity Liners—Glass Ionomer				
33-12 Placing Cavity Varnish				
33-13 Placement of Cement Bases				
34-1 Using Dental Amalgamator				
34-2 Complete Amalgam Restoration—Class II				
34-3 Complete Composite Restoration—Class III				
34-4 Placing and Removing Dental Dam				
34-5 Rubber Dam Application for Child Patient				
34-6 Quickdam Placement				
34-7 Assembly of Tofflemire Matrix				
34-8 Placement of Tofflemire Matrix				
34-9 Removal of Wedge and Tofflemire Matrix				
34-10 Placement of Strip Matrix				
34-11 Removal of Strip Matrix				
35-1 Mixing Alginate with Alginator II Mixing Device				
35-2 Preparing for Alginate Impression				

Assessment No. and Title	Workbook Page No.	Self-Evaluation Date/Initials	Student Evaluation Date/Initials	Instructor Evaluation Date/Initials
35-3 Taking Alginate Impression				
35-4 Removing Alginate Impression				
35-5 Disinfecting Alginate Impressions				
35-6 Taking Bite Registration				
35-7 Taking Polysulfide Impression				
35-8 Taking Silicone (Polysiloxane) Two-Step Impression				
35-9 Pouring Alginate Impression with Plaster				
35-10 Pouring Alginate Impression for Study Model				
35-11 The Art of Pouring a Plaster Study Model Using the Two-Pour Method				
35-12 Removing Plaster Model from Alginate Impression				
35-13 Trimming Diagnostic Casts/Study Models				
35-14 Taking the Records and Performing a Facebow Transfer				
35-15 Mount Models on Articulator After Facebow Records Have Been Completed				
35-16 Constructing Self-Cured Acrylic Resin Custom Tray				
35-17 Constructing Vacuum-Formed Acrylic Resin Custom Tray				
35-18 Sizing, Adapting, and Seating Aluminum Temporary Crown				
35-19 Cementing Aluminum Crown				
35-20 Sizing, Adapting, and Seating Preformed Acrylic Crown				
35-21 Adapting, Trimming, and Seating Matrix and Custom Temporary Restoration				
35-22 Preparing a Full Crown Provisional on a Lower Left Molar				
35-23 Cementing Custom Self-Curing Composite Temporary Crown				

Assessment No. and Title	Workbook Page No.	Self-Evaluation Date/Initials	Student Evaluation Date/Initials	Instructor Evaluation Date/Initials
36-1 Preparing for the Day's Patients				
36-2 Day Sheet Preparation for Posting				
36-3 Posting Charges and Payments on Pegboard				
36-4 Balancing Day Sheets and End-of-the-Month Figures				
36-5 Preparing a Deposit Slip				
36-6 Reordering Supplies				
36-7 Reconciling a Bank Statement				
36-8 Writing a Business Check				

Review of Textbook Chapters

Introduction

Introduction to the Dental Profession

SPECIFIC INSTRUCTIONAL OBJECTIVES

The student should strive to meet the following objectives and demonstrate an understanding of the facts and principles presented in this chapter:

1. Review dental disease and dentistry from the "beginning of time."
2. Identify the items on the timeline of dental history.
3. Name the individuals who had a great impact on the profession of dentistry.
4. Identify the people who promoted education and organized dentistry.
5. Explain what DDS and DMD stand for.
6. Identify the nine specialties of dentistry.
7. Describe, generally, the career skills performed by dental assistants, dental hygienists, and dental laboratory technicians.
8. List the education required for, and the professional organizations that represent, each dental career path.

SUMMARY

It is important to know the historic struggles that took place and contributions that were made to advance the dentistry profession into what it is today. Organized dentistry was formed with the intent to promote the sharing of information concerned with excellence in dentistry. To provide excellence in dentistry, additional dental team members (such as dental assistants, dental receptionists, dental hygienists, and dental laboratory technicians) would become recognized and add contributing roles to the field. Therefore, the dental assistant will need to be able to identify and define those who contribute to the dental profession and look forward to the future of dentistry.

EXERCISES AND ACTIVITIES

Multiple Choice

100%

1. Dr. Greene Vardiman Black was known as

   a. an inventor of numerous machines for testing alloys.

   b. an inventor of numerous instruments to refine the cavity prep.

   c. the "grand old man of dentistry."

   d. all of the above.

2. The ADA represents _____.

   a. hygienists

   b. assistants

   c. dentists

   d. laboratory technicians

3. The ADAA represents _____.

   a. hygienists

   b. assistants

   c. dentists

   d. laboratory technicians

4. An endodontist handles _____.

   a. oral care in children

   b. removal of third molars

   c. root canal therapy

   d. removal of calculus

5. Orthodontics is the specialty of performing _____.

   a. root canal therapy

   b. straightening of the teeth

   c. extraction of third molars

   d. treatment of surrounding tissues

6. Pediatric dentistry is the specialty concerned with _____.

   a. geriatric patients

   b. extraction of third molars

   c. oral care of children

   d. straightening teeth with braces

7. The specialty concerned with the diagnosis and treatment of the diseases of the tissues that support and surround the tooth is _____.

   a. endodontics

   b. orthodontics

   c. periodontics

   d. pediatric dentistry

8. The first dentist, whose name was recorded in 3000 BCE, was_____.

   a. Pierre Fauchard

   b. Hesi-Re

   c. John Greenwood

   d. Guy de Chauliac

9. _____ is considered to be one of the founders of professional dentistry in the United States.

   a. Horace Hayden

   b. Paul Revere

   c. Robert Woofendale

   d. Josiah Flagg

10. _____ helped to establish the first national association to represent the dental profession.

    a. James B. Morrison

    b. John Greenwood

    c. Josiah Flagg

    d. Chapin Harris

Matching

Match the individual with his contribution.

Individual

1. _C_ Hippocrates

2. _D_ Guy de Chauliac

3. _B_ Leonardo da Vinci

4. _G_ Pierre Fauchard

5. _A_ Wilhelm Conrad Roentgen

6. _E_ Paul Revere

7. _F_ Robert Woofendale

Contribution

a. Discovered x-rays

b. First to make the distinction between premolars and molars

c. Father of medicine

d. Wrote the "Hygienic Rules for Oral Hygiene"

e. Silversmith who made surgical instruments and advertised as a dentist

f. One of the first dentists to arrive in the colonies from England

g. Early advocate of treatment for diseased gingival tissue

 Critical Thinking

1. Name the four principles on which the American Dental Assistants Association was founded.

2. There are certain benefits to membership in the American Dental Assistants Association.

   a. Name the benefits.

   b. What is the ADAA's Web site address?

   c. How does this professional organization assist you?

3. Provide the year in which each of the following dentistry technologies was introduced or reported.

   a. First dental foot engine constructed.

   b. Development of the dental chair.

   c. Discovery that nitrous oxide can be used for dental pain relief.

   d. First commercially manufactured foot-treadle dental engine is patented.

   e. First fluoride toothpastes are marketed.

   f. Four-handed, sit-down dentistry is adopted.

   g. First synthetic bristle (nylon) toothbrush marketed.

   h. Hepatitis B vaccine becomes available.

   i. First reclining dental chair invented.

   j. Food and Drug Administration approves use of the laser in removing tooth decay.

   k. "Lost wax" casting machine is invented.

l. Tooth-whitening commercial products are marketed.

m. The x-ray is discovered.

CASE STUDY 1

Gwen, age 18, is a first-year college student. She has occasionally experienced swollen gums at the back of her last molar. Now, it is final exam week and the swelling will not go down.

1. What should Gwen do?

2. What specialist would Gwen be referred to for resolving this condition?

CASE STUDY 2

Meridith, age 45, has recently been diagnosed with various conditions. A specialist is indicated to treat each of these conditions. What specialist will be sought for each of the following conditions?

1. Gum and bone loss.

2. Decay that has infected both the pulp canal and root/apex of the anterior tooth.

3. An impacted third molar.

4. A lesion unknown in general dentistry.

CHAPTER 2

Psychology, Communication, and Multicultural Interaction

SPECIFIC INSTRUCTIONAL OBJECTIVES

The student should strive to meet the following objectives and demonstrate an understanding of the facts and principles presented in this chapter:

1. Define psychology and paradigm.

2. Describe the components of the communication process.

3. Describe how the baby boomer generation may differ from generations "X" and "Y."

4. List the skills used in listening.

5. Differentiate the terms used in verbal and nonverbal communication.

6. Demonstrate how the following body language is used in nonverbal communication behavior: spatial, posture, facial expression, gestures, and perception.

7. Discuss how Maslow's hierarchy of needs is used and how it relates to communication in today's dental office.

8. Discuss how defense mechanisms can inhibit communication.

9. Describe some general behaviors of multicultural patient populations.

SUMMARY

The role of the dental assistant includes making dental treatment comfortable for patients of any culture by understanding those patients' psychological backgrounds and their paradigms concerning dentistry. Appropriate communication is the key to successful interaction. A dental assistant should have skills in listening and in verbal and nonverbal communication, and should know how to overcome defense mechanisms to meet patient needs.

EXERCISES AND ACTIVITIES

True or False

Circle whether the answer is true of false. If false, rewrite the statement to make it true.

1. Abraham Maslow is considered the founder of a movement called *humanistic psychology.*

    a. True

    b. False

2. The dental assistant can communicate with and treat all patients in the same manner.

    a. True

    b. False

3. Encoding involves the use of specific signs, symbols, interpersonal communication, or language used in sending the message.

    a. True

    b. False

4. The kinesthetic channel of communication is hearing or listening to the verbal message.

    a. True

    b. False

5. Psychology is an acquired belief system that a person establishes through various life experiences.

    a. True

    b. False

Multiple Choice

1. _____ is the science of the mind and of the reasons people think and act as they do.

    a. A person's paradigm

    b. Psychology

    c. Communication

    d. Hierarchy of needs

2. Observation and perception use which channel(s) to receive a message?

    a. Auditory

    b. Visual

    c. Kinesthetic

    d. All of the above

3. The communication process begins with

    a. the message.

    b. the sender.

    c. the feedback.

    d. the receiver.

4. On average, how much time during the day do most college students spend talking?

    a. 15%

    b. 20%

    c. 25%

    d. 30%

5. What proportion of communication is verbal?

    a. 20%

    b. 40%

    c. 60%

    d. 80%

6. Which generation is often referred to as the "me generation"?

    a. Generation "X"

    b. Generation "Y"

    c. The MTV generation

    d. Baby boomers

7. The generation that statistically holds the highest education levels is commonly referred to as

    a. generation "X."

    b. generation "Y."

    c. brainy boomers.

    d. baby boomers.

8. This generation is thought of as being highly connected.

    a. Generation "X"

    b. Generation "Y"

    c. Generation "I"

    d. Baby boomers

9. Intimate touching often occurs within a distance of

    a. 3 inches.

    b. 6 inches.

    c. 9 inches.

    d. 12 inches.

10. If a patient is having difficulty breathing, which level of Maslow's hierarchy needs to be addressed?

    a. Belongingness and love

    b. Prestige and esteem

    c. Self-actualization

    d. Survival and physiological

Matching

Match each term with the appropriate definition.

Term	Definition
1. _____ Psychology	a. Act of passing along information, or transmitting any idea
2. _____ Paradigm	b. Humanistic psychology, self-actualization
3. _____ Communication	c. Life experiences that comprise personal belief systems
4. _____ Maslow's Hierarchy of Needs	d. Science of mind and of the reasons people think and act as they do

Communication consists of five major process components. Match each term with its process.

Term	Process
5. _____ Sender	a. Communication medium in which message is sent
6. _____ Message	b. Formulated response, after decoding
7. _____ Channel	c. Shapes the idea, often starts an image the sender visualizes
8. _____ Receiver	d. Stimuli produced by the sender in written, verbal, or non-verbal form
9. _____ Feedback	e. Takes the message and must make some sense of what the sender transmitted in the message

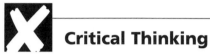 **Critical Thinking**

1. It is critical for a dental assistant to be a good listener and observer. During a dental procedure, the dental assistant notices that the patient is squeezing the dental chair arm and his knuckles are white. Name this method of communication. What can the dental assistant do in response to this communication to meet the patient's needs?

2. The dental assistant is speaking to a patient to explain proper flossing technique. While speaking to the patient, the dental assistant demonstrates the technique using a model of the teeth and some dental floss. What channel(s) of communication is the dental assistant using to send a message to the patient?

3. During a charting exercise, the dental assistant is uncertain about the tooth number, the surface, and the diagnosis to be charted. What communication skill is necessary for her to ensure a correct recording?

4. The dental assistant is speaking over the phone to a patient with a toothache who wishes to be seen as soon as possible. What actions can the dental assistant take to make sure the patient's needs are met and that the patient feels comfortable with how his or her needs are being addressed?

5. Some patients frequently use defense mechanisms to block communication. How would the dental assistant overcome this type of resistance to communication?

6. Maslow studied well-adjusted people and identified several levels of human needs. Provide an example for each level of need on Maslow's hierarchy of needs.

Self-Actualization

Prestige and Esteem Needs

Belongingness and Love Needs

Safety Needs

Survival or Physiological Needs

Ethics, Jurisprudence, and the Health Information Portability and Accountability Act

SPECIFIC INSTRUCTIONAL OBJECTIVES

The student should strive to meet the following objectives and demonstrate an understanding of the facts and principles presented in this chapter:

1. Identify the difference between civil and criminal law.

2. Define the Dental Practice Act and what it covers.

3. Identify who oversees the Dental Practice Act and how licenses for the dental profession are obtained.

4. Define expanded functions.

5. Identify the components of a contract.

6. Identify due care and give examples of malpractice and torts.

7. Define fraud and where it may be seen in the dental office.

8. Identify care that can be given under the Good Samaritan Law.

9. Identify the four areas of the Americans with Disabilities Act.

10. Identify the responsibilities of the dental team in regard to dental records, implied and informed consent, subpoenas, and the statute of limitations.

11. Define ethics and give examples of the American Dental Association and American Dental Assistants Association's principles of ethics.

12. State how dentistry follows ethical principles in regard to advertising, professional fees and charges, and professional responsibilities and rights.

13. State how the HIPAA law has impacted the dental office and identify the parameters of the law.

14. Identify how patient health information can be used and disclosed, as well as the rights of the patients.

15. Gain an understanding of requirements that the staff must follow to be compliant with the HIPAA laws.

16. Identify the CDT transactions and code sets.

SUMMARY

Each dental team member is faced with daily decisions that require judgments regarding legal and ethical principles. Maintaining professional ethical standards at all times is essential. The consequences for not doing what should be legally done or doing what should not be done can include fines or imprisonment. A license is granted to protect the public from unqualified individuals providing dental treatment. Some states require dental assistants to become licensed to perform specific dental tasks. The expanded functions are most often specified in the Dental Practice Act according to how they are to be delegated. They may be stipulated for general supervision, which means that

the procedure authorized in the Dental Practice Act can be legally performed on a patient of record by the dental assistant under the general supervision of the dentist, or they may be specified to be delegated under direct supervision. The dental assistant must thoroughly understand the law in order to protect the patient, the dentist, and the profession. Dental health care continues to change, and the assistant must understand how the law affects these changes and must stay within the law. HIPAA regulations are required to protect patient information. It is the responsibility of the dental team members to stay informed and comply with the standards.

EXERCISES AND ACTIVITIES

True or False

1. The office HIPAA manual must include a job description for each employee.

   a. True
   b. False

2. The office HIPPA manual must have a HIPAA training plan with dates of training for each employee.

   a. True
   b. False

3. In order to maintain security of personal health information, locks must be placed on all cabinets in the dental office.

   a. True
   b. False

4. The dental office does not have a right to charge for copying and transferring patient information.

   a. True
   b. False

5. The Security Rule mandates the safeguards required to control access and protect information from accidental disclosure to an unauthorized person.

  a. True
  b. False

Multiple Choice

1. The area of law that governs dentistry is
  a. civil law.
  b. criminal law.
  c. dental jurisprudence.
  d. common law.

2. Defining what is right and wrong is called
  a. civil law.
  b. criminal law.
  c. common law.
  d. ethics.

3. What is (are) enacted by each state legislative body to establish rules and regulations?
  a. State Board of Dentistry
  b. Statutes
  c. Dental Practice Act
  d. Reciprocity

4. What gives states the guidelines regarding eligibility for licensing and identifies the grounds by which this license can be suspended or repealed?
  a. Dental jurisprudence
  b. Dental Practice Act
  c. State Board of Dentistry
  d. Statutes

5. Delegated functions that require increased responsibility and skill are called
  a. expanded functions.
  b. dental jurisprudence.
  c. laws.
  d. contracts.

6. In some states, an individual who has passed the requirements for one state may apply for an agreement in another state to be allowed to perform dental skills without retaking a written or clinical exam. What is this called?
  a. contract
  b. consent
  c. reciprocity
  d. malpractice

7. Expanded functions are specific advanced functions that require increased skill and responsibility. Like all functions that the auxiliary performs, the expanded functions fall under the _____, which means "Let the master answer."
  a. American Dental Association
  b. Dental Practice Act
  c. Good Samaritan Law
  d. doctrine of respondeat superior

8. A binding agreement between two or more people is called
  a. a contract.
  b. informed consent.
  c. implied consent.
  d. a tort.

9. A contract that is written or verbal and that describes specifically what each party in the contract will do is called
  a. informed consent.
  b. an expressed contract.
  c. a breach of contract.
  d. a termination contract.

10. The _____ is the enforcement authority for transactions, code set identifiers, and security.
  a. PHI
  b. CDT
  c. CMS
  d. HHS

11. What is the legal term used for the situation in which a dentist fails to notify a patient that she or he can no longer provide services?

    a. Noncompliance

    b. Due care

    c. Negligence

    d. Abandonment

12. The dentist and the dental team members have the responsibility and duty to perform due care in treating all patients. What is failure to do this is called?

    a. Assault

    b. Sufficient care

    c. Malpractice

    d. Abandonment

13. A tort law protects against an individual causing injury to another person's reputation, name, or character. This injury is called

    a. invasion of privacy.

    b. defamation of character.

    c. assault and battery.

    d. fraud.

14. The area of law covering any wrongful act that is a breach in due care that results in an injury to another person is called

    a. malpractice.

    b. ethics.

    c. civil law.

    d. torts.

15. If a child refused treatment and the dental personnel threatened and restrained the child without parental consent, what charges could be brought?

    a. Civil law

    b. Criminal law

    c. Assault and battery

    d. Invasion of privacy

16. The general term for the situation in which care is given without intent to do bodily harm and without compensation for this care is called

    a. the Americans with Disabilities Act.

    b. invasion of privacy.

    c. Doctrine of Respondeat Superior.

    d. a Good Samaritan act.

17. What national mandate stipulates that individuals must not be discriminated against because of their disabilities?

    a. American Dental Association Principles of Ethics

    b. Statute of limitations

    c. Americans with Disabilities Act

    d. Doctrine of respondeat superior

18. Each patient has the right to know and understand any procedure that is performed. The form that patients sign indicating they understand and accept treatment is called

    a. an expressed contract.

    b. an implied contract.

    c. informed consent.

    d. implied consent.

19. When a dentist sits down and the patient opens his or her mouth, what type of consent does this indicate?

    a. Informed

    b. Implied contract

    c. Implied

    d. Expressed contract

20. In the dental care setting, what is the most frequently exercised law?

    a. Civil

    b. Criminal

    c. Common

    d. Ethics

21. Which of the following areas are referred to in the Americans with Disabilities Act?
    1. Immunity while providing emergency treatment
    2. Providing access for the disabled to public services
    3. Telecommunication services for the hearing and speech impaired
    4. Unwanted hug without consent
    5. Threat of unprivileged touching
    6. Employment discrimination due to disability
        a. 1, 4, 5
        b. 2, 4, 5
        c. 2, 3, 6
        d. 1, 2, 6

22. Which of the following are included in the American Dental Association's Principles of Ethics?
    1. Advertising
    2. Professional fees
    3. Service to the public and quality of care
    4. Education
    5. Research and development
    6. Enhancing personal gain
        a. 1, 2, 6
        b. 2, 4, 5
        c. 3, 4, 5
        d. 3, 4, 6

23. In accordance with the Health Insurance Portability and Accountability Act of 1996, if any part of the dental office chooses to transmit any transactions electronically, the office falls under the _____ Act
    a. ADA
    b. PHI
    c. HHS
    d. HIPAA

24. In a dental office, patient records need to be protected. Which of the following is considered identifiable information and is protected by PHI rules?
    1. Post-op instructions
    2. Name
    3. Aseptic techniques
    4. Birth date
    5. Telephone conversations
    6. Telephone number
        a. 1, 2, 3
        b. 2, 4, 6
        c. 1, 3, 5
        d. 2, 3, 5

25. HIPAA requires that dental patients receive written notice of information practices, and an accounting of disclosures. The _____ officer provides information to patients about their individual privacy rights and how their information may be used.
    a. civil rights
    b. privacy
    c. information
    d. public

Matching

Match each word or term with its definition.

Term	Definition
1. __C__ Libel	a. False and malicious spoken words
2. __A__ Slander	b. State law contrary to federal law
3. __d__ Res gestae	c. False and malicious written words
4. __b__ Preemption	d. "Part of the action"

Critical Thinking

1. Explain the intent of the HIPAA Act of 1996. Whom does it protect? Who must comply with HIPAA?

2. A new cleaning service has been hired for the dental office. Services will be performed after business hours and when no office personnel are present. The covered entities and business associates must comply with HIPAA. What compliance requirements will be necessary? Explain the PHI privacy rule. What effect does PHI have in the dental office? Name the reasonable steps to protect PHI.

3. What contracts, if any, are required for patient protection? A contract can be terminated by failure of a party to meet obligations. Name them. Give examples of termination of contract. State causes for a contract to be terminated.

4. When were the transaction codes set for dental offices put into place? Name the enforcement authority for transactions, code sets, and security. Who are the OCR and how do they differ from the CMS?

Prevention and Nutrition

Oral Health and Preventive Techniques

SPECIFIC INSTRUCTIONAL OBJECTIVES

The student should strive to meet the following objectives and demonstrate an understanding of the facts and principles presented in this chapter:

1. Describe how plaque forms and affects the tooth.

2. Identify oral hygiene tips that will aid each age group.

3. Identify oral hygiene aids, including manual and automatic, available to all patients.

4. Demonstrate the six toothbrushing techniques.

5. Identify types of dental floss and demonstrate flossing technique.

6. Describe fluoride and its use in dentistry.

7. Define fluoridation and describe its effectiveness on tooth development and the posteruption stage.

8. List and explain the forms of fluoride. Describe how to prepare a patient and demonstrate a fluoride application.

SUMMARY

To be effective in preventive dentistry, dental assistants must first care for their own teeth properly. Becoming knowledgeable about the oral disease process will aid the dental assistant in educating patients on how to prevent it. The dental assistant must have the knowledge to problem solve oral hygiene concerns, know what preventive aids are available, and then aid patients in maintaining their teeth and gums.

EXERCISES AND ACTIVITIES

True or False

1. When developing personal oral hygiene goals for patients, each patient should be treated as an individual.

   a. True

   b. False

2. Acute fluoride poisoning is very common.

   a. True

   b. False

3. A patient should drink milk as a demulcent when fluoride toxicity is suspected.

   a. True

   b. False

4. With increased exposure to fluoride, the enamel of the teeth may become cracked and pitted.

   a. True

   b. False

5. There can be a dual benefit of chewing fluoride tablets.

   a. True

   b. False

6. Topical fluoride can assist in the remineralization of decalcified areas.

   a. True

   b. False

7. There is only one method to properly remove plaque buildup on teeth.

   a. True

   b. False

8. Individuals with dental appliances should practice the same oral hygiene techniques as those without.

   a. True

   b. False

9. In order to protect users from the condition of fluoride toxicity, dentifrice should not contain fluoride.

   a. True

   b. False

10. Patients with congestive heart failure may experience discomfort if the dental chair is reclined.

    a. True

    b. False

Multiple Choice

1. Which of the following is *not* a preventive dentistry step for all individuals to follow?

   a. Daily brushing and flossing

   b. Good nutrition

   c. Routine dental visits and examination

   d. Sucking on hard candy daily

2. Dental plaque

   a. contains bacteria, which grows in colonies.

   b. is a soft, white, sticky mass.

   c. contains bacteria, which is fed by foods we eat.

   d. All of the above.

3. Which of the following is the dental decay (caries) equation?

   a. Sugar + Protein = Caries + Gingiva = Decay

   b. Sugar + Plaque = Acid + Gingiva = Decay

   c. Sugar + Plaque = Acid + Tooth = Decay

   d. None of the above

4. The use of disclosing agents will

   a. replace toothbrushing.

   b. replace flossing.

   c. make plaque visible.

   d. replace the use of dentifrice.

5. Which organization awards a Seal of Acceptance classification to products that are safe and effective for self-care?

   a. American Dental Hygienists' Association (ADHA)

   b. American Dental Assistants Association (ADAA)

   c. American Dental Association (ADA)

   d. Occupational Health and Safety Administration (OSHA)

6. Mouth rinsing is often used to

   a. loosen debris.

   b. temporarily eliminate bad breath.

   c. give patients a pleasant taste in the mouth.

   d. All of the above.

7. Correct toothbrush design includes

   a. bristles that are flexible.

   b. a firm handle.

   c. a lightweight handle.

   d. All of the above.

8. Dental floss is *not* available in

   a. waxed form.

   b. unwaxed form.

   c. coarse form.

   d. lightly waxed form.

9. How often should the teeth be flossed?

   a. Once a week

   b. Daily

   c. Every other day

   d. Every other week

10. Which prosthetic device requires special oral hygiene care?

    a. Amalgam

    b. Composite

    c. Root canal

    d. Fixed bridge

11. Orthodontic appliances must be kept plaque free by using

    a. just floss.

    b. soda pop.

    c. apples.

    d. a water irrigation device.

12. Chronic fluoride poisoning can result from

    a. ingestion of high fluoride levels in water.

    b. combinations of several fluoride sources over a period of time.

    c. fluoride levels of 1.8 ppm to 2.0 ppm.

    d. All of the above

13. What is the primary dental health benefit of fluoride?

    a. No plaque

    b. Reduction of caries

    c. No calculus

    d. No orthodontics ever needed

14. Fluoride compounds used today are
    a. sodium fluoride.
    b. stannous fluoride.
    c. acidulated fluoride.
    d. All of the above.

15. Which of the following dental aids help to clean between the teeth?
    1. Interproximal brush
    2. Rubber stimulator
    3. Wooden stimulator
    4. Dental floss
    5. Water irrigation device
    6. Toothbrush
    7. Disclosing tablet
    8. Chewing gum
        a. 1, 6, 7, 8
        b. 1, 2, 3, 7
        c. 3, 4, 5, 8
        d. 1, 2, 3, 4, 5

Matching

Patient motivation is critical for the successful prevention of dental disease. Match the age characteristic with the general characteristics of that group.

Age Group

1. _____ Infant up to 1 year
2. _____ Preschool
3. _____ Ages 5 through 8
4. _____ Ages 9 through 12
5. _____ Ages 13 through 15

General Characteristics

a. Can brush with parent supervision
b. Can brush and begin to floss
c. Oral hygiene performed by parent or caregiver
d. Routinely snacks; rate of decay rising
e. Brushes and flosses proficiently

Following are the various toothbrushing techniques and methods of use. Match the correct toothbrushing technique with its descriptive method.

Brushing Technique

6. _____ Bass or modified Bass
7. _____ Charters
8. _____ Modified Stillman
9. _____ Rolling stroke
10. _____ Modified scrub

Method of Use

a. Activate the brush back and forth (scrubbing motion)
b. Brush is parallel to tooth with bristles pointed apically
c. Removes plaque next to and directly beneath the gingival margin
d. Stimulates gingiva, both marginal and interdental
e. Bristles of brush are angled against the tooth surface, toward the root

Match the term with the best definition.

Term	Definition
11. _____ Acute fluoride poisoning	a. Ingestion of high fluoride levels from several fluoride sources over a period of time
12. _____ Chronic fluoride poisoning	b. Occurs when large amounts of fluoride are ingested or inhaled or absorbed at one time
13. _____ Antibacterial effect	c. Varying degrees of white areas and brown lines
14. _____ Enamel hypoplasia	d. Condition that inhibits the production of acids responsible for dental decay

Match the term with the best definition.

Term	Definition
15. _____ Fluoride	a. Also known as fluorosis
16. _____ Mottled enamel	b. Process of adding fluoride to water supply
17. _____Optimum level of fluoride in water	c. Essential to formation of healthy bones and teeth
18. _____ Fluoridation	d. Fluoride absorbed in excessive amounts
19. _____ Fluoride toxicity	e. 1 ppm

 Critical Thinking

1. If you have a dental implant, how can you maintain optimal home care?

2. Are metal scalers used in the dental office to remove calculus from dental implants?

3. Patients who are pregnant may require a special program in dental hygiene techniques. What are some causes of gingival irritation?

4. Problem solving with a pregnant patient will help her maintain her goal of proper oral hygiene. What are a couple of suggestions?

CASE STUDY 1

Claire, age 42, recently acquired dental coverage from her employer and is registering as a first-time dental patient. The dentist has completed her oral health diagnosis and found areas of plaque, gingivitis, and the beginning stages of periodontitis. Dental charting shows some restorations. Patient x-rays indicate that demineralization is also occurring in certain areas.

1. What steps will be taken to motivate this patient to better oral health?

2. How will the dental assistant assess the patient's attitude?

3. Developing solutions to the patient's needs requires the exercise of what skill?

4. Identify Claire's abilities and skills and any special considerations related to her age group that are important for meeting her oral hygiene goals.

5. What type of home care should be emphasized?

6. Discuss the dental decay (caries) equation. How does it relate to Claire's diagnosis?

SKILL COMPETENCY ASSESSMENT

4-1 Applying Disclosing Agent for Plaque Identification

Student's Name _____ Date _____

Instructor's Name _____

Skill: To identify plaque and its location for patient and operator.

Performance Objective: The student will demonstrate the application of the disclosing agent.

	Self-Evaluation	Student Evaluation	Possible Points	Instructor Evaluation	Comments
Equipment and Supplies					
1. Basic setup: mouth mirror, explorer, cotton pliers			1		
2. Saliva ejector, evacuator tip (HVE), and air-water syringe tip			1		
3. Cotton rolls, cotton-tip applicator, and gauze sponges			1		
4. Petroleum jelly (lubricant)			1		
5. Disclosing agent (liquid or tablet) and dappen dish			1		
6. Plaque chart and red pencil			1		
Competency Steps					
1. While seating the patient, the operator reviews the medical and dental health history with the patient.			3		
2. The operator washes hands, applies all PPEs, and examines the oral cavity.			2		
3. The operator applies the petroleum jelly (lubricant) to the patient's lips and to any tooth-colored restorations to prevent staining.			2		

	Self-Evaluation	Student Evaluation	Possible Points	Instructor Evaluation	Comments
4. The operator can apply the liquid using the dappen dish and a cotton-tip applicator. Every accessible surface of the teeth should be covered with the disclosing solution.			2		
5. If using the tablet, the patient chews and swishes around for 15 seconds.			2		
6. The remaining solution is rinsed and evacuated from the area.			2		
7. The patient uses a hand mirror to view the plaque and the operator uses a mouth mirror and an air-water syringe to identify the plaque.			2		
8. Overgloves are placed over treatment gloves to chart the plaque on the patient chart.			2		
9. The operator removes the overgloves, and then demonstrates for the patient methods of brushing and flossing for plaque removal.			3		

TOTAL POINTS POSSIBLE 26

TOTAL POINTS POSSIBLE—2nd attempt 24

TOTAL POINTS EARNED ____

Points assigned reflect importance of step to meeting objective: Important = 1, Essential = 2, Critical = 3. Students will lose 2 points for repeated attempts. Failure results if any of the critical steps are omitted or performed incorrectly. If using a 100-point scale, determine score by dividing points earned by total points possible and multiplying the results by 100.

SCORE: _____

SKILL COMPETENCY ASSESSMENT

4-2 Bass or Modified Bass Brushing Technique

Student's Name _____ Date _____

Instructor's Name _____

Skill: To remove plaque next to and directly beneath the gingival margin.

Performance Objective: The student will demonstrate application of this toothbrushing technique.

	Self-Evaluation	Student Evaluation	Possible Points	Instructor Evaluation	Comments
Equipment and Supplies 1. Toothbrush			1		
Competency Steps 1. Grasp the brush and place it so the bristles are at a 45-degree angle with the tips of the bristles directed straight into the gingival sulcus.			2		
2. Using the tips of the bristles, vibrate back and forth with short, light strokes for a count of 10, allowing the tips of the bristles to enter the sulcus and cover the gingival margin.			3		
3. Lift the brush and continue into the next area or group of teeth until all areas have been cleaned.			1		
4. The toe bristles of the brush can be used to clean the lingual (tongue) anterior area in the arch.			1		

	Self-Evaluation	Student Evaluation	Possible Points	Instructor Evaluation	Comments
5. Modified Bass. After the vibratory motion has been completed in each area, sweep the bristles over the crown of the tooth, toward the biting surface of the tooth.			1		

TOTAL POINTS POSSIBLE   9

TOTAL POINTS POSSIBLE—2nd attempt   7

TOTAL POINTS EARNED   ____

Points assigned reflect importance of step to meeting objective: Important = 1, Essential = 2, Critical = 3. Students will lose 2 points for repeated attempts. Failure results if any of the critical steps are omitted or performed incorrectly. If using a 100-point scale, determine score by dividing points earned by total points possible and multiplying the results by 100.

SCORE: _____

SKILL COMPETENCY ASSESSMENT

4-3 Charters Brushing Technique

Student's Name _____ Date _____

Instructor's Name _____

Skill: To loosen plaque and debris and to stimulate the gingiva, both marginal and interdental.

Performance Objective: The student will demonstrate the application of this toothbrushing technique.

	Self-Evaluation	Student Evaluation	Possible Points	Instructor Evaluation	Comments
Equipment and Supplies 1. Toothbrush			1		
Competency Steps 1. Grasp the brush and place it so that the back of the head is directed back apically (toward the end of the root), with the bristles placed downward on the maxillary and upward on the mandibular.			2		
2. The bristles should be placed over the gingiva, where the tooth and gingiva meet.			1		
3. Press the bristles into the space between the teeth.			1		
4. Vibrate gently back and forth while maintaining the position. Count to 10.			3		
5. Reposition and repeat the technique for each subsequent area.			2		

	Self-Evaluation	Student Evaluation	Possible Points	Instructor Evaluation	Comments
6. For anterior areas, hold the brush parallel to the teeth and use the sides of the toe bristles to clean the area. Count to 10.			3		

TOTAL POINTS POSSIBLE   13

TOTAL POINTS POSSIBLE—2nd attempt   11

TOTAL POINTS EARNED   ____

Points assigned reflect importance of step to meeting objective: Important = 1, Essential = 2, Critical = 3. Students will lose 2 points for repeated attempts. Failure results if any of the critical steps are omitted or performed incorrectly. If using a 100-point scale, determine score by dividing points earned by total points possible and multiplying by 100.

SCORE: ____

SKILL COMPETENCY ASSESSMENT

4-4 Modified Stillman Brushing Technique

Student's Name _____ Date _____

Instructor's Name _____

Skill: To provide a good overall cleaning, remove plaque, and stimulate and massage the gingiva.

Performance Objective: The student will demonstrate the application of this toothbrushing technique.

	Self-Evaluation	Student Evaluation	Possible Points	Instructor Evaluation	Comments
Equipment and Supplies 1. Toothbrush			1		
Competency Steps 1. Place the toothbrush so that the bristles are pointing apically and the handle of the brush is level with the biting surface of the tooth.			2		
2. Rotate the bristles downward and vibrate back and forth until the brush has rotated over the entire surface of the tooth. Do this motion slowly and count to 10.			3		
3. Repeat this motion over the same area at least five times.			2		

	Self-Evaluation	Student Evaluation	Possible Points	Instructor Evaluation	Comments
4. Continue until each area and every tooth has been cleaned in this manner.			2		

TOTAL POINTS POSSIBLE   10

TOTAL POINTS POSSIBLE—2nd attempt   8

TOTAL POINTS EARNED   _____

Points assigned reflect importance of step to meeting objective: Important = 1, Essential = 2, Critical = 3. Students will lose 2 points for repeated attempts. Failure results if any of the critical steps are omitted or performed incorrectly. If using a 100-point scale, determine score by dividing points earned by total points possible and multiplying by 100.

SCORE: _____

SKILL COMPETENCY ASSESSMENT

4-5 Rolling Stroke Brushing Technique

Student's Name _____ Date _____

Instructor's Name _____ _____

Skill: To remove food debris and plaque from teeth and to stimulate the gingival tissue.

Performance Objective: The student will demonstrate the application of this toothbrushing technique.

	Self-Evaluation	Student Evaluation	Possible Points	Instructor Evaluation	Comments
Equipment and Supplies 1. Toothbrush			1		
Competency Steps 1. Grasp the brush and place it parallel to the tooth so that the bristles are pointing apically, upward for the maxillary arch and downward for the mandibular arch.			2		
2. Firmly but gently press the bristles against the gingiva and roll them slowly over the tissue and the teeth, toward the biting surface.			3		
3. Repeat this rolling stroke over the same surface a total of five times.			2		
4. Move the brush to the next area and repeat the five rolling strokes.			2		

	Self-Evaluation	Student Evaluation	Possible Points	Instructor Evaluation	Comments
5. Use the heel or toe of the toothbrush to clean the lingual surfaces of the anterior teeth. The bristles will still need to be pressed gently into the area and rolled toward the biting surface.			2		

TOTAL POINTS POSSIBLE	10
TOTAL POINTS POSSIBLE—2nd attempt	12
TOTAL POINTS EARNED	____

Points assigned reflect importance of step to meeting objective: Important = 1, Essential = 2, Critical = 3. Students will lose 2 points for repeated attempts. Failure results if any of the critical steps are omitted or performed incorrectly. If using a 100-point scale, determine score by dividing points earned by total points possible and multiplying by 100.

SCORE: ____

SKILL COMPETENCY ASSESSMENT

4-6 Fones Brushing Technique

Student's Name _____ Date _____

Instructor's Name _____

Skill: To provide a good overall cleaning.

Performance Objective: The student will demonstrate the application of this toothbrushing technique.

	Self-Evaluation	Student Evaluation	Possible Points	Instructor Evaluation	Comments
Equipment and Supplies 1. Toothbrush			1		
Competency Steps 1. Close the teeth together and place the brush against the cheek. Starting with the posterior teeth, the brush is placed over the maxillary and mandibular teeth.			2		
2. The brush goes over the teeth in a circular motion as it progresses toward the anterior in a quick sweeping motion.			3		
3. The anterior teeth are placed in the biting position and the brush is used in a circular motion, quick sweeping from right to left.			3		

	Self-Evaluation	Student Evaluation	Possible Points	Instructor Evaluation	Comments
4. In-and-out strokes are used to cleanse the palatal and lingual areas.			2		

TOTAL POINTS POSSIBLE   11

TOTAL POINTS POSSIBLE—2nd attempt   9

TOTAL POINTS EARNED   ____

Points assigned reflect importance of step to meeting objective: Important = 1, Essential = 2, Critical = 3. Students will lose 2 points for repeated attempts. Failure results if any of the critical steps are omitted or performed incorrectly. If using a 100-point scale, determine score by dividing points earned by total points possible and multiplying by 100.

SCORE: ____

SKILL COMPETENCY ASSESSMENT

4-7 Modified Scrub Brushing Technique

Student's Name _____ Date _____

Instructor's Name _____

Skill: To remove plaque and stimulate the gingival tissue.

Performance Objective: The student will demonstrate the application of this toothbrushing technique.

	Self-Evaluation	Student Evaluation	Possible Points	Instructor Evaluation	Comments
Equipment and Supplies 1. Toothbrush			1		
Competency Steps 1. Grasp the brush and place the bristles at a right angle to the tooth surface.			2		
2. Use gentle but firm pressure and place the bristles over the area where the tooth and gingiva tissue come together.			2		
3. Activate the brush with back-and-forth scrubbing strokes.			3		

	Self-Evaluation	Student Evaluation	Possible Points	Instructor Evaluation	Comments
4. Repeat this action throughout the mouth until all areas have been cleaned.			2		

TOTAL POINTS POSSIBLE   10

TOTAL POINTS POSSIBLE—2nd attempt   8

TOTAL POINTS EARNED   ____

Points assigned reflect importance of step to meeting objective: Important = 1, Essential = 2, Critical = 3. Students will lose 2 points for repeated attempts. Failure results if any of the critical steps are omitted or performed incorrectly. If using a 100-point scale, determine score by dividing points earned by total points possible and multiplying by 100.

SCORE: ____

SKILL COMPETENCY ASSESSMENT

4-8 Dental Flossing Technique

Student's Name _____ Date _____

Instructor's Name _____

Skill: To remove bacterial plaque and other debris from otherwise inaccessible areas, the interproximal surfaces of the teeth.

Performance Objective: The student will demonstrate the application of this flossing technique.

	Self-Evaluation	Student Evaluation	Possible Points	Instructor Evaluation	Comments
Equipment and Supplies 1. Dental floss			1		
Competency Steps 1. Obtain appropriate dental floss and dispense 18 inches.			2		
2. Wrap the ends of the floss around the middle or ring finger as anchors.			3		
3. Grasp the floss between the thumb and index finger of both hands, allowing 1/2 to 1 inch to remain between the two hands.			2		
4. a. For the maxillary teeth, pass the floss over the two thumbs (or thumb and finger) and direct the floss upward.			2		
b. For the mandibular teeth, pass the floss over the two index fingers and guide it downward.			2		
5. Direct the floss to pass gently between the teeth, using a sawing motion. Try not to snap the floss through the contacts because it may damage the interdental papilla (gingival point between teeth).			2		

	Self-Evaluation	Student Evaluation	Possible Points	Instructor Evaluation	Comments
6. Curve the floss in a C-shape to wrap it around the tooth and allow access into the sulcus area. When a resistance is felt, the bottom of the gingival sulcus has been reached.			2		
7. Move the floss gently up and down the surface of the tooth to remove the plaque.			2		
8. Lift slightly and wrap the floss in the opposite direction in a C-shape over the adjacent tooth.			2		
9. Move the floss gently up and down the surface of this tooth before removing it from the area.			2		
10. Rotate the floss on the fingers to allow for a fresh section to be used each time, and continue to clean between each and every tooth. Be systematic so that no areas are missed.			1		
11. a. Use the dental floss around the distal surface of the most posterior tooth by wrapping it in a tight C-shape and moving it gently up and down with a firm pressure.			1		
b. Do the most posterior teeth in all four quadrants in the same manner.			1		

TOTAL POINTS POSSIBLE   25

TOTAL POINTS POSSIBLE—2nd attempt   23

TOTAL POINTS EARNED   ____

Points assigned reflect importance of step to meeting objective: Important = 1, Essential = 2, Critical = 3. Students will lose 2 points for repeated attempts. Failure results if any of the critical steps are omitted or performed incorrectly. If using a 100-point scale, determine score by dividing points earned by total points possible and multiplying the results by 100.

SCORE: ____

SKILL COMPETENCY ASSESSMENT

4-9 Fluoride Application

Student's Name _____ Date _____

Instructor's Name _____

Skill: To apply topical fluoride after either toothbrushing or a rubber-cup polish. Fluoride penetrates only the outer layer of the enamel if the tooth is clean.

Performance Objective: The student will demonstrate the application of this topical fluoride technique.

	Self-Evaluation	Student Evaluation	Possible Points	Instructor Evaluation	Comments
Equipment and Supplies					
1. Basic setup: mouth mirror, explorer, and cotton pliers			1		
2. Saliva ejector, evacuator tip (HVE), air-water syringe tip			1		
3. Cotton rolls, gauze sponges			1		
4. Fluoride solution			1		
5. Appropriately sized trays			1		
6. Timer (for 1 to 4 minutes)			1		
Competency Steps					
1. Seat the patient in an upright position, review health history, and confirm he or she has had no allergic reactions to fluorides.			2		
2. Explain the procedure to the patient. Inform the patient to try to not swallow the fluoride.			2		
3. Explain to the patient that for the fluoride to be most effective, he or she should not eat, drink, or rinse for 30 minutes after the fluoride treatment.			2		

	Self-Evaluation	Student Evaluation	Possible Points	Instructor Evaluation	Comments
4. Don glasses and mask. Wash hands and don treatment gloves.			3		
5. Select the trays and try them in the patient's mouth to ensure coverage of all the exposed teeth.			2		
6. Place the fluoride gel or foam in the tray. The tray should be about one-third full. Show the patient how to use the saliva ejector.			2		
7. Dry all the teeth with the air syringe. To keep the teeth dry while reaching for the tray, keep your finger in the patient's mouth and tell the patient to keep it open.			2		
8. Place the tray over the dried teeth. The maxillary and mandibular arches can be done at the same time or individually.			2		
9. Move the trays up and down to dispense the fluoride solution around the teeth.			2		
10. Place the saliva ejector between the arches and have the patient close gently.			2		
11. Set the timer for the designated amount of time.			2		
12. When the timer goes off, remove the saliva ejector and the trays from the patient's mouth.			1		

	Self-Evaluation	Student Evaluation	Possible Points	Instructor Evaluation	Comments
13. Quickly evacuate the mouth with the saliva ejector or the evacuator (HVE) to completely remove any excess fluoride.			1		
14. Remind the patient not to eat, drink, or rinse for 30 minutes.			1		
15. Don overgloves and make the chart entry, including the date, the fluoride solution applied, and any reactions.			2		

TOTAL POINTS POSSIBLE 34

TOTAL POINTS POSSIBLE—2nd attempt 32

TOTAL POINTS EARNED _____

Points assigned reflect importance of step to meeting objective: Important = 1, Essential = 2, Critical = 3. Students will lose 2 points for repeated attempts. Failure results if any of the critical steps are omitted or performed incorrectly. If using a 100-point scale, determine score by dividing points earned by total points possible and multiplying the results by 100.

SCORE: _____

CHAPTER 5

Nutrition

SPECIFIC INSTRUCTIONAL OBJECTIVES

The student should strive to meet the following objectives and demonstrate an understanding of the facts and principles presented in this chapter:

1. Describe how an understanding of nutrition is used in the profession of dental assisting.

2. Define nutrients found in foods, including carbohydrates, fiber, fats, proteins, and amino acids. Explain how they affect oral hygiene.

3. Define a calorie and the basal metabolic rate.

4. Identify and explain how vitamins, major minerals, and water function in the body.

5. Explain how to interpret food labeling.

6. Discuss the implications of eating disorders.

7. Identify the food sources, functions, and implications of deficiencies of fat-soluble vitamins, water-soluble vitamins, and the seven major minerals.

SUMMARY

Dental assistants need to have a background in nutrition to maintain good overall health as well as aid patients in decision making. Everyone can benefit from knowledge of how to read nutrition labels and what it means when a product is organic or organically grown. Having an understanding of eating disorders may prove beneficial in the work environment with other co-workers and patients.

EXERCISES AND ACTIVITIES

True or False

1. An adequate diet meets all the individual's nutritional needs.

   a. True

   b. False

2. People can eat large amounts of food yet still be undernourished, i.e., lacking the correct nutrients for the body.

   a. True

   b. False

3. Malnutrition is a disorder that results from being undernourished.

   a. True

   b. False

4. Carbohydrates primarily come from milk, eggs, and meat.

   a. True

   b. False

5. Care should be taken when eating fats and lipids because these foods are typically cariogenic.

   a. True

   b. False

6. Vitamins provide the body with energy.

   a. True

   b. False

7. Calcium and phosphorus are minerals that contribute to healthy tooth development.

   a. True

   b. False

8. Water makes up 60 to 70 percent of our body weight.

   a. True

   b. False

9. To maintain a healthy diet, people should use more energy than is supplied by the nutrients they consume.

   a. True

   b. False

10. To be labeled as organic, food must be grown without the use of herbicides, chemical pesticides, or fertilizers.

    a. True

    b. False

Multiple Choice

1. The most important nutrient(s) in the body is (are)

   a. water.

   b. vitamins.

   c. minerals.

   d. fluoride.

2. Nutrients are defined as

   a. cariogenic food and carbohydrates.

   b. any chemical substance in food that is necessary for growth.

   c. an undernourished diet.

   d. everything that is ingested via the mouth.

3. The number one cause of death of Americans over age 40 is heart disease, and a contributing factor may be the consumption of too many

   a. fats.

   b. proteins.

   c. carbohydrates.

   d. foods containing fiber.

4. How many major minerals are found in the body?

   a. Ten

   b. Two

   c. Three

   d. Seven

5. It requires more energy to fuel muscle than burn fat; therefore, the basal metabolic rate (BMR) will be higher for which of the following groups of people?

   a. Heavy individuals

   b. Women

   c. Lean individuals

   d. The elderly

6. Which of the following is a complete protein?

   a. Eggs

   b. Corn

   c. Beans

   d. Cereal

7. If a label states that a food product is "light" on fat, fat content is normally reduced by about _____ % less than normal.

   a. 25

   b. 50

   c. 20

   d. 45

8. Which vitamin aids in maintaining skin health?

   a. Vitamin A

   b. Vitamin B

   c. Vitamin C

   d. Vitamin D

9. Which nutrient is the most abundant in the body?

   a. Carbohydrates

   b. Fats

   c. Proteins

   d. Water

10. The percent of daily value is based upon how many calories for an adult?

   a. 500

   b. 1000

   c. 1500

   d. 2000

Matching

Match the vitamin with how the body uses it.

Vitamin

1. _____ Vitamin A
2. _____ Vitamin D
3. _____ Vitamin K
4. _____ Vitamin C

Use

a. Promotes blood clotting and coagulation

b. Gives strength to epithelial tissue

c. Acts to hold cells together

d. Promotes tooth development

 Critical Thinking

To remain healthy, dental assistants must first be knowledgeable about nutrition, the manner in which foods are used to meet the body's needs. Vitamins are a class of nutrients that do not provide the body with energy. Instead, they perform other necessary functions.

1 All vitamins fall in one of two groups. Name them: _____ and _____

2. Identify the correct chemical name for each vitamin listed. Then describe whether it is water-soluble or fat-soluble, its food source(s), and its function.

Chemical Name	Vitamin	Water/Fat Soluble	Food Source(s)	Function
	Vitamin A			
	Vitamin B_1			
	Vitamin B_2			
	Vitamin B_6			
	Vitamin B_{12}			
	Vitamin C			
	Vitamin D			
	Vitamin E			
	Vitamin K			
	Folacin			
	Niacin			

CASE STUDY

On a routine dental visit, Muriel's oral exam revealed several tissue indications of change since her last visit. These conditions included tissue irritation and swelling, and beginning areas of decalcification. While discussing these conditions with the dental team, Muriel informs them that she is in early pregnancy (her second child).

1. What information can the assistant discuss regarding cariogenic foods?

2. What suggestions can the assistant provide the patient to improve her oral hygiene?

3. Name two minerals that must be increased.

4. Name three reasons why Muriel needs to increase her intake of nutrition and calories.

5. What dietary supplement usually needs to be added to an infant's diet?

3

Basic Dental Sciences

General Anatomy and Physiology

SPECIFIC INSTRUCTIONAL OBJECTIVES

The student should strive to meet the following objectives and demonstrate an understanding of the facts and principles presented in this chapter:

1. List the body systems, body planes and directions, and cavities of the body, and describe the structure and function of the cell.

2. Explain the functions and divisions of the skeletal system, list the composition of the bone, and identify the types of joints.

3. List the functions and parts of the muscular system.

4. List the functions and the structure of the nervous system.

5. List the functions and the parts of the endocrine system.

6. Explain dental concerns related to the reproductive system.

7. Explain the functions of the circulatory system and list and identify the parts.

8. Explain the functions and parts of the digestive system.

9. List the functions and parts of the respiratory system.

10. List the functions and parts of the lymphatic system and the immune system.

11. List the functions and parts of the integumentary system.

SUMMARY

Specific terms are used to establish a means for health professionals to communicate more effectively. The body is divided into systems, planes, cavities, and basic units that provide common references and terms for studying and communicating information about the body.

54

The dental assistant needs to be familiar with the terminology of body systems and how each system functions to provide the quality of care that each patient deserves. Both the anatomy and physiology of all body systems will need to be understood.

90%

EXERCISES AND ACTIVITIES

True or False

1. The circulatory system carries life-sustaining substances such as nutrients and oxygen throughout the body.
   a. True
   b. False

2. Anatomy means the study of body structure.
   a. True
   b. False

3. Physiology is the study of how the body functions.
   a. True
   b. False

4. The sagittal plane divides the body into upper and lower sections. *in to left and right*
   a. True
   b. False

5. The frontal plane divides the body into left and right halves. *into front and back section*
   a. True
   b. False

6. The dorsal cavity is in the anterior portion of the body. *is in the posterior portion of the body.*
   a. True
   b. False

7. Cancellous bone consists of a meshwork of interconnecting bone called trabeculae.
   a. True
   b. False

8. Cardiac muscle is voluntary in action. *is involuntary action.*
   a. True
   b. False

9. There are diseases and conditions of the endocrine system that affect dental patients and how they respond to dental treatments.
   a. True
   b. False

10. Asthma is a muscular spasm of the walls of the bronchi that makes it difficult for a person to breathe.
   a. True
   b. False

Multiple Choice

1. _____ refers to the part of the body closest to the point of attachment.

   a. Inferior
   b. Superior
   c. Dorsal
   d. Proximal

2. Which of the following planes divides the body into left and right halves?

   a. Frontal
   b. Transverse
   c. Horizontal
   d. Sagittal

3. Which of the following planes divides the body into front and back sections?

   a. Transverse
   b. Frontal
   c. Mid-sagittal
   d. Sagittal

4. The dorsal cavity comprises the spinal cavity and the

   a. thoracic cavity.
   b. abdominal cavity.
   c. pelvic cavity.
   d. cranial cavity.

5. The basic unit of all biological systems and the smallest functioning unit of the body is called a(n)

   a. cell.
   b. tissue.
   c. organ.
   d. muscle.

6. The axial skeleton includes the

   a. bones of the cranium.
   b. spinal column.
   c. ribs.
   d. All of the above.

7. In an adult skeleton, there are _____ bones.

   a. 300
   b. 200
   c. 216
   d. 206

8. The periosteum contains

   a. blood vessels.
   b. lymph vessels.
   c. osteoblasts.
   d. All of the above.

9. _____ marrow contains mainly fat cells.

   a. Red
   b. Yellow
   c. White
   d. Clear

10. _____ bones support the teeth and surrounding tissues.

    a. Synovial
    b. Facial
    c. Osteoclastic
    d. Cartilaginous

11. _____ is a condition or disease of the skeletal system.

    a. Indigestion
    b. Fibromyalgia
    c. Homeostasis
    d. Osteoporosis

12. The loss of bony material, leaving bones brittle and soft, is called

    a. osteomyelitis.
    b. periosteum.
    c. osteoblasts.
    d. osteoporosis.

13. The_____muscles move food along the digestive tract and keep the heart beating.

    a. involuntary
    b. external
    c. voluntary
    d. anterior

14. What muscle type accounts for the largest amount of muscle tissue in the human body?

    a. Cardiac

    b. Striated

    c. Nonstriated

    d. Fascia

15. If muscles are not used, they begin to deteriorate. This condition is known as

    a. Atrophy

    b. Fibromyalgia

    c. Spasticity

    d. Gravis

16. The specialized group of peripheral nerves that mainly functions automatically is called the

    a. sympathetic nervous system (SNS).

    b. peripheral nervous system (PNS).

    c. central nervous system (CNS).

    d. autonomic nervous system (ANS).

17. The nerve fibers that conduct impulses to the cell body are called

    a. axons.

    b. dendrites.

    c. synapses.

    d. myelin.

18. Which of the following statements is *not* true of the spinal cord?

    a. It is part of the reproductive system.

    b. It is a center for reflex responses.

    c. It generally protects the body from stressful situations.

    d. It transmits stimuli from the body to the brain.

19. The _____ cranial nerves are related directly to the oral cavity.

    a. fourth and seventh

    b. seventh and twelfth

    c. second and fifth

    d. fifth and seventh

20. Which system is affected when the patient is administered a pain blocker?

    a. Skeletal

    b. Nervous

    c. Muscular

    d. Respiratory

21. _____ is a sudden onset of facial paralysis.

    a. Multiple sclerosis

    b. Parkinson's disease

    c. Neuritis

    d. Bell's palsy

22. The _____ endocrine system generally controls

    a. the production of insulin.

    b. the breakdown of glycogen.

    c. the impulses of muscles.

    d. circulatory congestion in bone marrow.

23. The _____ glands are among the major glands of the endocrine system.

    a. respiratory

    b. adrenal

    c. neuritis

    d. muscular

24. The condition in which the thyroid gland is underactive is called

    a. hypothyroidism.

    b. hyperthyroidism.

    c. pericardium.

    d. myocardium.

25. The pathway that carries the blood from the aorta to the smallest blood vessels and back to the heart is called _____ circulation.

    a. pulmonary

    b. systemic

    c. pericardium

    d. myocardium

26. The thin lining on the inside of the heart is called the
    a. pericardium.
    c. endocardium.
    b. myocardium.
    d. atrium.

27. _____ carry oxygenated blood from the heart to the capillaries.
    a. Veins
    c. Arterioles
    b. Capillaries
    d. Arteries

28. _____ carry blood drained from capillaries back to the heart.
    a. Veins
    c. Arterioles
    b. Capillaries
    d. Arteries

29. _____ are the connections between the arteries and the veins.
    a. Corpuscles
    c. Arterioles
    b. Capillaries
    d. Bronchioles

30. What is the liquid portion of the blood called?
    a. Plasma
    c. Capillaries
    b. Arteries
    d. Veins

31. What are the cells or solid portion of the blood called?
    a. Blood
    c. Capillaries
    b. Plasma
    d. Corpuscles

32. Red blood cells contain the protein called
    a. leukemia.
    c. hemostasis.
    b. thrombocytes.
    d. hemoglobin.

33. A disorder called _____ is the failure of the blood to clot.
    a. hypothyroidism
    c. leukemia
    b. hyperthyroidism
    d. hemophilia

34. The alimentary canal does not include the
    a. pharynx.
    c. stomach.
    b. esophagus.
    d. atrium.

35. The _____ transmit(s) the genetic information, is(are) in the nucleus, and contain(s) the DNA.
    a. cell membrane
    c. nucleus
    b. chromosomes
    d. cytoplasm

Matching

Identify each muscle with the matching muscle characteristic.

Muscle

1. __C__ Extensibility
2. __A__ Muscle tone
3. __D__ Isometric contraction
4. __B__ Isotonic contraction

Characteristic

a. Tension of the muscular system
b. Muscle tension remains the same but the muscles shorten
c. Muscle stretches or spreads in order to perform tasks
d. No change in muscle length but muscle tension increases

Critical Thinking

1. To be an effective dental assistant, maintaining physical fitness and overall health are advantageous. Therefore the function, condition, and diseases of the muscular system need to be understood. Identify each of the muscle types below.

Type of muscle	Muscle description/function
_____	Only group of muscles over which person has conscious control
_____	Involuntary in action; able to receive an impulse and respond and relax very rapidly
_____	Nonstriated, found in internal organs other than the heart, part of involuntary muscles

2. Muscle tissue abilities to respond to stimuli are called _____ and _____.

3. Identify each muscle by characteristic.

Muscle	Characteristic
_____	Muscle to stretch or spread in order to perform tasks
_____	Tension of muscular system
_____	Length of muscle is not changed, but tension increases
_____	Muscle tension remains the same but muscles shorten

4. Name five examples of common conditions and diseases of the muscular system.

5. Explain atrophy.

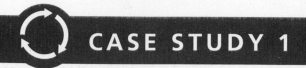

CASE STUDY 1

Jay, age 28, is a new dental patient. The patient is asked to complete a medical health history questionnaire. Jay noted that he has multiple sclerosis (MS). Jay will require several appointments for dental treatment. Several medical considerations will be required for compliance with the patient's needs during treatment.

1. What is MS?

2. In what age groups does this disease typically appear?

3. MS destroys which body systems? Describe what happens.

4. How will the above characteristics affect upcoming dental visits?

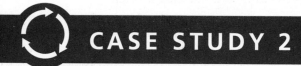

CASE STUDY 2

A scheduled dental appointment has brought Irene in today for a filling. Before treatment, in response to a query by the dental assistant about changes in her health history since the last appointment, Irene said that she is pregnant.

1. Which body systems are affected by pregnancy?

2. Explain the function of the endocrine system during pregnancy.

3. List the major glands of the endocrine system and their main functions.

4. State the main function of the reproductive system.

5. What, if any, dental treatment might be affected during pregnancy?

CHAPTER 7

Head and Neck Anatomy

SPECIFIC INSTRUCTIONAL OBJECTIVES

The student should strive to meet the following objectives and demonstrate an understanding of the facts and principles presented in this chapter:

1. List and identify the landmarks of the face and the oral cavity, including the tongue, floor of the mouth, and salivary glands.

2. Identify the bones of the cranium and the face and identify the landmarks on the maxilla and the mandible.

3. Identify the parts of the temporomandibular joint (TMJ) and describe how the joint works.

4. List and identify the muscles of mastication, facial expression, the floor of the mouth, the tongue, the throat, the neck, and the shoulders. Explain their functions.

5. List and identify the nerves of the maxilla and the mandible.

6. Identify the arteries and veins of the head and the neck.

SUMMARY

As a vital team member, the dental assistant needs to be able to recognize factors that may influence the general physical health of the patient. Understanding landmarks of the oral cavity, as well as being able to describe head and neck anatomy as it relates to location of structure and function, enables the dental assistant to recognize the abnormal. For this reason, accuracy is especially important when completing the patient's dental chart. This information provides a point of comparison for future visits.

EXERCISES AND ACTIVITIES

True or False

1. Between the bottom of the nose and the middle of the upper lip is a shallow, V-shaped depression known as the philtrum.

    a. True
    b. False

2. The reddish portion of the lips is covered by a thin layer of epithelium and is highly vascular; it is called the vermilion border.

    a. True
    b. False

3. The vermilion zone marks where the skin meets with and forms a line around the lips.

    a. True
    b. False

4. The tissue that lines the inner surface of the lips and cheeks is called papilla.

    a. True
    b. False

5. The corners of the mouth where the upper lip meets the lower lip are known as the labial commissures.

    a. True
    b. False

6. Inside the mouth, a pocket is formed by the soft tissue of the cheeks and the gingival; this pocket is called the oral vestibule.

    a. True
    b. False

7. The mucosa that covers the alveolar bone that supports the teeth is called the parotid papilla.

    a. True
    b. False

8. The plural form of frenum is frena.

    a. True
    b. False

9. Excessive dryness of the mouth is called xerostomia.

    a. True
    b. False

10. There are four pairs of salivary glands.

    a. True
    b. False

Multiple Choice

1. The lips are covered externally with
   a. skin.
   b. mucous membranes.
   c. lingual mucosa.
   d. gingival papilla.

2. The outer edge of the nostril is called the
   a. ala of the nose. — wing.
   b. philtrum.
   c. nasolabial groove.
   d. sulcus.

3. The portion of the lips called the labial commissures is examined for
   a. cracks.
   b. color change.
   c. variations in form.
   d. all of the above.

4. Which of the following landmarks is *not* a part of the oral cavity?
   a. Vestibule
   b. Lips
   c. Stensen's duct
   d. Gingiva

5. The deepest part of the oral vestibule is called the
   a. vestibule fornix.
   b. philtrum.
   c. vermilion.
   d. commissures.

6. The tissue that lines the inner surface of the lips and cheeks is called the
   a. papilla.
   b. gingiva.
   c. frenum.
   d. mucosa.

7. On the labial mucosa are yellowish glands just inside the commissures called (the)
   a. Fordyce's spots.
   b. fornix
   c. linea alba.
   d. uvula.

8. On the buccal mucosa is a raised white line that runs parallel to where the teeth meet, which is called the
   a. vestibule.
   b. frenum.
   c. fornix.
   d. linea alba.

9. The roof of the mouth is called the
   a. frenum.
   b. palate.
   c. tonsils.
   d. papilla.

10. The raised line that extends down the middle of the hard palate is called the
    a. palatine rugae.
    b. palatine raphe.
    c. palatine tonsils.
    d. palatine duct.

11. The occasional lump or prominence of bone in the maxillary palate is called a
    a. torus.
    b. uvula.
    c. fauces.
    d. frenum.

12. The projection(s) that extend(s) off the back of the maxillary soft palate is (are) the
    a. frenum.
    b. uvula.
    c. papilla
    d. commissures

13. Covering the dorsal side of the tongue, where the taste buds are located, are small raised projections called

    a. foliate.

    b. papilla.

    c. sulcus.

    d. fauces.

14. Covering the dorsal area of the tongue are hair-like projections called

    a. circumvallate papillae.

    b. filiform papillae.

    c. fungiform papillae.

    d. foliate papillae.

15. Name the sulcus that marks the end of the alveolar ridge and the beginning of the floor of the mouth.

    a. Sublingual caruncles

    b. Sublingual folds

    c. Sublingual sulcus

    d. Sublingual gland

16. The largest of the salivary glands are the

    a. parotids.

    b. submandibulars.

    c. subcaruncles.

    d. sublingual.

17. From which gland does the Wharton's duct empty saliva?

    a. Parotid

    b. Fauces

    c. Submandibular

    d. Terminalis

18. The mumps are a viral infection affecting the_____ gland.

    a. salivary

    b. parotid

    c. submandibular

    d. Wharton's

19. The bone that contains the mastoid process is the

    a. parietal.

    b. temporal.

    c. frontal.

    d. occipital.

20. Which bone forms part of the nose, orbits, and floor of the cranium?

    a. Sphenoid

    b. Ethmoid

    c. Pterygoid

    d. Styloid

21. The _____ bone is a single continuous bone that goes across the skull anterior to the temporal bones and is shaped like a bat with its wings spread.

    a. styloid

    b. occipital

    c. sphenoid

    d. pterygoid

22. Which bone forms the cheeks?

    a. Vomer

    b. Nasal

    c. Lacrimal

    d. Zygomatic

23. The tear ducts pass through which bones?

    a. Zygomatic

    b. Nasal

    c. Vomer

    d. Lacrimal

24. The largest of the facial bones, which has two sections, is the

    a. maxilla.

    b. mandible.

    c. palatine.

    d. rami.

25. The only movable bone of the face is the

    a. maxilla.

    b. mandible.

    c. rami.

    d. palatine.

26. The_____ process forms the bone that supports the maxillary teeth.

    a. alveolar
    b. palatine
    c. zygomatic
    d. median

27. The_____articulates with the temporal bones to form the temporomandibular joint.

    a. palatine
    b. condyle
    c. foramen
    d. symphysis

28. The function of the temporal muscles of mastication is to

    a. depress the mandible.
    b. depress the maxilla.
    c. expand the posterior fibers.
    d. elevate the mandible.

29. The masseter muscles belong to which group of muscles of the head and neck?

    a. Muscles of facial expression
    b. Muscles of the floor of the mouth
    c. Muscles of the tongue
    d. Muscles of mastication

30. This muscle is the medial surface of the lateral pterygoid plate, otherwise known as (the)

    a. external pterygoid.
    b. internal pterygoid.
    c. temporalis.
    d. masseter.

31. The buccinator muscle group belongs to which of the following?

    a. Muscles of facial expression
    b. Muscles of the floor of the mouth
    c. Muscles of the tongue
    d. Muscles of mastication

32. The function of this muscle is to wrinkle the skin of the chin.

    a. Buccinator
    b. Oris
    c. Orbicularis
    d. Mentalis

33. One of the muscles that serves to form the floor of the mouth is the

    a. digastric.
    b. gemoglossus.
    c. hypoglossus.
    d. styloglossus.

34. The largest cranial nerve, which innervates the maxilla and the mandible, is the

    a. ophthalmic.
    b. trigeminal.
    c. nasopalatine.
    d. infraorbital.

35. What nerve branch is composed of both sensory and motor nerves?

    a. Lingual
    b. Inferior alveolar
    c. Buccal
    d. Mandibular

36. The buccal nerve branch innervates which of the following?

    1. Lingual mucosa
    2. Buccal mucosa
    3. Posterior alveolar
    4. Buccal gingiva
    5. Buccal of the mandibular molars
    6. Mylohyoid

    a. 1, 3
    b. 2, 3, 4
    c. 2, 4, 6
    d. 2, 4, 5

37. The external jugular vein

    a. receives blood from the cranium.

    b. receives blood from the face.

    c. receives blood from the neck.

    (d.) drains blood from the superficial veins of the face and neck.

38. The internal jugular vein

    (a.) receives blood from the cranium.

    b. drains blood from the superficial veins of the face and neck.

    c. drains blood from the neck.

    d. drains blood from the cranium.

39. When the lips are pulled out, raised lines of mucosal tissue extend from the alveolar mucosa through the vestibule to the labial and buccal mucosa. These are called

    a. incisive papilla.

    (b.) frena.

    c. buccal mucosa.

    d. parotid papilla.

40. The largest papilla, which are mushroom shaped, are anterior to the sulcus terminalis in a row of 8 to 10. These are called

    a. filiform papillae.

    b. fungiform papillae.

    c. foliate papillae.

    (d.) circumvallate papillae.

Matching

Using the following diagram, match the landmarks with the correct terms.

1. B

2. D

3. E

4. C

5. A

a. Labial commissure

b. Nasolabial groove

c. Philtrum

d. Vermilion border

e. Labial mental groove

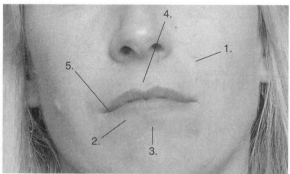

© Cengage Learning 2013

Match each landmark in the palatal area of the oral cavity with the correct description.

Landmark

6. __E__ Palate

7. __D__ Incisive papilla

8. __B__ Palatine raphe

9. __C__ Palatine rugae

10. __A__ Torus

Description

a. Prominence of bone in middle maxillary palate

b. Raised line at posterior, middle of hard palate

c. Ridges that run horizontal across hard palate

d. Raised area of tissue behind maxillary central incisors

e. Roof of the mouth

These nerve branches descend from the mandibular nerve. Match the nerve branch with its service.

Nerve Branch

11. __D__ Lingual

12. __A__ Inferior alveolar

13. __B__ Mental

14. __C__ Incisive

Service

a. Runs parallel to lingual nerve

b. Supplies chin and lower lip area

c. Innervates anterior teeth and labial gingiva

d. Descends to the underside of the tongue, the chin, and the lower lip area

Listed here are landmarks of the palatal and oral pharynx area. Match each term with its location on the diagram below.

15. __B__ Uvula

16. __C__ Incisive papilla

17. __D__ Palatine raphe

18. __A__ Anterior tonsillar pillars

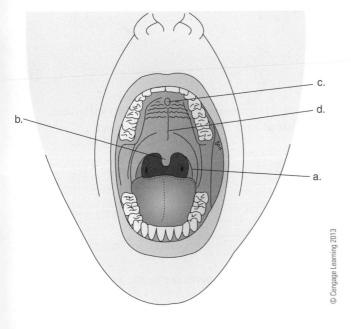

© Cengage Learning 2013

Match the following terms on the left with the definitions of the regions of the tongue on the right.

Term

Definition

19. __B__ Circumvallate papillae

a. Papillae that give the tongue its "strawberry effect"

20. __D__ Filiform papillae

b. Largest papilla, mushroom shaped

21. __A__ Fungiform papillae

c. Slightly raised, vertical folds of tissue on the lateral border of the tongue

22. __C__ Foliate papillae

d. Hair-like projections covering the dorsal side of the tongue

Critical Thinking

1. These landmarks are covered with skin consistent with skin in other parts of the face. These areas should be look at for scarring from accidents, surgeries, or physical conditions such as cleft lip. Name these landmarks.

2. Observations are made of cracks, color changes, and variations in form in this area of the mouth, where the upper lip meets the lower lip. Name this area.

3. Due to infection, the palatine tonsils are often marked with deep grooves and are red and inflamed. Name the landmarks of the soft palate and the oropharynx areas and describe their location.

4. This area of the oral cavity, which is sometimes under the tongue on the alveolar bone, is an excess bone formation. What is this excess bone formation called?

CASE STUDY 1

The dental office has made special efforts to ensure that alginate topical ointments have flavors that might win patients' approval. Lou is to have a dental impression, and the dental assistant states that the material she is using is strawberry flavored. Lou's response is "I have no sense of taste."

1. List the four fundamental taste senses.

2. List the basic taste bud locations by receptor.

3. Identify the sensation of taste.

4. How does the dental assistant access patient response?

CASE STUDY 2

Sara, a patient of record, is being prepared for dental treatment. The dental assistant questions Sara whether there has been any change in her health since her last appointment. Sara states that her mouth "is extremely dry lately."

1. List the function of the salivary glands.

2. Name the three major salivary glands and their functions.

3. Identify the color and viscosity of saliva.

4. Identify what may cause dry mouth.

5. What diseases may be related to dry mouth?

6. How will the dental assistant respond to the patient regarding dry mouth?

CASE STUDY 3

On a routine dental checkup, Martha complains of her glands just below and in front of the ear being sore to the touch. Upon further examination, the doctor indicates that Martha may have the mumps.

1. Name the glands in which mumps are most likely detectable.

2. List the characteristics of mumps.

3. List the age groups in which mumps most likely occur.

4. What other conditions cause swelling in these glands?

Labeling

Muscles of Mastication

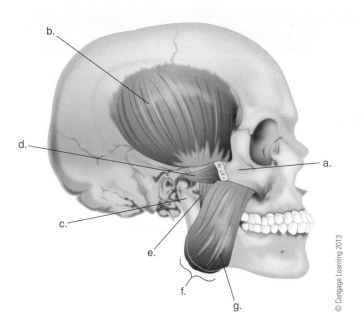

© Cengage Learning 2013

Identify the term and label its location on the diagram provided.

1. _____ Angle of the mandible

2. _____ External pterygoid muscle

3. _____ Internal pterygoid muscle

4. _____ Masseter muscle

5. _____ Neck of the condyle

6. _____ Temporal muscle

7. __F__ Zygomatic bone

Muscles of Facial Expression

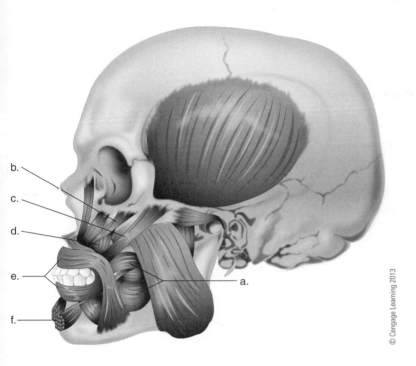

b.

c.

d.

e.

f.

a.

Identify the term and label its location on the diagram provided.

8. _____ Buccinator muscle

9. _____ Levator anguli oris muscle

10. _____ Mentalis

11. _____ Orbicularis oris

12. _____ Zygomatic major

13. _____ Zygomatic minor

Nerves of the Maxillary Arch

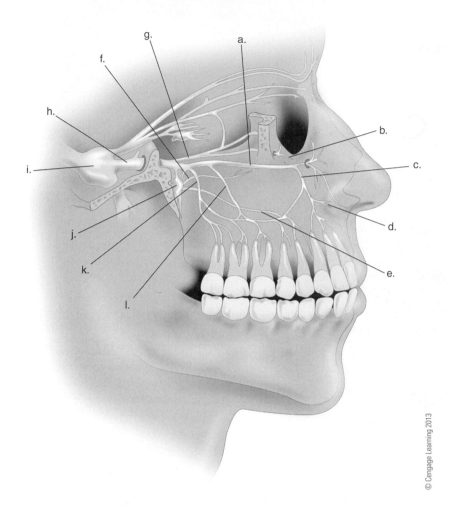

© Cengage Learning 2013

Identify the term and label its location on the diagram provided.

14. _____ Anterior superior alveolar nerve

15. _____ Infraorbital nerve

16. _____ Lateral nasal branches

17. _____ Maxillary division of trigeminal nerve

18. _____ Middle superior alveolar nerve

19. _____ Nasopalatine branch of pterygopalatine (sphenopalatine) nerve

20. _____ Posterior superior alveolar nerve

21. _____ Pterygopalatine ganglion

22. _____ Pterygopalatine nerve

23. _____ Trigeminal ganglion

24. _____ Zygomatic nerve

25. _____ Zygomaticofacial nerve

Mandibular Nerves

Identify the term and label its location on the diagram provided.

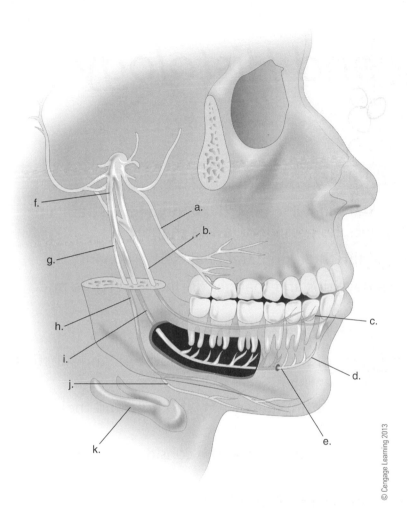

© Cengage Learning 2013

26. _____ Buccal nerve

27. _____ Hyoid bone

28. _____ Incisive nerves

29. _____ Inferior alveolar nerve (2) locations

30. _____ Lingual nerve

31. _____ Mental nerve at mental foramen

32. _____ Mylohyoid nerve (2) locations

33. _____ Posterior division of mandibular nerve

34. _____ Terminals of lingual nerve to tongue

CHAPTER **8**

Embryology and Histology

SPECIFIC INSTRUCTIONAL OBJECTIVES

The student should strive to meet the following objectives and demonstrate an understanding of the facts and principles presented in this chapter:

1. Identify the terms and times of the three prenatal phases of pregnancy.

2. Describe how the human face develops and changes during the zygote and embryo phases.

3. Describe the life cycle of a tooth and identify the stages.

4. Identify the four primary structures of the tooth and the location and function of each.

5. Identify the substances of enamel, dentin, cementum, and pulp and their identifying marks.

6. Identify the components of the periodontium and the considerations of the alveolar bone.

7. Describe the structures of the gingiva and the mucosa.

SUMMARY

It is vital for the entire dental team to be able to communicate about the structure and function of the oral cavity. Therefore, it is important for the dental assistant to understand the structure/function of tissue, the prenatal growth/development process of oral embryology, and the oral cavity that surrounds the teeth.

EXERCISES AND ACTIVITIES

Multiple Choice

1. _____ is the study of prenatal growth and development.

   a. Histology
   b. Microbiology

   c. Physiology
   d. Embryology

74

2. During the _____ phase, the development of various tissues takes place.

   a. morphodifferentiation
   b. cytodifferentiation
   c. histodifferentiation
   d. nasolacrimal

3. In which week of prenatal development will the face begin to form?

   a. Twelfth
   b. Fourth
   c. Sixteenth
   d. Ninth

4. In the facial development phase, which embryonic layer is responsible for forming the upper portion of the face, forehead, eyes, and nose?

   a. Medial nasal
   b. Mandibular process
   c. Frontonasal process
   d. Stomedeum

5. In the facial development phase, which embryonic layer is responsible for forming the cheeks, sides of the upper lip, and maxilla?

   a. Medial nasal
   b. Mandibular process
   c. Frontonasal process
   d. Stomedeum

6. Which factors can initiate malformation in the unborn child?

   a. Genetics
   b. Environment
   c. Infections
   d. All of the above

7. Fetal alcohol syndrome (FAS) in an infant is the result of the mother

   a. contracting infections.
   b. persisting in alcohol consumption.
   c. contracting syphilis.
   d. being exposed to measles.

8. If a cleft lip occurs on both sides of the lip, it is called

   a. unilateral.
   b. bilateral.
   c. complete.
   d. Parkal.

9. The first stage of the life cycle of the tooth is called

   a. initiation.
   b. lamina.
   c. odontogenesis.
   d. proliferation.

10. Enamel-forming cells are called

    a. odontoblasts.
    b. cementoblasts.
    c. ameloblasts.
    d. buds.

11. The last development stage before eruption is

    a. initiation.
    b. calcification.
    c. attrition.
    d. proliferation.

12. The final stage of the life cycle of the tooth is

    a. initiation.
    b. proliferation.
    c. calcification.
    d. attrition.

13. The study of the microscopic structure and function of tissues is

    a. physiology.
    b. histology.
    c. embryology.
    d. microbiology.

14. The hardest living tissue in the body is

    a. dentin.
    b. cementum.
    c. enamel.
    d. lamina.

15. Primary teeth may erupt with a covering over the enamel, called

    a. lines of Retzius.
    b. Tome's process.
    c. perikymata.
    d. Nasmyth's membrane.

16. Which of the following is softer than enamel but harder than cementum and bone?

    a. Dentin
    b. Fibroblast
    c. Osteoblast
    d. Osteoclast

17. _____ tubules pass through the entire surface of the dentin.

    a. Tertiary
    b. Mantle
    c. Circumpulpal
    d. Dentinal

18. The most pronounced stained contour line, which occurs due to the trauma of birth, is

    a. imbrication.
    b. contour.
    c. apposition.
    d. neonatal.

19. Which of the following are functions of pulp?

    1. To provide nourishment
    2. To support the dentin
    3. To provide maintenance for the dentin
    4. To transmit sensory information to the brain
    5. To identify temperature changes
    6. To identify chemical changes
    7. To pick up plaque easily
    8. To provide mineralization

       a. 1, 7, 8
       b. 1, 2, 3, 4, 5, 6
       c. 1, 2, 3, 7
       d. 3, 4, 6, 8

20. The pulp is partially made from _____, which are cells from which connective tissue evolves.

    a. pulpitis
    b. dentinal
    c. collagen
    d. fibroblasts

21. If the pulp is damaged due to an injury, the tissue may become inflamed, causing

    a. dentinal hypersensitivity.
    b. pulpitis.
    c. dysplasia.
    d. fibroblasts.

22. The _____ consists of portions of the tooth structure, supporting hard and soft dental tissues, and the alveolar bone.

    a. enamel
    b. dentin
    c. periodontium
    d. cementum

23. Which of the following are characteristics of cementum?

    1. Supports soft dental tissues
    2. Will regenerate like bone
    3. Lighter than dentin
    4. Darker than enamel
    5. Dull light pink in color
    6. Harder than dentin

       a. 1, 3
       b. 2, 4
       c. 3, 4
       d. 1, 4

24. The collagen fibers that act as anchors between the alveolar bone and teeth are called

    a. lines of Owen.
    b. lines of Von Ebner.

    c. Sharpey's fibers.
    d. Tome's process.

25. The bones of the mandible and the maxilla are formed by

    a. osteoblasts.
    b. osteoclasts.

    c. alveolus.
    d. lamina.

26. The cells that remodel and resorb bone are called

    a. osteoblasts.
    b. osteoclasts.

    c. alveolus.
    d. lamina.

27. The tooth-bearing extended areas of bone in each arch are called the

    a. alveolar crest.
    b. alveolus.

    c. alveolar process.
    d. lamina dura.

28. At the _____, two cortical bone plates come together between each tooth.

    a. alveolar crest
    b. alveolus

    c. alveolar process
    d. lamina dura

29. On a dental radiograph the radiopaque line, or _____, represents the thin, compact alveolus bone lining the socket.

    a. alveolar crest
    b. periodontal ligament

    c. alveolar process
    d. lamina dura

30. The periodontal ligament, like all connective tissue, is formed by _____ cells.

    a. odontoblast
    b. fibroblast

    c. osteoblast
    d. osteoclast

31. Which of the following are characteristics of healthy gingiva?

    1. Firm tissue surrounding teeth
    2. Stippled texture
    3. Can be attached to underlying bone
    4. Surrounds the root
    5. Thicker at root
    6. Mass attached to dentin

    a. 1, 3, 5
    b. 2, 3, 5

    c. 3, 4, 5
    d. 1, 2, 3

32. Free gingiva is also known as _____ gingiva.

    a. interdental
    b. epithelial

    c. attached
    d. marginal

33. The mucogingival junction is the line of demarcation between the _____ gingiva and the _____ mucosa.

    a. free, dentinal
    b. attached, alveolar

    c. interdental, alveolar
    d. sulcus, dentinal

34. The space between the unattached gingiva and the tooth is the

    a. attached gingiva.
    b. marginal gingiva.

    c. interdental gingiva.
    d. gingival sulcus.

35. In the floor of the gingival sulcus, _____ the attachment attaches to the enamel surface of the teeth.

    a. sulcus
    b. marginal

    c. interdental
    d. epithelial

36. In a healthy mouth, the gingival sulcus space would not exceed _____ millimeters in depth.

   a. 2 to 3

   b. 3 to 4

   c. 4 to 5

   d. 2 to 4

Matching

Dentin will differ according to area and is not uniform throughout. Identify the types of dentin and their functions.

Types of Dentin

1. __c__ Intertubular
2. __e__ Circumpulpal
3. __d__ Primary
4. __b__ Secondary
5. __a__ Tertiary

Function

a. Repairs and is reactive to irritations

b. Forms after completion of apical foramen

c. Found between the tubules

d. Forms the bulk of the tooth

e. Layer of dentin that surrounds pulp

Match the terms for pregnancy phases by time period.

Terms

6. __c__ Zygote
7. __a__ Embryo
8. __b__ Fetus

Time Period

a. Two weeks through the eighth week

b. Nine weeks through birth

c. Conception through the first two weeks

Critical Thinking

1. A patient complains of extreme pressure and inflammation around his maxillary second premolar. What clinical considerations would be reviewed?

   a. Treatment

   b. Causes

   c. Prevention

   d. Other

2. When the air-water syringe is used in an area that is not anesthetized and it causes discomfort to the patient:

  a. What is the cause for discomfort?

  b. What clinical considerations may apply?

3. A patient is diagnosed with periodontal disease. Several clinical concerns focus on supporting structures.

  a. Name the supporting structures that are likely involved.

  b. State their involvement in this disease

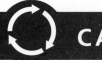 CASE STUDY 1

Ariel is concerned about the yellow staining on her teeth, and she has brought this concern to the dentist's attention. She has noticed the staining for some time, but as yet no one has suggested a cause.

1. Why would the dentist inquire whether tetracycline was taken?

2. What are the clinical considerations regarding permanent yellow staining?

 CASE STUDY 2

The patient expresses concern about the appearance of her tooth surface, stating, "These are pitted and grooved, can anything be done to improve them?" In the life cycle of the tooth, certain developmental disturbances can occur. What may have happened in this case?

1. What are the likely causes of pitting and grooving of tooth surfaces?

2. State the developmental stage at which pitting and grooving most likely occur.

3. Describe the life-cycle stage of this process.

4. Can this surface be restored?

5. How can demineralization be prevented?

Labeling

On the illustration showing the facial processes on an embryo, label the following:

- Medial nasal process
- Mandibular process
- Frontonasal process

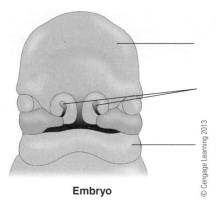

Embryo

© Cengage Learning 2013

On the illustration showing the facial processes on a child, label the following:

- Medial nasal (maxillary)
- Labial commissures
- Mandibular process
- Upper lip
- Philtrum
- Frontonasal process
- Nasolacrimal groove

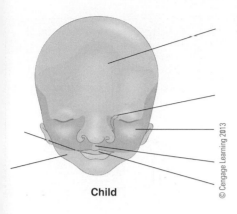

Child

On the illustration showing the facial processes on an adult, label the following:

- Labial commissures
- Mandibular process
- Philtrum
- Maxillary process
- Frontonasal process

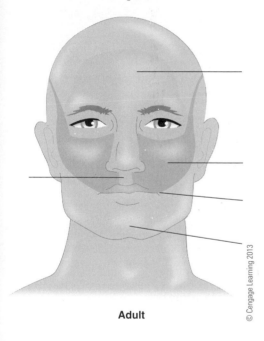

Adult

On the illustration showing the developing palate, label the following landmarks:

- Developing mandible
- Developing tongue
- Maxillary process
- Palatal shelf
- Stomodeum

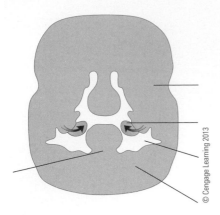

On the illustration showing the developing palate, label the following landmarks:

- Developing mandible
- Fusing palate
- Maxillary process
- Nasal cavity developing
- Nasal septum
- Oral cavity
- Tongue

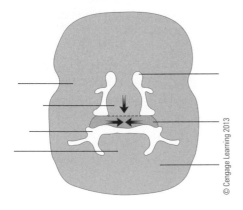

On the illustration showing the developing palate, label the following landmarks:

- Hard palate
- Incisive suture
- Median palatine suture
- Primary palate with central and lateral incisors
- Secondary palate with canines, premolars, and molars
- Soft palate
- Transverse palatine suture
- Uvula

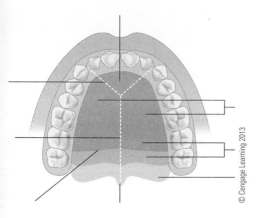

© Cengage Learning 2013

On the illustration of tooth tissues, label the following landmarks:

- Cementum

- Dentin

- Enamel

- Pulp

- Pulp canal

- Pulp chamber

- Pulp horns

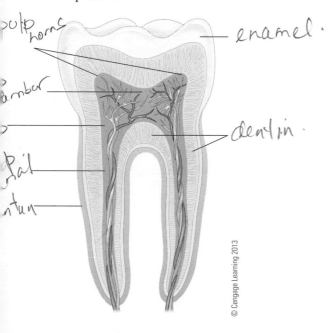

pulp horns

enamel.

chamber

dentin.

pal

ntun

© Cengage Learning 2013

Using the figure, label this section of the mandibular molar by identifying all periodontal ligaments and group fibers of alveolar crest, horizontal, oblique, apical, interradicular, and interdental bone.

- Alveolar bone

- Alveolar crest

- Alveolar crest fiber group

- Alveolus (lamina dura)

- Apical fiber group

- Cementum
- Dentin
- Horizontal fiber group
- Interdental bone
- Interdental fiber group
- Interradicular fiber group
- Interradicular septum
- Oblique fiber group

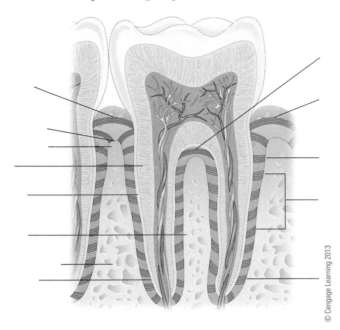

© Cengage Learning 2013

Utilizing the figure, label and identify the landmarks of the periodontium.

- Alveolar bone
- Attached gingiva
- Cementum
- Dentin
- Enamel
- Epithelial attachment
- Gingival crest
- Gingival groove (free gingival groove)
- Gingival sulcus
- Lamina dura
- Marginal gingiva (free gingiva)
- Mucogingival junction
- Periodontal ligaments

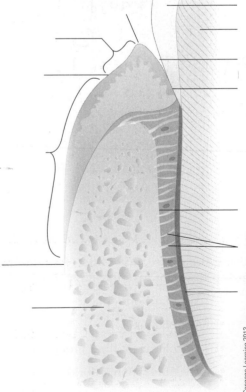

© Cengage Learning 2013

Using the figure, label and identify the sections of the tooth and the surrounding structures.

- Alveolar process
- Apex
- Apical foramen
- Cementoenamel junction (CEJ)
- Cementum
- Dentin
- Dentinoenamel junction (DEJ)
- Enamel
- Gingiva
- Lamina dura
- Pulp

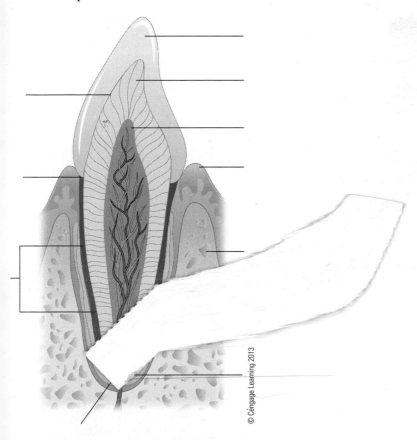

© Cengage Learning 2013

Using the figure, label and identify all the sections of the tooth and all fibers.

- Alveolar crest of alveolar bone proper
- Cementoenamel junction (CEJ)
- Cementum
- Dentinocementum junction (DCJ)
- Enamel
- Epithelial attachment

- Gingival fiber group
- Lamina propria of the marginal gingiva
- Mantle dentin
- Periodontal ligament
- Pulp
- Sharpey's fibers

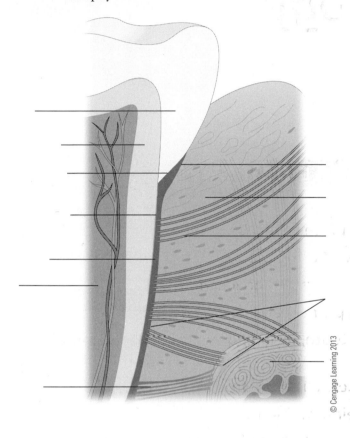

© Cengage Learning 2013

CHAPTER 9

Tooth Morphology

SPECIFIC INSTRUCTIONAL OBJECTIVES

The student should strive to meet the following objectives and demonstrate an understanding of the facts and principles presented in this chapter:

1. Identify the dental arches and quadrants using the correct terminology.

2. List the primary and permanent teeth by name and location.

3. Explain the eruption schedule for the primary and permanent teeth.

4. Identify the different divisions of the tooth, including clinical and anatomical divisions.

5. Identify the surfaces of each tooth and their locations.

6. List the anatomical structures and their definitions.

7. Describe each permanent tooth according to location, anatomical features, morphology, function, position, and other identifying factors.

8. Describe each deciduous (primary) tooth according to its location, anatomical features, morphology, function, position, and other identifying factors.

SUMMARY

Understanding tooth morphology will prepare the assistant to record accurately for the dentist or hygienist, contributing in a vital way to help those team members make a more accurate diagnosis. Therefore, the dental assistant will need to be able to identify each tooth from its anatomical form.

EXERCISES AND ACTIVITIES

True or False

1. The anterior sextant is made from the six front teeth.

   a. True
   b. False

2. The area between the apical third of the root and the cervical third of the root is called the middle third of the root.

   a. True
   b. False

3. A developmental groove that has an imperfect union where the lobes join is called a fissure.

   a. True
   b. False

4. A convex surface means that the surface is recessed.

   a. True
   b. False

5. A marginal ridge is an elevated area of enamel that forms the mesial and distal borders of the occlusal surface of the posterior teeth.

   a. True
   b. False

Multiple Choice

1. The _____ surface is toward the midline.

   a. labial   c. mesial
   b. distal   d. lingual

2. The _____ surface is away from the midline.

   a. lingual   c. mesial
   b. distal   d. facial

3. The anatomical crown is the portion of the tooth that is covered with

   a. dentin.   c. enamel.
   b. cementum.   d. fiber.

4. The anatomical root is the portion of the tooth that is covered with

   a. enamel.   c. apex.
   b. cementum.   d. mamelons.

5. The primary (deciduous) dentition consists of

   a. 32 teeth, 18 in each arch, and 9 in each quadrant.   c. 16 teeth, 8 in each arch, and 4 in each quadrant.
   b. 20 teeth, 10 in each arch, and 5 in each quadrant.   d. 12 teeth, 6 in each arch, and 3 in each quadrant.

6. The primary first molar is replaced by an adult

   a. canine.   c. first molar.
   b. premolar.   d. lateral.

7. These teeth are used to pulverize food, (i.e., they break the food down into small pieces).

   a. Canine

   b. Premolar

   c. Molars

   d. Wisdom teeth

8. These teeth are used for the chewing process.

   a. Canine

   b. Premolars

   c. Molars

   d. Centrals

9. These are the teeth that are farthest from the midline.

   a. Canine

   b. Premolars

   c. Molars

   d. Wisdom teeth

10. There are _____ posterior sextants in each arch.

    a. two

    b. one

    c. six

    d. four

11. The area on the crown of the tooth that is closest to the incisal edge on the anterior tooth is called the

    a. occlusal third.

    b. cervical third.

    c. incisal third.

    d. apical third.

12. The area on the crown of the tooth between the incisal third and the cervical third is called the

    a. occlusal third.

    b. middle third.

    c. occlusal surface.

    d. contact area.

Matching

Match each term with its definition.

Term

1. ___b___ Midline

2. ___d___ Quadrant

3. ___a___ Maxillary

4. ___c___ Mandibular

Definition

a. Upper arch

b. Division between two equal halves

c. Lower arch

d. One-fourth of the complete dentition

Match the following terms with the deciduous teeth in the following diagram.

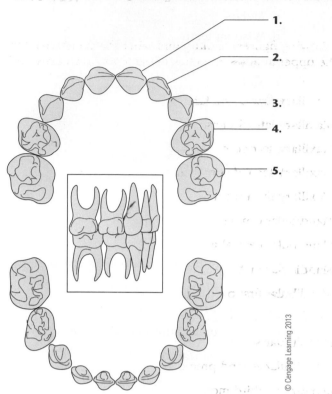

5. Canine

6. Central incisor

7. First molar

8. Second molar

9. Lateral incisor

1. _6_

2. _9_

3. _5_

4. _7_

5. _8_

Critical Thinking

1. In our lifetime, we have two sets of teeth. On the following figures, identify and label the deciduous dentition and the permanent dentition. Next, identify the upper and lower arches of each set—maxillary and mandibular.

- Maxillary canine
- Maxillary central incisor
- Maxillary first molar
- Maxillary lateral incisor
- Maxillary second molar
- Mandibular canine
- Mandibular central incisor
- Mandibular first molar
- Mandibular lateral incisor
- Mandibular second molar
- Maxillary canine
- Maxillary central incisor
- Maxillary first molar

- Maxillary first premolar
- Maxillary lateral incisor
- Maxillary second molar
- Maxillary second premolar
- Maxillary third molar
- Mandibular canine
- Mandibular central incisor
- Mandibular first molar
- Mandibular first premolar
- Mandibular lateral incisor
- Mandibular second molar
- Mandibular second premolar
- Mandibular third molar

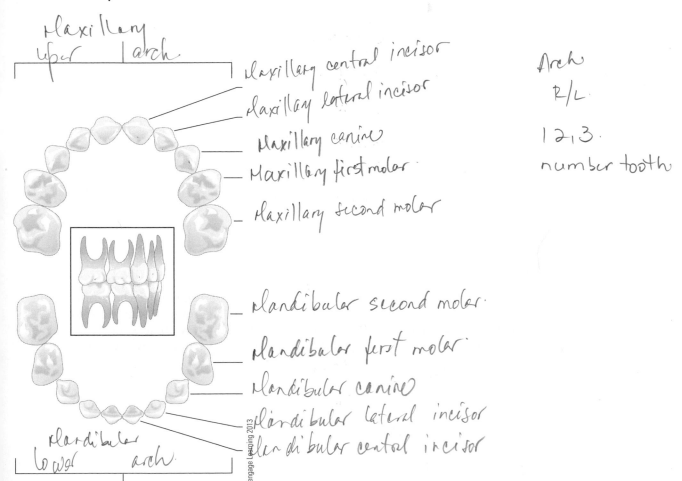

Maxillary
Upper   arch

Maxillary central incisor
Maxillary lateral incisor
Maxillary canine
Maxillary first molar
Maxillary second molar

Arch
R/L.
1 2 3.
number tooth

Mandibular second molar.
Mandibular first molar.
Mandibular canine
Mandibular lateral incisor
Mandibular central incisor

Mandibular
lower   arch.

© Cengage Learning 2013

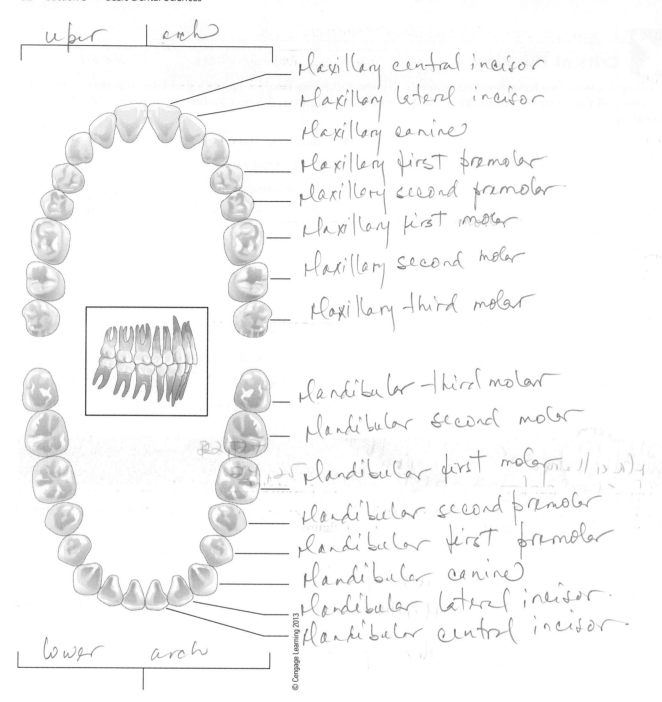

upper | arch

Maxillary central incisor

Maxillary lateral incisor

Maxillary canine

Maxillary first premolar

Maxillary second premolar

Maxillary first molar

Maxillary second molar

Maxillary third molar

Mandibular third molar

Mandibular second molar

Mandibular first molar

Mandibular second premolar

Mandibular first premolar

Mandibular canine

Mandibular lateral incisor

Mandibular central incisor

lower | arch

© Cengage Learning 2013

2. Jessica, age 6, is seeing her dentist about a loose anterior tooth. An understanding of the eruption and exfoliation dates will aid in explaining this to Jessica and her mother. The normal pattern for losing deciduous teeth to be replaced by permanent teeth will be better understood by completing Table 9-1. Fill in the eruption dates (months), exfoliation dates (years), and the order of eruption by arch (maxillary/mandibular).

Table 9.1 Eruption and Exfoliation Dates for Primary Teeth

Tooth	Eruption Date (Months)	Exfoliation Date (Years)	Maxillary Order
Central incisor			
Lateral incisor			
Canine			
First molar			
Second molar			
			Mandibular Order
Central incisor			
Lateral incisor			
Canine			
First molar			
Second molar			

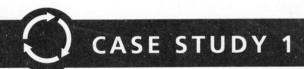

CASE STUDY 1

Cory, age 7-1/2, may lose his maxillary or mandibular deciduous second molar prematurely due to decay. He would likely have a mixed dentition as in the next figure.

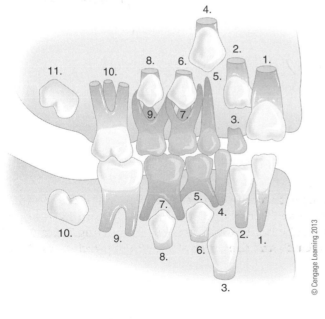

© Cengage Learning 2013

1. Using the figure, identify the following teeth:

Maxillary

a. Deciduous canine <u>C, H, M, R</u>

b. Deciduous lateral incisor <u>D, G, N, Q</u>

c. Deciduous first molar <u>B, I, L, S</u>

d. Deciduous second molar <u>A, J, K, T</u>

e. Permanent central incisor <u>8, 9, 24, 25</u>

f. Permanent lateral incisor <u>7, 10, 23, 26</u>

g. Permanent first molar <u>3, 14, 19, 30</u>

h. Permanent first premolar <u>5, 12, 21, 28</u>

i. Permanent second molar <u>2, 15, 18, 31</u>

j. Permanent second premolar <u>4, 13, 20, 29</u>

k. Permanent canine <u>6, 11, 22, 27</u>

Mandibular

a. Deciduous canine <u>M R</u>

b. Deciduous first molar <u>L, S</u>

c. Deciduous second molar <u>K T</u>

d. Permanent canine <u>22, 27</u>

e. Permanent central incisor <u>24, 25</u>

f. Permanent lateral incisor <u>23, 26</u>

g. Permanent first molar <u>19, 30</u>

h. Permanent first premolar <u>21, 28</u>

i. Permanent second molar <u>18, 31</u>

j. Permanent second premolar <u>20, 29</u>

2. If one of the deciduous molars is lost, which adult tooth will replace it?

   #4, 13, 20, 29.

3. What age will Cory be when he would expect his second premolar to erupt?

   11-12 years old.

CASE STUDY 2

Mixed dentition is common at ages 6 to 13. Some individuals may have congenitally missing teeth. When assisting in dental charting, it is essential to understand and be knowledgeable of the eruption dates and order of eruption of the adult dentition. Use Table 9-2 to present the eruption dates and order of eruption of the maxillary and mandibular adult teeth.

Table 9.2 Eruption Dates for the Maxillary and Mandibular Permanent Teeth

Tooth	Eruption Date (Years)	Order of Eruption (Maxillary)
Central incisor	7-8	#2
Lateral incisor	8-9	#3
Canine	11-12	#6
First premolar	10-11	#4
Second premolar	6-7	#5
First molar	6-7	#1
Second molar	12-13	#7
Third molar	17-21	#8

Tooth	Eruption Date (Years)	Order of Eruption (Mandibular)
Central incisor	6-7	#2
Lateral incisor	7-8	#3
Cuspid	9-10	#4
First premolar	10-11	#5
Second premolar		
First molar	6-7	#1
Second molar	11-13	#7
Third molar	17-21	#8

Preclinical Dental Skills

CHAPTER 10

Microbiology

SPECIFIC INSTRUCTIONAL OBJECTIVES

The student should strive to meet the following objectives and demonstrate an understanding of the facts and principles presented in this chapter:

1. Identify Anton Van Leeuwenhoek, Ferdinand Cohn, Louis Pasteur, Robert Koch, and Richard Petri according to their contributions to microbiology.

2. Explain the groups of microorganisms and staining procedures used to identify them.

3. Identify characteristics pertaining to bacteria.

4. List the characteristics of protozoa.

5. Identify the characteristics of *Rickettsia*.

6. Explain the characteristics of yeasts and molds.

7. List the characteristics of viruses.

8. Describe the diseases of major concern to the dental assistant and explain why they cause concern.

9. Identify how the body fights disease. Explain types of immunity and routes of microorganism infection.

SUMMARY

To safeguard against microorganism exposure in a dental office, one must understand how these pathogens pass from an infected person to a susceptible person. Therefore, within this chapter you have been given information about pathogenic microorganisms along with the diseases they cause and how the body can defend against them.

EXERCISES AND ACTIVITIES

100%

True or False

1. Pediculosis is the state of being infected with anthrax.

   a. True
   b. False ✓

2. The seroconversion rate is the amount or level at which a vaccine causes development of immunity.

   a. True ✓
   b. False

3. Tuberculosis is caused by a virus.

   a. True
   b. False ✓

4. Robert Koch is known as the "Father of Microbiology."

   a. True
   b. False ✓ bacteria.

5. Periodontal disease may be caused by protozoa.

   a. True ✓
   b. False

6. West Nile Virus is transmitted through the bites of lice.

   a. True ✓
   b. False

7. Dental assistants should consider hepatitis vaccinations.

   a. True ✓
   b. False

8. A pathogen that stimulates the production of antibodies is called an antigen.

   a. True ✓
   b. False

9. Humans are not born with any sort of immunity.

   a. True
   b. False ✓

10. Anaphylactic shock can be fatal.

   a. True ✓
   b. False

Multiple Choice

1. The study of microorganisms is called

   a. pathogens.
   b. microbiology. ✓
   c. bacteria.
   d. virus.

2. _____ was acknowledged for being the first to see microorganisms.

   a. Van Leeuwenhoek   c. Koch

   b. Pasteur   d. Rickettsia

3. _____ determined the etiologic agent for tuberculosis. *Robert*

   a. Van Leeuwenhoek   c. Koch

   b. Pasteur   d. Rickettsia

4. When a specific type of bacteria causes a specific disease, it is called the _____ agent.

   a. bacteria   c. spore

   b. virus   d. etiologic

5. A staining procedure that differentiates bacteria into two major groups is (the)

   a. gram positive.   c. gram negative.

   b. Gram stain.   d. sporulating.

6. In the Gram staining process, if the bacteria appear dark purple under the microscope, they are

   a. gram negative.   c. spores.

   b. gram positive.   d. viruses.

7. In the Gram staining process, if the bacteria appear colorless under the microscope, they are

   a. gram negative.   c. viruses.

   b. gram positive.   d. spores.

8. _____ bacteria are destroyed in the presence of oxygen.

   a. Aerobic   c. Facultative anaerobic

   b. Anaerobic   d. Sporulating

9. Under a microscope, _____ bacteria will appear rod shaped.

   a. cocci   c. vibrios

   b. spirilla   d. bacilli

10. Under a microscope, _____ bacteria will appear round or bead shaped.

   a. cocci   c. vibrios

   b. spirilla   d. bacilli

11. Bacteria grown in colonies or clusters like grapes are called

   a. diplococci.   c. streptococci.

   b. staphylococci.   d. bacilli.

12. What type of bacteria is identified by a chain shape or form?

   a. Diplococci   c. Streptococci

   b. Staphylococci   d. Bacilli

13. Which of the following represent symptoms of tuberculosis?

   1. Severe throat infection   4. Whooping cough

   2. Tiredness   5. Persistent cough

   3. Night sweats   6. Stiffness of jaw

     a. 2,3,5   c. 1,3,4

     b. 1,2,3   d. 1,4,6

14. Name the group of bacteria that have been known to contribute to dental caries and endocarditis, as well as lead to pneumonia or rheumatic fever.

    a. Staphylococcal

    b. *Streptococcus mutans*

    c. Bacilli

    d. Protozoa

15. _____ microorganisms are often called amoebas, and they reproduce by binary fission.

    a. Staphylococcal

    b. *Streptococcus mutans*

    c. Bacilli

    d. Protozoa

16. Amoebic dysentery is connected with which of the following?

    a. Infection

    b. Severe diarrhea as a symptom

    c. Can cause abscesses in the liver in severe cases

    d. All of the above

17. Protozoa and bacteria together cause a dental condition called _____ that is found in the inflamed tissue around the tooth

    a. dental decay

    b. calculus/tartar

    c. periodontal disease

    d. candidiasis

18. Two diseases caused by *Rickettsia* bacteria are

    a. candidiasis and dysentery.
    b. malaria and periodontal disease.

    c. Rocky Mountain spotted fever and typhus.
    d. candidiasis and tinea.

19. Candidiasis is an infection caused by (a)

    a. virus.

    b. fungus.

    c. influenza.

    d. herpes.

20. The fungus tinea corporis is commonly called

    a. athlete's foot.

    b. thrush.

    c. ringworm.

    d. measles.

21. _____ are the smallest microorganisms known to date and can be visualized only under an electron microscope.

    a. Bacteria

    b. Tinea

    c. Typhus

    d. Viruses

22. Which of the following diseases are caused by a virus?

    1. Measles

    2. Typhus

    3. Malaria

    4. Chicken pox

    5. Poliomyelitis

    6. Dysentery

    a. 1,3,6

    b. 1,4,5

    c. 1,2,3

    d. 2,3,6

23. Which viral disease is usually associated with infections of the lips, mouth, and face?

    a. Herpetic whitlow

    b. Conjunctivitis

    c. Herpes simplex virus type 2

    d. Herpes simplex virus type 1

24. _____ (a virus) is extremely contagious and can spread by direct contact with the lesion or the fluid from the lesion.

    a. HIV

    b. Hepatitis C

    c. Herpes simplex

    d. Hepatitis B

25. Name high-risk behaviors for acquiring hepatitis B.

    1. Injuries with sharp objects contaminated with blood
    2. Usage of latex gloves
    3. Wearing a mask
    4. Multiple unprotected sexual partners
    5. Using eyewear
    6. Exposure to an open wound with contaminated body fluid

        a. 1,4,5
        b. 2,3,5
        c. 1,3,6
        d. 1,4,6

26. Hepatitis _____ is transmitted by ingestion of contaminated food.

    a. E
    b. B
    c. A
    d. C

27. Hepatitis _____ is commonly called serum hepatitis.

    a. C
    b. B
    c. A
    d. C

28. Hepatitis _____ has a range of symptoms, including loss of appetite and jaundice.

    a. C
    b. B
    c. A
    d. C

29. The _____ vaccine shows effectiveness against hepatitis B.

    a. Heptavax-B
    b. Recombivax HB
    c. DPT
    d. L-Lysen

30. An individual who is a carrier of a disease but is not aware of it is called

    a. a delta agent.
    b. a contaminate.
    c. asymptomatic.
    d. a case.

31. Name the retrovirus disease that attacks T-lymphocytes, which are an important element of the immune system, and then multiplies.

    a. HBV
    b. HIV
    c. CDC
    d. MMR

32. Which of the following are full-blown AIDS conditions?

    1. Cancers
    2. Infections
    3. Diarrhea
    4. Constipation
    5. Lockjaw
    6. Rheumatic fever

        a. 3,4,5
        b. 1,2,3,4,5
        c. 1,5,6
        d. 3,4,6

33. A(n) _____ is a group of symptoms that characterizes a disease.

    a. syndrome
    b. etiologic agent
    c. spore
    d. bacterium

34. The body responds to disease in a number of ways. First, _____ must pass the body's first line of defense.

    a. antitoxins
    b. antibodies
    c. antigens
    d. pathogens

35. The _____ membrane is a wall that contains the infection and does not allow it to spread.

    a. periodontal

    (b.) pyogenic

    c. antigen

    d. toxin

36. As its final line of defense, the body forms _____ to produce immunities against a foreign substance.

    a. antigens

    (b.) antibodies

    c. antitoxins

    d. pathogens

37. If immunity develops as a result of exposure to a pathogen, the immunity is called

    a. normal.

    b. passive.

    (c.) acquired.

    d. active.

38. An individual who has the ability to resist pathogens is called

    a. an allergen.

    b. hypersensitive.

    (c.) immune.

    d. erythemic.

39. If a person's antigen-antibody response stimulates a massive secretion of histamine, the result would cause a severe reaction called

    a. active immunity.

    b. artificial immunity.

    c. passive immunity.

    (d.) anaphylactic shock.

40. If an antigen causes an allergic response, it is called

    a. immune.

    (b.) an allergen.

    c. inoculated.

    d. hypersensitive.

41. Which of the following release airborne particles that can spread tuberculosis to others?

    a. While coughing

    b. From saliva contact

    c. Cross-contamination by dental treatment

    (d.) All of the above

42. Identify the colony shown in this figure.

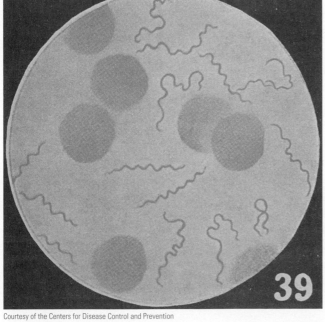

Courtesy of the Centers for Disease Control and Prevention

a. Bacilli

b. Cocci

(c.) Spirilla

d. Vibrios

43. Identify the colony shown in this figure.

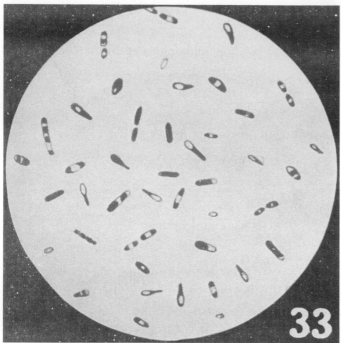

a. Spirilla   c. Vibrios
b. Bacilli   d. Cocci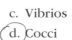

44. Identify the colony shown in this figure.

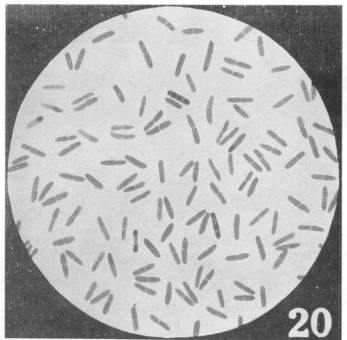

a. Spirilla   c. Bacilli
b. Cocci   d. Vibrios

Matching

Match each important person with his contribution to microbiology.

Important People	Contribution
1. _B_ Anton Van Leeuwenhoek	a. Proved that bacteria cause disease
2. _a_ Louis Pasteur	b. Father of microbiology
3. _A_ Robert Koch	c. Found that bacteria could be destroyed by heat

Match each type of microorganism with a disease and symptoms.

Microorganism	Disease or Symptom
4. _D_ Bacteria	a. MMR, poliomyelitis
5. _C_ Rickettsiae	b. Fungal infection
6. _B_ Yeasts and molds	c. Typhus
7. _A_ Virus	d. TB, DPT

Match each of the following diseases of major concern to the dental assistant with its respective infection.

Disease	Infection
8. _C_ Herpes simplex virus type 1	a. Serum hepatitis
9. _D_ Herpes simplex virus type 2	b. Class of retrovirus
10. _a_ Hepatitis B	c. Infections of lips, mouth, and face
11. _B_ HIV	d. Associated with genital area

Critical Thinking

1. Ferdinand Julius Cohn, a biologist, studied the life cycle of *Bacillus*. Why have his findings had such an impact on how dental offices perform sterilization?

2. Pasteur discovered a method of using an artificially generated weak form of a disease to fight the disease or prevent its occurrence. His work laid the foundation for many of these now being produced. Name this disease-fighting development.

3. Within the transmissible spongiform encephalopathy group is a disease called Creutzfeldt-Jakob disease. What age group is affected by it? What are the symptoms?

4. What do hepatitis A and hepatitis E have in common?

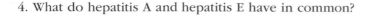

CASE STUDY 1

Bloodborne diseases are of major concern to the dental assistant. One of these diseases is transmitted directly through blood-contaminated body fluids.

1. Name the five different types of viral hepatitis.

2. Name four high-risk behaviors for acquiring hepatitis B, HIV, and AIDS.

CASE STUDY 2

Dental assistants must protect themselves against bacteria and also from the patient transmitting bacteria. One of the most common bacterial diseases infecting humans is strep throat.

1. Name the bacteria type.

2. Describe the bacteria simple fusion theory.

3. List the symptoms of strep throat.

4. Name some of the conditions that this bacteria can cause.

CASE STUDY 3

Individually, the health care worker must take action to enhance his or her ability to resist pathogens and thus disease.

1. Name and describe the two general types of immunity.

2. Identify borrowed immunity and how this occurs.

3. Name the two types of active acquired immunity.

4. List examples of each of the active acquired immunity types.

5. Explain what happens when there is an overreaction to an antigen.

C H A P T E R **11**

Infection Control

SPECIFIC INSTRUCTIONAL OBJECTIVES

The student should strive to meet the following objectives and demonstrate an understanding of the facts and principles presented in this chapter:

1. Identify the rationale, regulations, recommendations, and training that govern infection control in the dental office.

2. Describe how pathogens travel from person to person in the dental office.

3. List the three primary routes of microbial transmission and the associated dental procedures that affect the dental assistant.

4. Demonstrate the principles of infection control, including medical history, hand-washing, personal protective equipment (PPE), barriers, chemical disinfectants, ultrasonic cleaners, sterilizers, and instrument storage.

5. List various disinfectants and their applications as used in dentistry.

6. Identify and demonstrate the usage of different types of sterilizers.

7. Demonstrate the usage of several types of sterilization monitors, such as biological and process indicators.

8. Identify and show the proper usage of preprocedure mouth rinses, high-volume evacuation, dental dams, and disposable items.

9. Identify and demonstrate the correct protocol for disinfecting, cleaning, and sterilizing prior to seating the patient, as well as at the end of the dental treatment, in the dental radiography area, and in the dental laboratory.

SUMMARY

Staff must be trained for a safe workplace. Compliance with all regulations must be accomplished to ensure that the process of infection control will be adequate. Training will occur at initial employment, when job tasks change, and annually thereafter.

EXERCISES AND ACTIVITIES

True or False

1. BSI is a system that requires wearing PPE to prevent contact with all body fluids.

    a. True
    b. False

2. Asepsis means the creation of an environment free of disease-causing microorganisms.

    a. True
    b. False

3. Employers must protect their employees from exposure to blood and OPIM during the time when employees are at work.

    a. True
    b. False

4. When a disinfecting solution meets all the claims listed and the safety concerns are noted, the FDA will assign an EPA number that must appear on the solution's label.

    a. True
    b. False

5. Microorganisms may be missed because they appear as a mist or dry clear on the surfaces that are touched.

    a. True
    b. False

6. OSHA states that when removing protective clothing, special care is to be taken with items that are considered potentially infectious.

    a. True
    b. False

7. Latex allergies can result in contact dermatitis.

    a. True
    b. False

8. Low-level disinfection will kill bacterial spores.

    a. True
    b. False

9. Solutions used to disinfect instruments can be universally used in all types of disinfecting machines.

    a. True
    b. False

10. A heat-sensitive tape used to identify when materials have been sterilized is a type of biological monitor.

    a. True
    b. False

Multiple Choice

1. _____ is the principal professional organization for dentistry in the United States.

   a. CDC
   b. OSHA
   c. U.S. Public Health Service
   d. ADA

2. Name the agency that is part of the U.S. Public Health Service, a division of the U.S. Department of Health and Human Services, and is a source of many regulations.

   a. CDC
   b. OSHA
   c. ADA
   d. OPIM

3. In 1992, OSHA established the Bloodborne Pathogens Standard. It mandates that facilities must do which of the following?

   1. Provide a sterile environment

   2. Protect workers from infectious hazards

   3. Provide automatic handwashing systems

   4. Provide antimicrobial soap

   5. Protect workers from chemical hazards

   6. Protect workers from physical hazards

   a. 1, 5, 6
   b. 2, 5, 6
   c. 2, 3, 4
   d. 1, 3, 4

4. An employee who would have any occupational exposure to blood would be a category _____ employee by job classification.

   a. 1
   b. 2
   c. 3
   d. 4

5. Items in the dental office, such as sterilizers and PPE, are regulated by the _____, which holds manufacturers responsible for problems that develop.

   a. ADA
   b. FDA
   c. EPA
   d. ADAA

6. Name the agency that regulates disposal of hazardous waste after it leaves the office.

   a. CDC
   b. OSHA
   c. FDA
   d. EPA

7. What cycle is perpetuated when pathogens are allowed to pass from dentist to patient or from patient to dentist?

   a. Material safety data
   b. Cross-contamination
   c. Pathogens standard
   d. Standard exposure

8. If a dental assistant is hired, but has not already had the hepatitis B immunization, who pays for the vaccine series?

   a. Dentist
   b. Assistant
   c. Accountant
   d. OSHA

9. Patients could be infected with HBV and HIV and have no symptoms. This condition is called

   a. cross-contamination.
   b. antimicrobial.
   c. asymptomatic.
   d. transient.

10. One of the primary concerns of handwashing is to remove the _____ microorganisms because they constitute the group that includes hepatitis.

    a. transient
    b. causative
    c. bloodborne
    d. saliva

11. During the handwashing procedure, proper chemical antisepsis is accomplished with

    a. chlorhexidine digluconate.
    b. triclosan.
    c. parachlorometaxylenol.
    d. All of the above.

12. Handwashing before and after patient care requires a minimum of _____ seconds.

    a. 60
    b. 30
    c. 15
    d. 90

13. Barriers that prevent potential pathogens encountered during patient care from gaining access to dental personnel include which of the following?

    1. Material safety data sheets (MSDS)
    2. EPA
    3. Regulations
    4. Gloves
    5. Mask
    6. Eyewear

    a. 1, 2, 3
    b. 4, 5, 6
    c. 1, 4, 5
    d. 2, 3, 5

14. The _____ developed a standard for the design and characteristics of occupational protective eyewear/glasses.

    a. CDC
    b. OSHA
    c. EPA
    d. ANSI

15. The _____ regulates the gloves used in the health care industry.

    a. FDA
    b. EPA
    c. OSHA
    d. CDC

16. _____ gloves are used for patient treatment whenever the dental assistant anticipates contact with saliva or blood.

    a. Polynitrile
    b. Nitrile
    c. Utility
    d. Vinyl

17. _____ are worn by dental assistants whenever the possibility of aerosol mist exists.

    a. Overgloves
    b. Masks
    c. Rubber dams
    d. Lead aprons

18. The dental _____ also protects the patient and assistant from the transmission of communicable diseases.

    a. handpiece
    b. scaler
    c. mask
    d. ultrasonic

19. Special protective clothing worn only in the dental office is regulated by OSHA and includes

    a. uniforms.
    b. lab coats.
    c. gowns.
    d. All of the above

20. When the gown or uniform is on, the glove fits _____ it.

    a. over
    b. under

    c. behind
    d. on top of

21. Special protective clothing is regulated by OSHA. Which of the following are OSHA regulations regarding special protective clothing?

    1. Worn only in the dental offices
    2. Can be changed weekly
    3. Must be laundered in the office or by a laundry service
    4. Must close tightly at neck and around cuff
    5. Must be knee length when sitting during high-risk procedures
    6. Must bear ornamental designs
    7. Must be removed if going out to lunch or into the lunchroom
    8. Must be removed at end of day prior to going home
    9. Gown can be short-sleeved for summer
    10. Cuffs of gown do not need to overlap with cuffs of gloves

    a. 2, 5, 6, 8, 9, 10
    b. 1, 3, 6, 7, 9, 10

    c. 1, 3, 4, 5, 7, 8
    d. 2, 3, 7, 8, 9, 10

22. Concerning the asepsis requirement, some surfaces do not lend themselves to the use of barriers. Those surfaces will need to be

    a. suctioned.
    b. sterilized.

    c. autoclaved.
    d. disinfected.

23. According to EPA ratings, which disinfection level will kill most bacterial spores?

    a. High
    b. Intermediate

    c. Low
    d. Holding

24. Which of the following is considered to be a high-level disinfectant?

    a. Alcohol
    b. Glutaraldehyde

    c. Iodopher
    d. Sodium hypochlorite

25. Which of the following is considered an intermediate-level disinfectant?

    a. Alcohol
    b. Chlorine dioxide

    c. Glutaraldehyde
    d. Iodopher

26. The _____ is a device that uses sound waves that travel through glass and metal while using a special solution to clean debris from dental instruments.

    a. sterilizer
    b. autoclave

    c. ultrasonic cleaner
    d. holding bath

27. All forms of microorganisms are destroyed in the process of

    a. disinfection.
    b. asepsis.

    c. sterilization.
    d. sanitization.

28. If immersion sterilization is used, items are placed in the disinfecting solution for _____ hour(s) to ensure that all microorganisms are destroyed.

    a. 1
    b. 5

    c. 10
    d. 3

29. Most dental offices sterilize their dental handpieces exclusively in the _____ sterilizer.

    a. chemical vapor

    b. dry heat

    c. steam autoclave

    d. dishwasher-disinfector

30. _____ monitors offer the most accurate way to assess sterilization.

    a. Cavitation

    b. Biological

    c. Cleaning

    d. Sanitizing

31. _____ indicators are printed on packaging materials for sterilization and contain dyes that change color on quick exposure to sterilizing cycles.

    a. Biological

    b. Process

    c. Sanitizing

    d. Disinfecting

32. _____ indicators are placed inside sterilization packing and indicate whether the correct conditions were present for sterilization to take place.

    a. Biological

    b. Dosage

    c. Process

    d. Disinfecting

33. Which preprocedure reduces the total number of microorganisms in the oral cavity?

    a. Antiseptic mouth rinse

    b. Rubber dam

    c. Evacuation system

    d. Disinfectant

34. If an acrylic appliance needs to be sent from the dental office to an outside lab, the appliance will need to be placed in

    a. diluted sodium hypochlorite.

    b. dry heat.

    c. chemical vapor.

    d. steam.

35. The OSHA Bloodborne Pathogens Standard applies to which of the following facilities where employees can or have the potential to be exposed to body fluids?

    a. Research laboratories

    b. Emergency medical services

    c. Dental offices

    d. All of the above

36. Which of the following are anticipated occupational exposures?

    a. Needlestick

    b. Puncture

    c. Any contact with blood

    d. All of the above

37. OSHA-mandated training for dental office employees can be accomplished by which of the following methods?

    a. Only by videos

    b. Only by interactive computer training programs

    c. By an individual who has the background necessary to answer questions and to supplement the training with information specific to the office

    d. None of the above

38. An individual contacts a microorganism through contaminated instruments; this is an example of _____.

    a. indirect contact

    b. direct contact

    c. vectorborne-transmission

    d. airborne transmission

39. An individual contacts a microorganism when the high-speed handpiece is used in the dental office; this is an example of _____.

    a. direct contact

    b. inhalation/aerosol transmission

    c. bloodborne transmission

    d. indirect contact

40. According to dental unit waterline guidelines, waterlines should be disinfected _____ to remove biofilms.

a. daily   c. monthly

(b.) weekly   d. bimonthly

Matching

To provide complete infection control in a dental office, a number of steps must be followed. Match the following standards with the protection that they provide for both the patient and assistant.

Standard

1. _B_ Immunization
2. _C_ Handwashing
3. _D_ Gloves
4. _A_ Mask

Protection Benefit

a. Protects mucous membrane from aerosol
b. Hepatitis B vaccine
c. Removes transient microorganisms
d. Five primary types, and are regulated by FDA

Numerous gloves are available that meet FDA regulations. Following are four of the primary types of gloves. Match the glove with its designed use for the dental team member.

Glove Type

5. _D_ Latex
6. _A_ Overglove
7. _B_ Utility
8. _C_ Polynitrile

Glove Use

a. Known as food handlers' glove
b. Can be washed and reused
c. Can be sterilized in autoclave after each use
d. Called the examination glove

To ensure that all items used in intraoral procedures are sterile, there are several sterilization choices available. Match the sterilization method with its use.

Sterilization Method

9. _C_ Liquid chemical disinfectant
10. _A_ Dry heat
11. _D_ Chemical vapor
12. _B_ Steam autoclave

Use

a. Uses heat at 340°F
b. Uses 250°F
c. Requires 10 hours in solution
d. Must be 270°F

 Critical Thinking

1. Who establishes regulations for infection control in the dental office?

2. When an OSHA requirement is not met, what can happen?

3. Who can make a report regarding a noncompliance with an OSHA standard?

4. Define OPIM. Describe the role of OPIM.

5. List who in the dental office is mandated for OSHA training. Is there a cost for this training? When should training be implemented under this classification?

CASE STUDY 1

Lisa is a new employee in a dental office. A review of OHSA office compliance instructions discussed PPEs and sharps containers. Several notices had been given to the office regarding the use (wearing in/out of the office) and disposal of the uniform gowns that had been provided (a uniform service was to have been provided and was not). The sharps container was overflowing and no new replacements had arrived. Observation and how to report noncompliance are contained within the written exposure plan.

1. Which regulating body enforces the requirement that employers protect their employees from blood and OPIM during the time when employees are at work?

2. What standard indicates that every facility must provide PPE?

3. Name two of the Bloodborne Pathogens Standards that indicate protection from needlestick injuries.

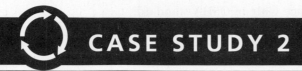

CASE STUDY 2

As a new chairside dental assistant employee in this office, the employer will be providing you instruction on OSHA Bloodborne Standards.

1. What do the written standards include?

2. What three categories determine occupational exposure?

3. List the recommendations in Category 1 for exposure determination.

4. List the recommendations in Category 2 for exposure determination.

5. List the recommendations in Category 3 for exposure determination.

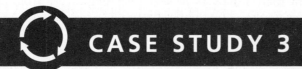

CASE STUDY 3

Pathogens can travel from personnel to patients. Routes of microbial transmission by most microorganisms can exist and can be missed. Thus, the dental assistant is the primary caretaker of infection control practices.

1. List the three possible routes of microbial transmission.

2. What should the dental assistant do in order to fight off pathogens encountered due to the close proximity of patients during dental treatment?

3. What is one of the most important ways to prevent the transfer of microorganisms from one person or object to another person?

SKILL COMPETENCY ASSESSMENT

11-1 Handwashing

Student's Name _____ Date _____

Instructor's Name _____

Skill: At the beginning of each day, two consecutive 30-second handwashings should be performed. Each should consist of a vigorous rubbing together of well-lathered soapy hands (ensuring friction on all surfaces), and conclude with a thorough rinsing under a stream of water and proper drying. Handwashing is both a mechanical cleaning and chemical antisepsis. *Routine handwashing* must occur before and after patients, donning gloves, and taking breaks. Each consists of a 15-second handwashing. Routine handwashing must be completed at the end of each day and any other time that the hands become contaminated.

Performance Objective: The student will remove jewelry, adjust the water flow, wet hands thoroughly, and apply antimicrobial soap and bring to a lather while rubbing all areas of the hands, getting between fingers and cleaning beneath fingernails. Rinse and dry thoroughly.

	Self-Evaluation	Student Evaluation	Possible Points	Instructor Evaluation	Comments
Equipment and Supplies 1. Liquid antimicrobial hand-washing agent			1		
2. Soft, sterile brush or sponge (optional)			1		
3. Sink with hot and cold running water			1		
4. Paper towels			1		
Competency Steps *At the beginning of every day (two consecutive 30-second handwashes)* 1. Remove jewelry (rings and watch).			2		
2. Adjust water flow and wet hands thoroughly.			2		
3. Apply about one teaspoon of antimicrobial handwashing agent with water; bring to a lather.			2		

	Self-Evaluation	Student Evaluation	Possible Points	Instructor Evaluation	Comments
4. Scrub hands together or with a sterile brush or sponge, making sure to get between each finger, the surface of the palms and wrists, and under the fingernails.			3		
5. Rinse, and repeat Steps 3 and 4.			2		
6. Final rinse with cool to lukewarm water for 10 seconds to close the pores.			1		
7. Dry with paper towels—hands first and then the wrist area.			1		
8. Use paper towels to turn off the hand-controlled faucets.			2		
TOTAL POINTS POSSIBLE			19		
TOTAL POINTS POSSIBLE—2nd attempt			17		
TOTAL POINTS EARNED			____		

Points assigned reflect importance of step to meeting objective: Important = 1, Essential = 2, Critical = 3. Students will lose 2 points for repeated attempts. Failure results if any of the critical steps are omitted or performed incorrectly. If using a 100-point scale, determine score by dividing points earned by total points possible and multiplying the results by 100.

SCORE: ____

SKILL COMPETENCY ASSESSMENT

11-2 Putting on Personal Protective Equipment (PPE)

Student's Name _____ Date _____

Instructor's Name _____

Skill: Barriers such as protective eyewear, face masks, disposable gloves, and appropriate uniforms should be used routinely to minimize exposure to infectious microorganisms.

Performance Objective: The student will properly don gloves, eyewear, mask, and gown.

	Self-Evaluation	Student Evaluation	Possible Points	Instructor Evaluation	Comments
Equipment and Supplies 1. Protective clothing			1		
2. Surgical mask			1		
3. Protective eyewear			1		
4. Procedure gloves			1		
Competency Steps 1. Don a lab coat, clinic gown, or clinic jacket.			2		
2. Don a surgical mask, making sure it is properly adjusted around the nose.			2		
3. Wash hands and properly don treatment gloves.			3		
4. Don protective eyewear.			2		
TOTAL POINTS POSSIBLE			13		
TOTAL POINTS POSSIBLE—2nd attempt			11		
TOTAL POINTS EARNED			____		

Points assigned reflect importance of step to meeting objective: Important = 1, Essential = 2, Critical = 3. Students will lose 2 points for repeated attempts. Failure results if any of the critical steps are omitted or performed incorrectly. If using a 100-point scale, determine score by dividing points earned by total points possible and multiplying the results by 100.

SCORE: ____

SKILL COMPETENCY ASSESSMENT

11-3 Removing Personal Protective Equipment (PPE)

Student's Name _____ Date _____

Instructor's Name _____

Skill: All PPE should be properly removed and disposed of to prevent cross contamination.

Performance Objective: The student will properly remove eyewear, gloves, mask, and gown and properly dispose of contaminated materials.

	Self-Evaluation	Student Evaluation	Possible Points	Instructor Evaluation	Comments
Equipment and Supplies 1. Protective clothing			1		
2. Surgical mask			1		
3. Protective eyewear			1		
4. Procedure gloves			1		
Competency Steps 1. Properly remove and dispose of treatment gloves.			2		
2. Wash and dry hands.			3		
3. Remove protective eyewear.			2		
4. Remove mask and properly dispose of it.			3		
5. Remove the gown and properly dispose of it.			2		
TOTAL POINTS POSSIBLE			16		
TOTAL POINTS POSSIBLE—2nd attempt			14		
TOTAL POINTS EARNED			____		

Points assigned reflect importance of step to meeting objective: Important = 1, Essential = 2, Critical = 3. Students will lose 2 points for repeated attempts. Failure results if any of the critical steps are omitted or performed incorrectly. If using a 100-point scale, determine score by dividing points earned by total points possible and multiplying the results by 100.

SCORE: ____

SKILL COMPETENCY ASSESSMENT

11-4 Preparing the Dental Treatment Room

Student's Name _____ Date _____

Instructor's Name _____

Skill: Routine steps should be followed for all treatment areas to maintain absolute clinical asepsis.

Performance Objective: The procedure is performed by the dental assistant prior to seating the dental patient in the treatment room. The dental assistant will follow a routine procedure that meets the regulations and the protocol set forth by the dentist and regulatory agencies. The dental assistant prepares the operatory and equipment.

	Self-Evaluation	Student Evaluation	Possible Points	Instructor Evaluation	Comments
Equipment and Supplies					
1. Patient's medical and dental history (including dental radiographs)			2		
2. Barriers for dental chair, hoses, counter, light switches, and controls			3		
3. PPE for dental assistant (protective eyewear, mask, gloves, and overgloves)			3		
4. Patient napkin, napkin chain, and protective eyewear			3		
5. Sterile procedure tray			3		
Competency Steps (*follow aseptic procedures*)					
1. Wash hands.			3		
2. Review the patient's medical and dental history, place radiographs on viewbox, and identify procedure to be completed at this visit. Patient's medical and dental history can be placed in a plastic envelope or under a surface barrier.			3		

	Self-Evaluation	Student Evaluation	Possible Points	Instructor Evaluation	Comments
3. Place new barriers on all possible surfaces that can be contaminated (e.g., dental chair, hoses, counter, light switches, and controls).			3		
4. Bring the instrument tray with packaged sterile instruments into the operatory with patient's napkin and protective eyewear.			3		
5. Prepare dental assistant PPE (protective eyewear, mask, gloves, and overgloves).			3		

TOTAL POINTS POSSIBLE 29

TOTAL POINTS POSSIBLE—2nd attempt 27

TOTAL POINTS EARNED ____

Points assigned reflect importance of step to meeting objective: Important = 1, Essential = 2, Critical = 3. Students will lose 2 points for repeated attempts. Failure results if any of the critical steps are omitted or performed incorrectly. If using a 100-point scale, determine score by dividing points earned by total points possible and multiplying the results by 100.

SCORE: ____

SKILL COMPETENCY ASSESSMENT

11-5 Completion of Dental Treatment

Student's Name _____ Date _____

Instructor's Name _____

Skill: Routine steps should be followed for all treatment areas upon completion of dental treatment. Maintain absolute clinical asepsis and prevent cross-contamination.

Performance Objective: The procedure is performed by the dental assistant at the completion of the dental treatment. The dental assistant will follow a routine procedure that meets the regulations and the protocol set forth by the dentist and regulatory agencies. The dental assistant completes the procedure and dismisses the patient.

	Self-Evaluation	Student Evaluation	Possible Points	Instructor Evaluation	Comments
Equipment and Supplies					
1. Patient's medical and dental history (including dental radiographs)			3		
2. Barriers for dental chair, hoses, counter, light switches, and controls			3		
3. Dental handpiece			1		
4. Air-water syringe tip (disposable)			1		
5. Patient napkin			1		
6. Contaminated instruments on tray, including HVE tip			3		
Competency Steps (*follow aseptic procedures*)					
1. Remove handpieces, HVE tip, and air-water tip and place on treatment tray.			3		
2. Don overgloves to document on chart or on the computer and assemble radiographs and chart, preventing cross-contamination.			3		
3. Remove patient napkin and place over the treatment tray before dismissing the patient.			1		

	Self-Evaluation	Student Evaluation	Possible Points	Instructor Evaluation	Comments
With gloves in place, complete the following: 4. Place the handpiece, HVE, and air-water syringe back on unit and run for 20 to 30 seconds to clean the lines or flush the system. Remove handpiece and air-water syringe and place back on the treatment tray.			3		
5. Place sharps in puncture-resistant sharps disposal containers (in treatment room when possible).			3		
6. Remove chair cover from the patient dental chair, inverting it so that any splatter or debris remains inside the bag.			1		
7. Remove all barriers and place them in inverted bag. Any disposables can be placed in the bag as well.			2		
8. Carry treatment tray with all items from the treatment area to sterilizing area. Nothing must be left in operatory at this time that is to be sterilized.			2		
9. Remove the treatment gloves and place them in the inverted bag. Dispose of the bag.			1		
10. Wash hands.			1		

TOTAL POINTS POSSIBLE   32

TOTAL POINTS POSSIBLE—2nd attempt   30

TOTAL POINTS EARNED   ____

Points assigned reflect importance of step to meeting objective: Important = 1, Essential = 2, Critical = 3. Students will lose 2 points for repeated attempts. Failure results if any of the critical steps are omitted or performed incorrectly. If using a 100-point scale, determine score by dividing points earned by total points possible and multiplying the results by 100.

SCORE: ____

SKILL COMPETENCY ASSESSMENT

11-6 Final Treatment Room Disinfecting and Cleaning

Student's Name _____ Date _____

Instructor's Name _____

Skill: The process of cleaning (physical removal of organic matter such as blood, tissue, and debris) decreases the number of microorganisms in the area and removes substances that may hinder the process of disinfection. As long as all surfaces are disinfected, asepsis requirements are met.

Performance Objective: The procedure is performed by the dental assistant after the treatment has been completed and the patient has been dismissed. The dental assistant will follow a routine procedure that meets the regulations and the protocol set forth by the dentist and regulatory agencies. The dental assistant completes the procedure.

	Self-Evaluation	Student Evaluation	Possible Points	Instructor Evaluation	Comments
Equipment and Supplies					
1. Utility gloves			2		
2. Necessary disinfecting solutions (intermediate level)			2		
3. Wiping cloths			1		
4. 4 × 4 gauze			1		
Competency Steps (*follow aseptic procedures*)					
1. Wash hands, don utility gloves. • Obtain the necessary solutions/wiping cloths, including 4 × 4 gauze. (Items could be in a small utility carry tote.)			2		
2. All surfaces need to be sprayed and cleaned first, and then wiped to remove debris.			2		
3. The initial spray wipe can be done by using saturated "wiping devices" (prepare by spraying 4 × 4 gauze with disinfectant) and wiping each surface carefully/thoroughly.			2		

	Self-Evaluation	Student Evaluation	Possible Points	Instructor Evaluation	Comments
4. Spray disinfectant on a second time and leave for the correct time to accomplish disinfection (normally 10 minutes).			2		
5. Rewipe all surfaces.			3		
6. Review that all surfaces that could have been contaminated are disinfected (i.e., amalgam cradle, chair adjustments, curing light, and radiographic viewbox switch).			2		

TOTAL POINTS POSSIBLE   19

TOTAL POINTS POSSIBLE—2nd attempt   17

TOTAL POINTS EARNED   ____

Points assigned reflect importance of step to meeting objective: Important = 1, Essential = 2, Critical = 3. Students will lose 2 points for repeated attempts. Failure results if any of the critical steps are omitted or performed incorrectly If using a 100-point scale, determine score by dividing points earned by total points possible and multiplying the results by 100.

SCORE: ____

SKILL COMPETENCY ASSESSMENT

11-7 Treatment of Contaminated Tray in the Sterilization Center

Student's Name _____ Date _____

Instructor's Name _____

Skill: Once the treatment tray has been removed from the operatory and into the sterilization center, the dental assistant is ready to process the instruments. At this time, all the debris, blood, saliva, and tissue are removed from the instruments to ensure that sterilization can be completed on all surfaces.

Performance Objective: The student will follow a routine procedure that meets the regulations and the protocol set forth by the dentist and OSHA regulatory agencies.

	Self-Evaluation	Student Evaluation	Possible Points	Instructor Evaluation	Comments
Equipment and Supplies					
1. Utility gloves			2		
2. Necessary disinfecting solutions			2		
3. Wiping cloths			1		
4. 4 × 4 gauze			1		
5. Contaminated procedure tray			1		
Competency Steps (follow aseptic procedures)					
1. Place treatment tray in contaminated area of sterilization center immediately following dental treatment by the dental assistant. Return later for processing.			2		
2. Place instruments into holding solution as soon as possible to prevent debris from drying.			2		
3. Wear utility gloves during the entire procedure of caring for contaminated instrument tray.			3		

	Self-Evaluation	Student Evaluation	Possible Points	Instructor Evaluation	Comments
4. Place sharps into sharps container if not already accomplished in the dental operatory.			2		
5. All disposable items are discarded. Biohazard waste must be placed in an appropriately labeled waste container.			3		
6. Instruments from the holding solution are rinsed and placed in the ultrasonic cleaner. Small strainers will hold small items (burs, dental dam clamps). After the timed cleaning is completed (usually 3 to 10 minutes), rinse items off thoroughly.			3		
7. After rinsing the instruments, towel dry, bag, date, and place into appropriate sterilizer. If cassette is used versus bagging, instruments can be dipped into alcohol bath and left to air dry before placing in sealed bag and in sterilizer.			3		
8. Dental high-speed handpiece is rinsed off with isopropyl alcohol, lubricated, bagged in an instrument pouch (with indicator tape), and placed in the appropriate sterilizer (follow manufacturer's directions).			3		
9. The instrument tray and other items left on the tray need to be spray wiped, sprayed again, left for 10 minutes (follow manufacturer's directions), and wiped again before assembling them for another tray setup.			2		

	Self-Evaluation	Student Evaluation	Possible Points	Instructor Evaluation	Comments
10. Clean up area used in the sterilization center, wash and dry utility gloves, remove them, and wash and dry hands.			1		
11. When sterilizer indicates that the instruments are sterile, the pressure is released, and the door or tray is opened. The instruments can be removed from the sterilizer with forceps.			3		

TOTAL POINTS POSSIBLE   34

TOTAL POINTS POSSIBLE—2nd attempt   32

TOTAL POINTS EARNED   ____

Points assigned reflect importance of step to meeting objective: Important = 1, Essential = 2, Critical = 3. Students will lose 2 points for repeated attempts. Failure results if any of the critical steps are omitted or performed incorrectly. If using a 100-point scale, determine score by dividing points earned by total points possible and multiplying the results by 100.

SCORE: ____

SKILL COMPETENCY ASSESSMENT

11-8 Dental Radiography Infection Control Protocol

Student's Name _____ Date _____

Instructor's Name _____

Skill: Routine steps should be followed for all treatment areas, including the radiographic area, while performing radiographic exposures. Maintain absolute clinical asepsis and prevention of cross-contamination both in the radiography room and in the darkroom (or other processing area). Radiographs may be exposed in a dental radiography/special room and/or a dental/clinical operatory or treatment room.

Performance Objective: The student will follow a routine procedure that meets the regulations and the protocol set forth by the dentist and regulatory agencies. The dental assistant completes the procedure in the dental radiography room, if it is a separate area, or at the dental unit where the dental treatment is being performed.

Standard Precaution: X-ray room must have lead-lined door and walls.

	Self-Evaluation	Student Evaluation	Possible Points	Instructor Evaluation	Comments
Equipment and Supplies 1. Utility gloves			2		
2. Barriers			2		
3. Necessary disinfecting solutions			1		
4. Wiping cloths			1		
5. 4 × 4 gauze			1		
Competency Steps (follow aseptic procedures) 1. Wash hands, place barriers (dental chair bag over x-ray head).			2		
2. Barriers a. On either side of door handle to darkroom. b. On switch of dental radiography machine c. The chair can be covered in the event the patient vomits.			2 2 2		
3. Dental x-rays can be placed into barriers or use film that already has a barrier.			3		

	Self-Evaluation	Student Evaluation	Possible Points	Instructor Evaluation	Comments
4. PPE is placed as patient is seated. Place lead apron on patient.			2		
5. After each x-ray is taken, place x-ray in disposable cup outside the x-ray room.			3		
6. After the procedure is completed and the patient is dismissed, remove the barriers and dispose of them carefully. Remove the barrier from the exposed film, and let the film drop into a clean disposable cup before removing treatment gloves.			3		
7. Disinfect any areas not covered by the barriers, including the lead apron.			2		
8. Process x-rays. New gloves are used if x-ray film was not wrapped. Observe all aseptic techniques so as to ensure that x-rays being processed do not recontaminate any surface areas or equipment. Follow two-cup method.			3		
9. Daylight processor • Contaminated film (unwrapped film), two-cup method, one cup with contaminated film and one with nothing in it (new gloves are put on before entry to processor):			2		
a. Remove outer cover.			2		
b. Slide film out of sleeve cover. Place film in clean cup. Remove the gloves and place them in the contaminated cup.			3		
c. With clean hands place the uncontaminated dental film through the processor. Place film into processor slot. (Continue preceding process until slots are full.)			3		

	Self-Evaluation	Student Evaluation	Possible Points	Instructor Evaluation	Comments
d. Activate processor slot for drop. (Processing will start. Another group of films will follow Steps a through d until all films are processed.)			3		
• Wrapped film, now un-wrapped and new gloves, use of over-gloves are acceptable. (Dispose of wrapped outer surface before leaving treatment room.) Follow Steps b through d.			3		
• Remove clean hands from the processor and lift the lid.			2		
• Remove wrappings and disposable cups from the daylight loader by touching only the outside of the cup.			1		

TOTAL POINTS POSSIBLE 51

TOTAL POINTS POSSIBLE—2nd attempt 49

TOTAL POINTS EARNED ____

Points assigned reflect importance of step to meeting objective: Important = 1, Essential = 2, Critical = 3. Students will lose 2 points for repeated attempts. Failure results if any of the critical steps are omitted or performed incorrectly. If using a 100-point scale, determine score by dividing points earned by total points possible and multiplying the results by 100.

SCORE: ____

CHAPTER 12

Management of Hazardous Materials

SPECIFIC INSTRUCTIONAL OBJECTIVES

The student should strive to meet the following objectives and demonstrate an understanding of the facts and principles presented in this chapter:

1. Identify the scope of the OSHA Bloodborne/Hazardous Materials Standard.

2. Identify physical equipment and mechanical devices provided to safeguard employees.

3. Demonstrate safe disposal of sharps.

4. Describe MSDS manuals.

5. Demonstrate the use of the colors and numbers in hazardous chemical identification.

6. Describe employee training required to meet the OSHA standard for hazardous chemicals.

SUMMARY

OSHA regulations, including the hazard communication standard, are intended to require the employer to provide a safe work environment for all employees. The dental assistant must understand the complete standard and how compliance is accomplished. Staff must be trained for a safe workplace. Compliance with all standards must be accomplished to ensure a safe workplace.

EXERCISES AND ACTIVITIES

Multiple Choice

1. Dental office employees need to know and comply with the OSHA safety standards. Which of the following is not the subject of an OSHA safety standard?

   a. Employee training
   b. Labeling/MSDS
   c. Housekeeping/laundry
   d. ADA

2. The physical equipment and mechanical devices that employers provide to safeguard and protect employees are known as

   a. MSDSs.
   b. engineering/work practice controls.
   c. housekeeping/laundry.
   d. labeling.

3. Which of the following items are considered engineering/work practice controls?

   1. Splash guards on model trimmers
   2. Puncture-resistant sharps containers
   3. Etiologic agent
   4. Ventilation hoods for hazardous fumes
   5. Eye-wash station
   6. Gram stain
   7. Amoebic dysentery
   8. Tinea

   a. 1, 2, 4, 5
   b. 3, 6, 7, 8
   c. 3, 4, 6, 7
   d. 1, 2, 3, 5

4. Which of the following is not included in the definition of human fluids?

   a. Blood and anything that is visually contaminated with blood
   b. Saliva in dental oral procedures
   c. Synovial fluid
   d. Distilled water

5. _____ is a means of piercing mucous membranes or the skin barrier through such events as needlesticks, cuts, and abrasions.

   a. OPIM
   b. Parenteral
   c. Synovial
   d. Biohazardous

6. Which of the following would not go into the sharps container?

   a. Orthodontic wire
   b. Contaminated needles
   c. Surgical knives or blades
   d. Rubber dam

7. The sharps container must meet very strict standards. Which of the following descriptors is not part of the sharps standard?

   a. Labeled
   b. Leakproof
   c. Wide-mouth opening
   d. Puncture resistant

8. If an occupational exposure occurs for any employee, which of the following is(are) required?

   a. The employee must report the incident immediately.
   b. Employer must immediately provide medical evaluation and follow-up.
   c. Medical evaluation and follow-up are made available to the employee at no cost.
   d. All of the above.

9. Documentation of an exposure incident must include testing for

   a. tetanus.
   b. MMR.

   c. HBV.
   d. TB.

10. If employees choose to decline testing after an exposure incident, they can delay testing up to _____ days.

    a. 90
    b. 60

    c. 30
    d. 28

11. A postexposure prophylaxis is provided according to the current recommendations of (the)

    a. OSHA.
    b. U.S. Public Health Service.

    c. CDC.
    d. ADA.

12. In accordance with OSHA's standard on access to employee exposure and medical records, the employer must maintain employee records for _____ year(s).

    a. 15
    b. 24

    c. 1
    d. 30

13. Gloves that are contaminated with blood are required to go into

    a. regular waste.
    b. a biohazard container.

    c. the laundry.
    d. a leakproof sharps container.

14. _____ regulations are intended to ensure a safe work environment regarding the risks of using hazardous chemicals.

    a. ADA
    b. EPA

    c. OSHA
    d. Bloodborne

15. Within _____ days of employment, employee training must occur regarding the identification of hazardous chemicals and the use of personal protective equipment (PPE).

    a. 90
    b. 15

    c. 30
    d. 60

16. The _____ color and number method is used to signify a warning to employees using chemicals.

    a. Centers for Disease Control and Prevention

    b. National Fire Protection Association

    c. Occupational Safety and Health Administration
    d. American Dental Association

17. The color _____ identifies a health hazard.

    a. red
    b. yellow

    c. white
    d. blue

18. Within _____ days of employment, all dental employees must complete a safety training program before assuming responsibilities that involve exposure to body fluids or chemicals.

    a. 10
    b. 30

    c. 60
    d. 90

19. Under the 2001 revision to OSHA's Bloodborne Pathogen Standard, the employer must maintain a sharps injury log. This log must contain the following incident information:

    1. Reference to minutes of training
    2. Description of injury type
    3. Recommendations to employees from patients
    4. Brand of device involved

5. Description of the act

6. Location of the act
   a. 1, 3, 5, 6
   b. 2, 3, 4, 5
   c. 2, 4, 5, 6
   d. 1, 4, 5, 6

Matching

OSHA and the CDC define the following human fluids as blood and OPIM. Match the fluid with its excretion.

Fluid

1. __C__ Synovial

2. __D__ Saliva

3. __E__ Pleural

4. __A__ Peritoneal

5. __B__ Pericardial

Excretion

a. Abdominal fluid

b. Heart fluid

c. Joint and tendon fluid

d. Intraoral dental

e. Lung fluid

The National Fire Protection Association's color-coding method is used to signify a warning to employees using chemicals. Match the color with its hazard type/warning.

Color

6. __B__ Blue

7. __D__ Red

8. __A__ Yellow

9. __C__ White

Hazard

a. Reactivity or instability

b. Health

c. PPE needed

d. Fire

Critical Thinking

1. Contaminated syringe sharps injuries occur most frequently during postoperative handling of the anesthetic syringe. What recommendations are made by OSHA regarding needle disposal?

2. Engineering/work practice controls are established to provide safeguards and protect employees at work. Wearing eye protection is a key element of maintaining a safe environment for the dental assistant. When is eyewear to be worn? What if you have prescription glasses?

3. Data collection indicates a high number of contaminated sharps exposure incidents. If an employee has an occupational exposure, state the steps required for reporting the incident.

CASE STUDY 1

Lucy is the office safety coordinator. A new dental material has arrived, which is part of a new procedure that this office will provide. The MSDS is enclosed in the packing.

1. Does the staff require a safety update on this new product?

2. Are there universal practices to be learned?

3. Are specific PPE to be utilized?

4. Where is the MSDS log kept?

5. Is the training to be certified and logged?

CASE STUDY 2

A chemical spill occurs while an inventory of stored supplies is under way. Cleanup cannot proceed until the chemical is identified.

1. Where would the dental employee find the chemical composition and related warnings?

2. Cleaning can begin after the chemical MSDS information has been reviewed. Identify the four chemical labels.

3. Name one item from each of the four chemical categories that would apply.

CASE STUDY 3

OSHA provides safety standards regarding the use of gloves that are specific according to glove type.

1. State glove usage in accordance with the OSHA standard.

2. Name the type of gloves required for employee use.

3. What glove alternatives are available?

CHAPTER 13

Preparation for Patient Care

SPECIFIC INSTRUCTIONAL OBJECTIVES

The student should strive to meet the following objectives and demonstrate an understanding of the facts and principles presented in this chapter:

1. Explain how the patient record is developed and the importance of the personal registration form, medical and dental information, clinical evaluation, and the extraoral and intraoral examinations.

2. Describe how the patient record may be called into litigation or used in a forensic case.

3. Perform or assist the dentist in an extraoral and an intraoral evaluation including lips, tongue, glands, and oral cavity.

4. Explain how a diagnosis and treatment plan is developed.

5. Perform vital signs on the patient, including both oral and tympanic temperature, pulse, respiration, and blood pressure.

6. Document the vital signs and be alert to any signs that are abnormal.

7. Identify the five Korotkoff sounds, the two that are used in recording blood pressure, and the man who described them in 1905.

SUMMARY

The health condition of a dental patient must be kept private and confidential and updated at each visit. To treat a patient effectively, the patient's chart should include personal history, medical information, dental history, clinical observation, clinical evaluation, and vital signs.

EXERCISES AND ACTIVITIES

True or False

1. A clinical examination of the patient's lips involves checking for cracking.
   - a. True
   - b. False

2. During a clinical examination of the patient, the cervical lymph nodes are examined only on the patient's right side.
   - a. True
   - b. False

3. To estimate systolic pressure, overinflating the blood pressure cuff is recommended.
   - a. True
   - b. False

4. It is not necessary to update the patient's medical history at each visit.
   - a. True
   - b. False

5. The strength of a pulse may be described as irregular, slow, or rapid.
   - a. True
   - b. False

Multiple Choice

1. A patient is requested to fill out a personal history questionnaire. Which of the following is not a part of this history?
   - a. Full name
   - b. Vital signs
   - c. Address
   - d. Phone number

2. Which of the following health history questions is critical in that it could affect treatment?
   - a. Allergies
   - b. Systemic diseases
   - c. Injuries
   - d. All of the above

3. Which of the following allergies would concern the dentist as it relates to patient treatment?
   - a. Reactions to anesthesia
   - b. Seasonal allergies (ragweed)
   - c. Pet dander
   - d. Insect stings

4. If a patient indicates an epileptic condition, this information would be found in what section of the patient's chart?
   - a. Personal
   - b. Medical history
   - c. Vital response
   - d. Clinical observation

5. The dentist has a _____ responsibility to gain information about a patient's medical history before dental treatment.
   - a. clinical
   - b. legal
   - c. health
   - d. personal

6. The dental assistant can observe patients as they are escorted to the treatment room and can note which of the following?
   - a. Walk or gait
   - b. Speech
   - c. Facial symmetry
   - d. All of the above

7. The vermilion border is defined as (the)

   a. smile line.
   b. commissures.
   c. line around the lips.
   d. cracking or dryness.

8. During the external clinical examination, the area of the neck from the ear to the collar bone that is examined is (are) called the

   a. TMJ.
   b. floor of the mouth.
   c. lips.
   d. lymph nodes.

9. During the clinical exam, which area does the dental assistant palpate as the patient opens and closes the mouth?

   a. TMJ
   b. Floor of the mouth
   c. Lips
   d. Lymph nodes

10. Which of the following is not assessed during an internal oral examination?

    a. Lesions in the mouth
    b. Abscessed teeth
    c. Color changes in oral mucosa
    d. Noise from clicking or catching in jaw

11. The_____ are called the basic signs of life.

    a. statistics
    b. essential signals
    c. vital signs
    d. natural elements

12. An adult average baseline body temperature is

    a. 99.5°F.
    b. 98.6°F.
    c. 96.0°F.
    d. 37.5°C.

13. Body temperature can vary from patient to patient and at different times of the day. Which of the following can cause an increase in temperature?

    a. Exercise
    b. Eating
    c. Emotional excitement
    d. All of the above

14. When a manual thermometer is used, it will be placed

    a. between the buccal mucosa.
    b. only between the lips.
    c. under the tongue.
    d. None of the above.

15. If a digital thermometer is used to obtain a patient's temperature, how should the probe cover be disposed of?

    a. Regular waste
    b. Biohazard waste
    c. Sharps container
    d. It can be washed and reused.

16. Which is not a recorded pulse site?

    a. Radial
    b. TMJ
    c. Carotid
    d. Temporal

17. Respiration is one breath taken in, called_____ , and one breath let out.

    a. tachypnea
    b. bradypnea
    c. exhalation
    d. inhalation

18. A normal pulse rate for adults is_____ beats per minute.

    a. 90 to 120
    b. 12 to 18
    c. 60 to 90
    d. 20 to 40

19. A normal respiration rate for children is_____ respirations per minute.

    a. 90 to 120
    b. 12 to 18
    c. 60 to 90
    d. 20 to 40

20. Blood pressure is an important indicator of a patient's

    a. dental condition.
    b. cardiovascular condition.
    c. body temperature.
    d. respiration rate.

21. The brachial artery is located

    a. inside the wrist.
    b. under the chin.
    c. in the neck area.
    d. inside the elbow.

22. The blood pressure cuff is placed_____ inch(es) above the bend of the elbow and secured.

    a. 2
    b. 1
    c. 3
    d. 4

23. The normal blood pressure range for an adult is

    a. 100 to 140 mm Hg/60 to 90 mm Hg.
    b. 60 to 100 mm Hg/33 to 66 mm Hg.
    c. 68 to 118 mm Hg/46 to 76 mmHg.
    d. None of the above.

24. What length of time is recommended to wait before reinflating the blood pressure cuff?

    a. 30 minutes
    b. 1 minute
    c. 30 seconds
    d. No waiting is recommended

25. Which of the Korotkoff signs have no clinical significance?

    a. First and second
    b. Second and third
    c. Third and fifth
    d. Fourth and fifth

Matching

Body temperature is an essential component of every patient's vital signs. Match the term with its definition.

Term

1. C Fever
2. D Hypothermic
3. A Antipyretic
4. B Fahrenheit

Use

a. Used to reduce fever
b. Above the normal temperature range
c. Measure of temperature
d. Below the normal temperature range

The pulse is another component of the patient's vital signs. Match the term with the best definition.

Term

5. D Pulse
6. C Radial site
7. B Carotid site
8. A Temporal site

Definition

a. Front of ear/level of eyebrow
b. Large artery in neck
c. Thumb side of wrist
d. Intermittent beating sensation

Respiration is another vital sign of record. Match the term with the best definition.

Term

9. B Inhalation
10. C Exhalation
11. D Tachypnea
12. A Bradypnea

Definition

a. Abnormally slow resting rate
b. One breath taken in
c. One breath let out
d. Abnormally rapid resting rate

Blood pressure is an important indicator of the health of a patient's cardiovascular system. Match the term with the definition.

Term

13. _B_ Sphygmomanometer

14. _E_ Brachial artery

15. _D_ Stethoscope

16. _A_ Systolic pressure

17. _C_ Diastolic pressure

Definition

a. First sound as heart contracts and forces blood through arteries

b. Inflatable bladder to control blood flow to artery

c. Pulsation sound disappears as arteries relax

d. Instrument used to hear and amplify sounds of the heart

e. First palpated inside of elbow

Critical Thinking

1. The dental assistant must be as thorough as possible in the patient interview to ensure that the best possible care is provided. List five questions that the dental assistant might ask while taking a patient's health history.

2. Following the health history data review by the dental assistant, a clinical evaluation is performed in two stages. Name these two examination stages.

3. The dental assistant performs a clinical observation evaluation. Any deviations from normal are noted in the patient's chart. Name three specific areas that are examined and their anatomic locations.

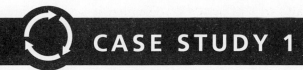

CASE STUDY 1

On Kate's initial visit to the dental office, the health history is completed by the patient and reviewed by the dental assistant. Kate has indicated that she is being treated for high blood pressure. The dental assistant explains that all vitals are taken to ensure successful planning of patient treatment. Sometimes vital signs can also point to previously undetected abnormalities.

1. Explain the method for taking a patient's blood pressure by estimating systolic pressure.

2. What is considered an important indicator of the health of a patient's cardiovascular system?

3. Name the categories of vital signs.

4. Are vital signs to be taken on all patients?

5. Explain baseline vital signs.

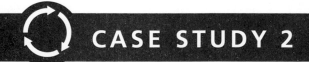

CASE STUDY 2

After an hour workout at the gym, Fred rushed to avoid arriving late for his dental appointment. Fred seemed to be out of breath. It is this dental office's policy to take vitals on all patients.

1. Will Fred's body temperature be elevated? Why or why not?

2. What is considered the normal temperature range, both in Fahrenheit and Celsius?

3. Name situations that can elevate body temperatures.

4. Will young children and infants' body temperature vary more than adults?

CASE STUDY 3

As a dental assistant you can expect to take patients' vital signs as a regular part of your daily work routine. You will make decisions about the equipment you use and the methods used to take these measurements. You will be required to know all aspects of vital signs.

1. What is considered a normal pulse range?

2. What is considered a normal respiration range?

3. What is considered a normal temperature range?

4. What is considered a normal blood pressure range?

Labeling

Identify the structures inspected during a visual examination that are indicated in the following diagram.

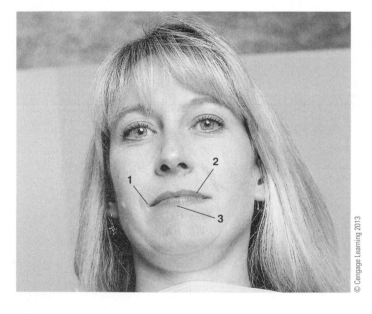

© Cengage Learning 2013

1. _____

2. _____

3. _____

SKILL COMPETENCY ASSESSMENT

13-1 Taking an Oral Temperature Using a Digital Thermometer

Student's Name _____ Date _____

Instructor's Name _____

Skill: Identifying patient body temperature compared to normal body temperature for every patient health evaluation. Temperatures will vary in young children and infants.

Performance Objective: The student will follow a routine procedure that meets the guidelines and protocol to obtain the patient's body temperature. The dental assistant completes the procedure in the dental operatory.

	Self-Evaluation	Student Evaluation	Possible Points	Instructor Evaluation	Comments
Equipment and Supplies 1. Digital thermometer			2		
2. Probe covers			1		
3. Biohazard waste container			1		
Competency Steps *(follow aseptic procedures)* 1. Wash hands.			2		
2. Verify thermometer is correctly assembled and functioning properly.			1		
3. Seat patient in the dental treatment room and position him or her comfortably in an upright position.			3		
4. Verify that the patient has not had a hot/cold drink or smoked within the last 30 minutes.			2		
5. Explain the procedure to the patient.			3		

	Self-Evaluation	Student Evaluation	Possible Points	Instructor Evaluation	Comments
6. Position the new probe cover on the digital thermometer.			2		
7. Insert the probe under the tongue to either side of the patient's mouth.			2		
8. Instruct the patient to carefully close his or her lips around the probe, not biting down on it.			2		
9. Leave probe in position until the digital thermometer beeps.			3		
10. Remove the probe from the patient's mouth.			1		
11. Read the results from the digital thermometer display window.			3		
12. Dispose of the probe cover in the hazardous waste container.			1		
13. Wash hands.			2		
14. Document the procedure and results in the patient's chart.			3		

TOTAL POINTS POSSIBLE   34

TOTAL POINTS POSSIBLE—2nd attempt   32

TOTAL POINTS EARNED   _____

Points assigned reflect importance of step to meeting objective: Important = 1, Essential = 2, Critical = 3. Students will lose 2 points for repeated attempts. Failure results if any of the critical steps are omitted or performed incorrectly. If using a 100-point scale, determine score by dividing points earned by total points possible and multiplying the results by 100.

SCORE: _____

SKILL COMPETENCY ASSESSMENT

13-2 Taking Tympanic Temperature

Student's Name _____ Date _____

Instructor's Name _____

Skill: Identifying patient body temperature compared to normal body temperature for every patient health evaluation. Temperatures will vary in young children and infants.

Performance Objective: The student will follow a routine procedure that meets the guidelines and protocol to obtain the patient's body temperature. The dental assistant completes the procedure in the dental operatory.

	Self-Evaluation	Student Evaluation	Possible Points	Instructor Evaluation	Comments
Equipment and Supplies 1. Tympanic thermometer			2		
2. Probe covers			1		
3. Biohazard waste container			1		
Competency Steps (*follow standard precautions*) 1. Wash hands.			2		
2. Assemble thermometer and probe cover.			1		
3. Seat patient in the dental treatment room and position him or her comfortably in an upright position.			3		
4. Gently position the ear and place the probe in the ear canal—it should not touch the ear drum.			3		
5. Press the button on the thermometer.			3		

	Self-Evaluation	Student Evaluation	Possible Points	Instructor Evaluation	Comments
6. After the beep remove the probe from the ear and record the displayed temperature.			2		
7. Dispose of the probe cover.			2		

TOTAL POINTS POSSIBLE   20

TOTAL POINTS POSSIBLE—2nd attempt   18

TOTAL POINTS EARNED   _____

Points assigned reflect importance of step to meeting objective: Important = 1, Essential = 2, Critical = 3. Students will lose 2 points for repeated attempts. Failure results if any of the critical steps are omitted or performed incorrectly. If using a 100-point scale, determine score by dividing points earned by total points possible and multiplying the results by 100.

SCORE: _____

SKILL COMPETENCY ASSESSMENT

13-3 Taking a Radial Pulse and Measuring the Respiration Rate

Student's Name _____ Date _____

Instructor's Name _____

Skill: To identify patient body pulse and respiration compared to the normal rates for every patient health evaluation. Rates will vary depending on the patient's age, gender, and physical and mental condition.

Performance Objective: The student will follow a routine procedure that meets the guidelines and protocol to obtain the patient's vital signs. The dental assistant completes the procedure in the dental operatory.

	Self-Evaluation	Student Evaluation	Possible Points	Instructor Evaluation	Comments
Equipment and Supplies 1. Watch with a second hand			3		
Competency Steps *(follow standard precautions)* 1. Wash hands.			2		
2. Position the patient in a comfortable, upright position (same as for temperature).			2		
3. Explain the procedure.			3		
4. Have the patient position the wrist resting on the arm of the dental chair or counter.			2		
5. Locate the radial pulse by placing the pads of the first three fingers over the patient's wrist.			3		
6. Gently compress the radial artery so that the pulse can be felt.			2		

	Self-Evaluation	Student Evaluation	Possible Points	Instructor Evaluation	Comments
7. Using the watch with the second hand, count the number of pulsations for one full minute.			2		
8. Record the number of pulsations.			2		
9. Note any irregular rhythm patterns.			2		
10. While keeping finger pads on the radial pulse, count the rise and fall of the chest for one minute.			2		
11. Record the number of respirations. Note any irregularities in the breathing.			2		
12. Wash hands.			1		
13. Document the procedure and the pulse and respiration rate on the patient's chart.			2		

TOTAL POINTS POSSIBLE   30

TOTAL POINTS POSSIBLE—2nd attempt   28

TOTAL POINTS EARNED   _____

Points assigned reflect importance of step to meeting objective: Important = 1, Essential = 2, Critical = 3. Students will lose 2 points for repeated attempts. Failure results if any of the critical steps are omitted or performed incorrectly. If using a 100-point scale, determine score by dividing points earned by total points possible and multiplying the results by 100.

SCORE: _____

SKILL COMPETENCY ASSESSMENT

13-4 Measuring Blood Pressure

Student's Name _____ Date _____

Instructor's Name _____

Skill: Identifying the patient's blood pressure compared to the normal blood pressure range is an important indicator of a patient's health. Blood pressures will vary in ranges much like other vital signs. Children normally have lower pressure; as adults age, blood pressure goes up.

Performance Objective: The student will follow a routine procedure that meets the guidelines and protocol to obtain the patient's blood pressure. The dental assistant completes the procedure in the dental operatory.

	Self-Evaluation	Student Evaluation	Possible Points	Instructor Evaluation	Comments
Equipment and Supplies 1. Stethoscope			2		
2. Sphygmomanometer			2		
3. Disinfectant and gauze			1		
Competency Steps *(follow standard precautions)* 1. Wash hands.			2		
2. Assemble the stethoscope and the sphygmomanometer and disinfect the earpieces of the stethoscope.			3		
3. Position the patient in a comfortable position, upright in the dental chair (same as for temperature).			1		
4. Explain the procedure.			2		
5. Have the patient position the arm resting at heart level on the counter or the arm of dental chair.			2		

	Self-Evaluation	Student Evaluation	Possible Points	Instructor Evaluation	Comments
6. Have the patient remove any outer clothing that restricts the upper arm. Bare the upper arm and palpate the brachial artery.			2		
7. Center the bladder of the cuff securely, about two inches above the bend of the elbow.			2		
8. Inflate the cuff slowly, and palpate the radial pulse until the pulse is obliterated.			3		
9. Release pressure.			3		
10. Add 30 mmHg to number representing the pulse obliteration point.			3		
11. Wait one minute before reinflating the cuff.			3		
12. Position the earpieces of stethoscope in a forward manner into the ears.			2		
13. Place the diaphragm of the stethoscope over the brachial artery, holding in place with the thumb. Place the other fingers under the elbow to hyperextend the artery (access is easier and enables better reading).			3		
14. Inflate the cuff using the bulb and control valve of the sphygmo-manometer. If the cuff is not inflating, recheck control valve on sphyg-momanometer to ensure it is closed. Air should not escape.			3		
15. Inflation level should include the palpate, inflate, obliterate, and deflate technique.			3		

	Self-Evaluation	Student Evaluation	Possible Points	Instructor Evaluation	Comments
16. Deflate the cuff at a rate of 2 to 4 millimeters of mercury per second by rotating control valve slightly.			3		
17. Listen for first sound and note its measurement on the scale.			1		
18. Continue to deflate the cuff and listen to the pulsing sounds. Note when all sounds disappear. Continue deflating for another 10 millimeters to ensure the last sound has been heard.			2		
19. Deflate the cuff rapidly and remove it from the patient's arm.			3		
20. Disinfect the earpieces of stethoscope.			1		
21. Wash hands and record the procedure and the measurement on the patient's chart. (Blood pressure is recorded in even numbers in a fraction format with the systolic measurement on top.)			3		

TOTAL POINTS POSSIBLE   55

TOTAL POINTS POSSIBLE—2nd attempt   53

TOTAL POINTS EARNED   _____

Points assigned reflect importance of step to meeting objective: Important = 1, Essential = 2, Critical = 3. Students will lose 2 points for repeated attempts. Failure results if any of the critical steps are omitted or performed incorrectly. If using a 100-point scale, determine score by dividing points earned by total points possible and multiplying the results by 100.

SCORE: _____

Dental Charting

The student should strive to meet the following objectives and demonstrate an understanding of the facts and principles presented in this chapter:

1. Explain why charting is used in dental practices.

2. Identify charts that use symbols to represent conditions in the oral cavity.

3. List and explain the systems used for charting the permanent and deciduous dentitions.

4. Define G.V. Black's six classifications of cavity preparations.

5. List common abbreviations used to identify simple, compound, and complex cavities.

6. Describe basic dental charting terminology.

7. Explain color indicators and identify charting symbols.

SUMMARY

Dental charting provides legal documentation of the patient's oral cavity. The correct numbering system and charting symbols ensure proper documentation. Therefore, accuracy in charting is critical.

EXERCISES AND ACTIVITIES

True or False

1. Charting in most dental offices is the method of recording conditions in the patient's oral cavity.

    a. True

    b. False

2. The initial charting or recording of the condition of the patient's oral cavity is normally accomplished during the patient's first examination.

   a. True
   b. False

3. Class V caries were not a part of the original classifications developed by G. V. Black.

   a. True
   b. False

4. A chart that shows the crown of the tooth, or the crown and a small portion of the root, or the crown and the complete root is called geometric.

   a. True
   b. False

5. The most commonly used chart is one with diagrams of the teeth that may show an anatomic or geometric representation of the teeth.

   a. True
   b. False

6. The space between two adjacent teeth in the same dental arch is called a diastema.

   a. True
   b. False

7. Class II caries are on the interproximal surface of the anterior teeth and include the incisal edge.

   a. True
   b. False

8. Disto-incisal is abbreviated in charting as DO.

   a. True
   b. False

9. Use of the color red in charting indicates dental work that needs to be completed.

   a. True
   b. False

10. A cantilever bridge is attached on two sides.

    a. True
    b. False

Multiple Choice

1. Which numbering system is most commonly used in the United States?

   a. Universal/National System
   b. Federation Dentaire Internationale System
   c. Palmer System
   d. ADA System

2. Most dental charts will show

   1. anatomic representation of teeth.
   2. geometric representation of teeth.
   3. cavity classification.
   4. primary dentition.

5. abbreviated tooth surfaces.

6. permanent dentition.

    a. 1, 2, 3, 5   c. 1, 2, 3, 4
    b. 1, 2, 4, 6   d. 2, 3, 4, 6

3. How many original standard classifications of cavities were first developed by G.V. Black?

    a. Two   c. Four
    b. Three   d. Five

4. A _____ cavity involves the incisal and/or an occlusal surface worn away due to abrasion.

    a. Class I   c. Class IV
    b. Class II   d. Class VI

5. Which of the following cavities would be referred to as simple?

    1. Class I

    2. Class II

    3. Class III

    4. Class V

    5. Class VI

    6. Class IV

        a. 1, 2, 5   c. 1, 3, 4
        b. 1, 4, 5   d. 2, 3, 6

6. What is the abbreviation notation for mesio-occluso-disto-bucco-lingual?

    a. MODL   c. MODBL
    b. MIDB   d. MDOI

7. The attaching sides of a bridge are called

    a. pontics.   c. cantilevers.
    b. plates.   d. abutments.

8. The portion of a bridge that replaces the missing tooth is called a(n)

    a. abutment.   c. plate.
    b. pontic.   d. denture.

9. _____ is a term used to identify a localized area of infection.

    a. Incipient   c. Sealant
    b. Decay   d. Abscess

10. All teeth support one another. _____ can occur when a tooth is removed and a space is created.

    a. Drifting   c. Periodontal disease
    b. Overhang   d. Abscess

11. _____ refers to an area that does not yet show decay, but the surface has begun to decalcify.

    a. Gold foil   c. Sealant
    b. Incipient   d. Cavity

12. (A) _____ is the result of excessive restorative material.

    a. Pocket   c. Sealant
    b. Overhang   d. Root canal

13. What prosthetic device replaces missing teeth with a metal framework and artificial teeth?

    a. Upper plate

    b. Full denture

    c. Partial denture

    d. Bridge

14. A sulcus depth of _____ millimeter(s) is considered periodontal disease.

    a. 1

    b. 2

    c. 3

    d. 6

15. Which charting color indicates work to be done?

    a. Black

    b. Yellow

    c. Blue

    d. Red

16. Which charting color indicates that work has been completed?

    a. Black

    b. Yellow

    c. Blue

    d. Red

17. Which numbering system assigns the primary teeth a letter or a "d" with a number?

    a. Fédération Dentaire Internationale

    b. Palmer

    c. Universal/National

    d. International Standards Organization

18. A(n) _____ restoration would be charted as outlined and filled solidly with blue.

    a. gold

    b. porcelain

    c. amalgam

    d. composite

19. Which restoration would be charted as outlined with swervy lines?

    a. Gold crown

    b. Stainless steel

    c. Amalgam

    d. Composite

20. Composite restorations are charted by using which of the following charting schematics?

    a. Outlining

    b. Outlining and filling in

    c. Outlining with diagonal lines

    d. Crosshatch lines

21. A restoration charted as outlined with dots drawn would represent a(n) _____ restoration.

    a. amalgam

    b. composite

    c. gold

    d. porcelain

22. The space between the maxillary central incisors in humans is called a(n)

    a. fistula.

    b. abscess.

    c. pocket.

    d. diastema.

23. The abbreviation for a compound cavity restoration is

    a. O

    b. MOD.

    c. DO.

    d. MODBL.

24. A mesio-occluso-distal restoration is a technical term for a _____ cavity restoration.

    a. compound

    b. complex

    c. simple

    d. single

25. The software programs for computer charting(s) can record the following periodontal charting:

    a. conditions of dentition.

    b. conditions of occlusion.

    c. conditions of tissue.

    d. All of the above

26. Which of the following are required to record on a dental chart the conditions in the patient's oral cavity?

    a. Symbols

    b. Numbers

    c. Colors

    d. All of the above

27. The patient's dental record (chart) is used for

    a. billing purposes.

    b. diagnosis.

    c. consultation.

    d. All of the above

28. In this numbering system, the permanent teeth are numbered 1–8 in each quadrant.

    a. ISO

    b. Palmer

    c. FDI

    d. Universal/National System

29. A classification I cavity can occur on which of the following surfaces?

    a. Occlusal surface on posterior teeth

    b. Buccal or lingual pits on the molars

    c. Lingual pit near the cingulum of the maxillary incisors

    d. All of the above

30. Patients refer to these as "fillings"; what term is used in the field of dentistry?

    a. amalgamation

    b. restoration

    c. denturation

    d. composition

Matching

Cavity classifications aid in recording the type of dental caries. Match the cavity classification with the surface area(s).

Classification

1. __D__ Class I

2. __A__ Class II

3. __B__ Class III

4. __E__ Class IV

5. __C__ Class V

Surface Area(s)

a. Two or more surfaces posterior

b. Interproximal surface of anterior

c. Cervical third facial or lingual surface

d. Caries in pits and fissures

e. Interproximal surface and incisal edge of anterior

All patient records in a given office are documented using one of several numbering systems. Match the system with its corresponding coding.

System

6. __C__ Universal/National

7. __A__ Fédération Dentaire Internationale

8. __B__ Palmer

Corresponding Coding

a. 1 for the upper right quadrant

b. 1–8 in each quadrant

c. 1–16, 17–32

Understanding the use of charting symbols is required for accuracy in charting. Use the following charting conditions and match the corresponding charting symbol.

9. _____ Missing teeth

a.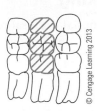

10. _____ Teeth impacted or unerupted

b.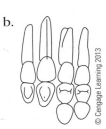

11. _____ Teeth that need root-canal therapy

c.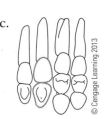

12. _____ Tooth with full gold crown

d.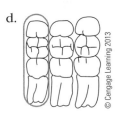

13. _____ Tooth with porcelain crown

e.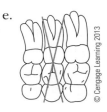

Critical Thinking

1. A tooth with a present mesial occlusal restoration now needs a mesio-occluso-distal restoration. Use the following figure.

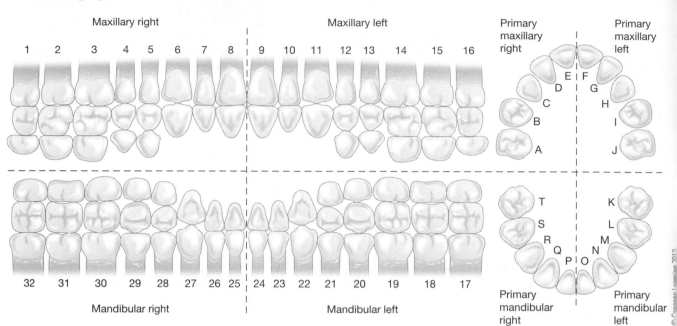

a. Chart both restorations.

b. What cavity classification will this new restoration be?

2. A change has occurred in the gingival health of Drew. The following conditions were noted on Drew's chart; state which teeth identify these conditions.

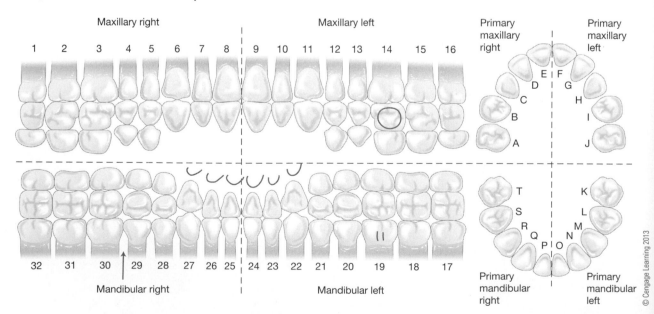

a. Pocket on tooth number

b. Mobility on tooth number

c. Temporary

d. Heavy calculus on which teeth

3. The dental assistant is a new employee in the dental office. This office uses the ISO numbering system. Label the following permanent and primary dentition arches using the ISO system and the Fédération Dentaire Internationale system.

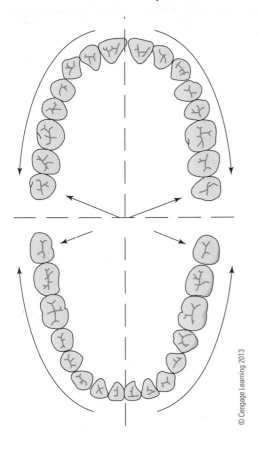

© Cengage Learning 2013

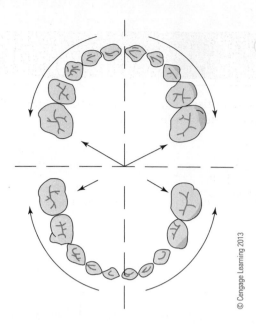

© Cengage Learning 2013

4. Sensitivity by pressure is causing this patient to see the dentist. An x-ray reveals overhangs on which of the following teeth?

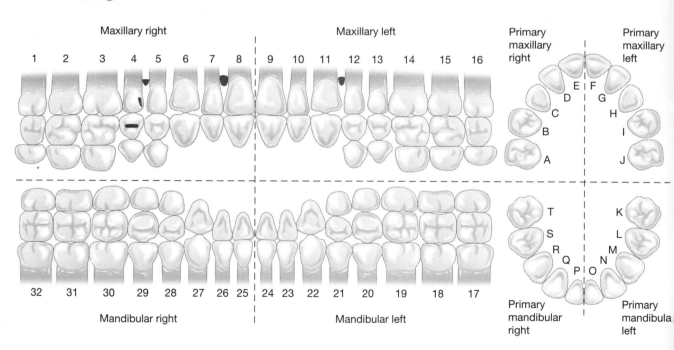

CASE STUDY 1

Since Ester's last dental visit, a change has occurred in her gingival tissue. In this diagram, several periodontal conditions are noted. Identify the following conditions as noted on the chart.

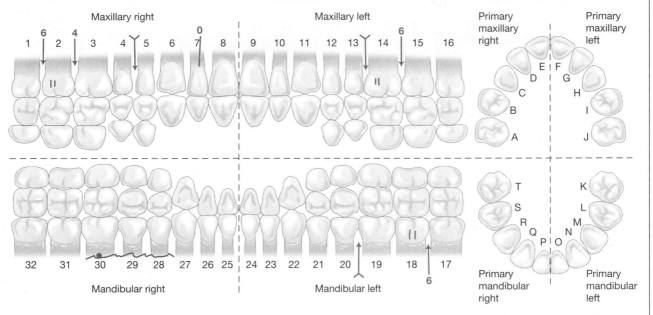

1. Food impactions

2. Perio pockets

3. Root canal and reoccuring abscess

4. Gingival furca

5. Mobility

CASE STUDY 2

A patient with mixed dentition is in for a dental examination. Using the figure, identify the following:

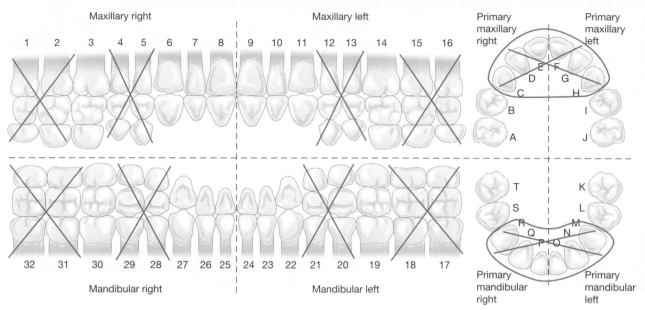

1. Which primary teeth are missing?

2. Which primary teeth are present?

3. Which adult teeth are present?

4. Which adult teeth are missing?

CASE STUDY 3

During the dental examination of a new patient, various conditions are noted. Identify these conditions using the chart provided.

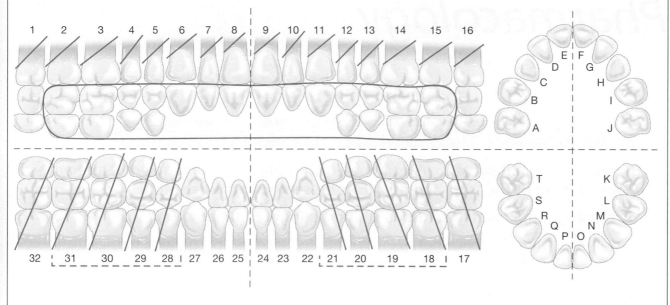

1. Teeth to be extracted.

2. Teeth to be replaced with a partial.

3. Teeth to be replaced with a denture.

© Cengage Learning 2013

CHAPTER 15

Pharmacology

SPECIFIC INSTRUCTIONAL OBJECTIVES

The student should strive to meet the following objectives and demonstrate an understanding of the facts and principles presented in this chapter:

1. Identify terms related to drugs, pharmacology, and medicines.
2. Identify the difference between drug brand names and generic names.
3. Identify the parts of a written prescription.
4. Identify the texts pertinent to pharmacology.
5. Provide the English meanings of the Latin abbreviations used for prescriptions.
6. Specify the drug laws and who enforces them.
7. Identify the schedules for the Comprehensive Drug Abuse Prevention and Control Act of 1970.
8. Identify the routes through which drugs can be administered.
9. Demonstrate an understanding of the drugs used in dentistry and the ways in which they are used.
10. Summarize the uses and effects of nicotine, caffeine, alcohol, marijuana, and cocaine.
11. Summarize information about heroin, morphine, and codeine.
12. Supply information about amphetamines.
13. Demonstrate an understanding of hallucinogenic drugs such as LSD, PCP, and mescaline.
14. Demonstrate an understanding of barbiturates.

SUMMARY

At no other time have drugs been as widely used and misused as they are today. The dental assistant will need to pay attention to the patient's medical and dental history and carefully document the drugs used by the patient. The dental assistant will have to become knowledgeable about pharmacology, the side effects of drugs, and drug interactions. Dental assistants are concerned with prescribed drugs, but they must also have knowledge about illegal drugs that patients may be using and what will happen if the two types of drugs interact. It is also important to know the signs and symptoms that individuals may experience if under the influence of drugs. Background knowledge about drugs and their effects aids the dental assistant in providing better patient care.

EXERCISES AND ACTIVITIES

Multiple Choice

1. _____ is the study of all drugs.
   a. Medicine
   b. Addiction
   c. Pharmacology
   d. Parenteral

2. When a person becomes physically dependent on a drug, that person has a(n)
   a. interaction.
   b. addiction.
   c. withdrawal.
   d. prescription.

3. Drugs that cause psychological dependence are called
   a. broad spectrum.
   b. brand name.
   c. drug interaction.
   d. habit forming.

4. The _____ gathers information about drugs used in dentistry.
   a. CDC
   b. OSHA
   c. Council on Dental Therapeutics
   d. FDA

5. Individuals who dispense drugs must have a(n) _____ -issued number to prescribe drugs.
   a. FDA
   b. DEA
   c. PDR
   d. OTC

6. A prescription is written in several parts. The _____ includes the dentist's name and credentials, office address, and phone number.
   a. heading
   b. DEA
   c. closing
   d. Rx body

7. In the _____ of the prescription, the dentist inscribes or writes the name and strength of the drug being prescribed, the dose, and in what form the drug is to be dispensed.
   a. heading
   b. DEA
   c. closing
   d. Rx body

8. In English, the Latin abbreviation b.i.d. means
   a. before meals.
   b. daily.
   c. twice a day.
   d. take.

9. An oral drug that is enteric-coated indicates which of the following?
   a. Will break apart more easily
   b. Resists breaking down by gastric juices
   c. Time-released capsule
   d. Gelatin

10. The _____ is the federal regulatory agency that has control of all food, cosmetics, and drugs sold in the United States.

    a. DEA

    c. FDA

    b. PDR

    d. Controlled Substance Act

11. Alcohol is a _____, a drug that slows body processes.

    a. stimulant

    c. depressant

    b. narcotic

    d. sedative

12. _____ is an illegal drug that contains THC and affects the nervous system.

    a. Nicotine

    c. Heroin

    b. Cocaine

    d. Marijuana

13. _____ is the most addictive of the narcotics.

    a. Cocaine

    c. Heroin

    b. Marijuana

    d. Caffeine

14. One of the best-known narcotic analgesic drugs is

    a. codeine.

    e. amphetamines.

    b. marijuana.

    d. morphine.

15. Drugs that relieve pain can be non-narcotic, such as

    a. codeine.

    c. amphetamines.

    b. aspirin.

    d. morphine.

16. Antibiotics that are effective against a wide range of bacteria are called

    a. broad spectrum.

    c. drug interaction.

    b. brand names.

    d. OTC.

17. Schedule _____ drugs, such as marijuana, heroin, and LSD, have a high potential for abuse.

    a. I

    c. III

    b. II

    d. IV

18. Schedule _____ drugs, such as cocaine and morphine, have a high potential for abuse and lead to physical and psychological dependence.

    a. I

    c. III

    b. II

    d. IV

19. Schedule _____ drugs, such as Tylenol III, have a lower potential for abuse and are prescribed routinely in the dental office.

    a. I

    c. III

    b. II

    d. IV

20. The most common method of taking medications is

    a. topically.

    c. rectally.

    b. orally.

    d. sublingually.

21. One of the drugs used in dentistry is nitrous oxide. This drug can be administered

    a. sublingually.

    c. orally.

    b. topically.

    d. by inhalation.

22. _____ is an antifungal drug used in dentistry to treat candidiasis.

    a. Nystatin

    c. Atropine

    b. Anticholinergic

    d. Erythromycin

23. Which drug administration route is used when a medication is placed under the tongue?

    a. Subvenous

    b. Subcutaneous

    c. Sublingual

    d. Subdermal

24. Which type of medication prevents blood from clotting?

    a. Antihistamine

    b. Anticoagulant

    c. Antihypertensive

    d. Antilipemic

25. Which type of drug aids in the secretion of water from the body and is used to treat edema?

    a. Diuretic

    b. Decongestant

    c. Hemostatic

    d. Antihypertensive

Matching

Match each term with its definition.

Term

1. ___d___ Pharmacology

2. ___e___ Prescription

3. ___a___ Side effect

4. ___b___ Drug interaction

5. ___c___ Addiction

6. ___g___ Synergistic

7. ___f___ Stimulant

Definition

a. An unintended result of a drug

b. One drug changes the effect of another drug

c. Physical dependence on a drug

d. The study of all drugs

e. Written order for a particular drug

f. A substance that speeds up metabolic activities

g. The risk of combining drugs

Match administration by route of injection.

Administration

8. ___c___ Intravenous

9. ___d___ Intramuscular

10. ___b___ Subcutaneous

11. ___a___ Intradermal

Route of Injection

a. Under the epidermis (top layer of skin)

b. Under the skin above the muscle

c. Directly into the vein

d. Into the muscle

Critical Thinking

1. The doctor provides directions to the pharmacist within the body of the prescription. The directions include abbreviations of the name and strength of the drug dose. This information is often in the form of a Latin abbreviation. Define the following Latin abbreviations.

    a. a.c.

    b. q.i.d.

c. q.h.

d. q.4.h.

e. p.c.

2. When a prescription is taken to the pharmacist for filling, what instruction will the pharmacist look for regarding the brand of drug?

3. The dental assistant and dentist must check the patient's medical and dental histories carefully prior to the writing of a prescription. Beginning with the Drug Schedule for the Comprehensive Abuse and Prevention Control Act of 1970, define the five drug schedules and provide an example of the drugs included in each schedule.

4. A prescription is written in several parts. All information must be complete to ensure that the correct drug will be dispensed. Therefore, being thorough and writing clearly will assist the pharmacist in filling the prescription correctly. The dental assistant may be asked to review the prescription before the patient leaves the office. Define the nine parts of the blank prescription.

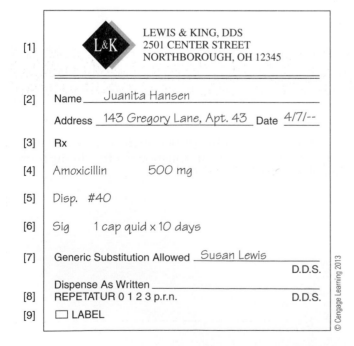

[1] LEWIS & KING, DDS
2501 CENTER STREET
NORTHBOROUGH, OH 12345

[2] Name Juanita Hansen

Address 143 Gregory Lane, Apt. 43 Date 4/7/--

[3] Rx

[4] Amoxicillin   500 mg

[5] Disp. #40

[6] Sig   1 cap quid × 10 days

[7] Generic Substitution Allowed Susan Lewis
                                                    D.D.S.

Dispense As Written _____
[8] REPETATUR 0 1 2 3 p.r.n.   D.D.S.
[9] ☐ LABEL

© Cengage Learning 2013

5. The route of drug administration is critical. Identify the various layers for delivery of an intravenous drug by using the following figure. What type of injection is this?

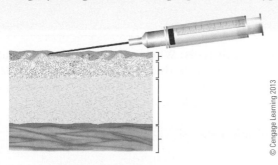

© Cengage Learning 2013

 # CASE STUDY 1

Stan arrives at the dental office and checks in with the receptionist. The receptionist notices that the patient reeks of alcohol. The patient is scheduled for a lengthy dental treatment, including various impressions. The patient will be required to keep his mouth open for long periods of time, and to be alert enough to make important decisions along the course of the treatment, such as the shade and color selections for the crown and veneers to be manufactured.

1. Is alcohol habit forming?

2. Can alcohol increase the effects of a stimulant?

3. What other symptoms could be demonstrated besides odor?

CASE STUDY 2

Beth's treatment scheduled for today is for deep root planning and ultrasonic scaling. Her health history indicates she has had a hip replacement.

1. Would Beth be a likely patient to take some type of broad-spectrum antibiotic?

2. Can a patient become resistant to antibiotics?

3. Name adverse effects of antibiotics.

CASE STUDY 3

Jana complains during a dental cleaning about how dry her mouth feels. When asked whether she has experienced health-related changes since her last appointment, she reports that she has allergies. The assistant then informs Jana that taking an antihistamine drug to deal with allergy symptoms could have a dry-mouth effect. At this time, the assistant also determines that Jana is taking an antidepressant.

1. What section in the patient's chart would indicate her medication status?

2. List the drugs that can cause dryness of the mouth.

3. Are there any other side effects to the drugs this patient is taking?

CHAPTER 16

Emergency Management

The student should strive to meet the following objectives and demonstrate an understanding of the facts and principles presented in this chapter:

1. Describe several emergency situations that may take place in the dental office. Explain how dental assistants can be prepared for these possibilities.

2. Describe the "CAB" approach to CPR and demonstrate the associated skills.

3. Define the terms and anatomy used in CPR delivery. Determine if the patient is unconscious and demonstrate knowledge of opening the airway and when and how to deliver chest compressions.

4. Identify several causes of airway obstructions in the dental office. Demonstrate the ability to open the airway and to perform the Heimlich maneuver.

5. Identify the causes, signs, and treatments for syncope, asthma, allergic reactions, anaphylactic reaction, hyperventilation, epilepsy, diabetes mellitus, hypoglycemia, angina pectoris, myocardial infarction, congestive heart failure, and stroke/cerebrovascular accident.

6. Identify several dental emergencies that a patient may have, such as abscessed tooth, alveolitis, avulsed tooth, broken prosthesis, soft tissue injury, broken tooth, and loose crown.

7. Gain an understanding of how a pulse oximeter, capnography, and electrocardiography work and how they can be used in the dental office.

SUMMARY

Even though the number of emergencies is not high in a dental office, the dental assistant must always observe the patient and be prepared to deal with emergencies. Emergencies may also happen to the dentist and to other dental auxiliaries.

When an emergency arises, the dental team must react automatically. Any hesitation at such a time may cost a life. It is best if a routine is established so that everyone can ensure that everything is addressed. The assistant has a vital role in the prevention of emergencies and in emergency care. Patient observation at all times assists in the prevention evaluation.

EXERCISES AND ACTIVITIES

Multiple Choice

1. Which of the following is *not* part of the assistant's role in observing the patient for emergency management?

   a. Is the patient having difficulty moving?

   b. Do the patient's eyes respond to light?

   c. Is the patient's speech slurred?

   d. Does the patient need an injection of epinephrine?

2. Having a well-defined emergency plan will provide the best treatment for the patient. Which of the following is *not* part of an emergency plan?

   a. Everyone knowing the oxygen location

   b. Who will perform CPR

   c. Who will call for help

   d. Who will reschedule the patient's next dental appointment

3. Which of the following are observations made by the dental assistant while escorting the patient from the waiting room to the treatment room?

   a. Does the patient have difficulty moving?

   b. Is the patient's speech slurred?

   c. Does the patient indicate anxiety about the dental treatment?

   d. All of the above.

4. If the patient reaches an unconscious state and progresses to a sudden cardiac arrest, what will the first step be?

   a. Start CPR.

   b. Phone for help.

   c. Perform the Heimlich maneuver.

   d. Remove any artificial appliances.

5. Assume that after determining that the patient is unconscious, you have called for help. What is the next step?

   a. Look for breathing.

   b. Give two breaths.

   c. Move the patient to the floor.

   d. Tilt the head and lift the chin.

6. Once it is determined that a patient is not breathing and emergency services has been called, the dental assistant should

   a. begin chest compressions.

   b. give two breaths.

   c. check for a pulse.

   d. attach the AED pads.

7. The rescuer administers two slow breaths of _____ seconds each for an adult.

   a. 1.5 to 2

   b. 1 to 1.5

   c. 5

   d. 3

8. During an adult CPR, the _____ pulse is checked during compression cycles.

   a. brachial

   b. femoral

   c. carotid

   d. radial

9. If the adult patient does not have a pulse, compressions at a rate of _____ per minute should be delivered.

   a. 100 to 110

   b. 80 to 100

   c. 90 to 100

   d. 80 to 90

10. The heels of the rescuer's hands are placed on the _____ of the sternum and compressions begin.

    a. lower third

    b. middle third

    c. upper third

    d. end

11. After every 30 compressions, deliver _____ more slow breath(s).

    a. four

    b. two

    c. one

    d. five

12. What is the most common effective method used to open the airway?

    a. jaw thrust

    b. insertion of mouth props

    c. head tilt, chin lift.

    d. chin lift.

13. The electrodes for the defibrillator are placed only if the patient

    a. is unconscious.

    b. is not breathing.

    c. has no pulse.

    d. All of the above.

14. In the dental office, _____ incidents are more common than other emergencies.

    a. airway obstruction

    b. asthma attack

    c. partial seizure

    d. cerebral hemorrhage

15. The universal distress signal for airway obstruction is

    a. syncope.

    b. clutching the throat.

    c. convulsing.

    d. clutching the chest.

16. The term for a foreign object lodged in the airway is

    a. Heimlich maneuver.

    b. CPR.

    c. FBAO (foreign body airway obstruction).

    d. anaphylactic.

17. During an airway obstruction, the patient becomes unconscious. You place the patient on the floor. Which of the following is the next critical step?

    a. Remove the foreign body.

    b. Activate emergency medical service.

    c. Attempt to give patient breaths.

    d. Reposition head and chin.

18. The most common and least life-threatening emergency that may occur in the dental office is

    a. allergic reaction.

    b. anaphylactic shock.

    c. syncope.

    d. angina pectoris.

19. In the dental office, a vasodepressor syncope occurred. This incident is also known as

    a. allergic reaction.

    b. anaphylactic shock.

    c. fainting.

    d. seizure.

20. A patient unable to respond to any sensory stimulation is defined as

    a. allergic.

    b. urticaria.

    c. hyperplasia.

    d. unconscious.

21. Symptoms of syncope may include

    a. dizziness.

    b. nausea.

    c. a feeling of weakness.

    d. All of the above.

22. A supine position with the feet elevated above the chest level is called the _____ position.

    a. Heimlich

    b. Trendelenburg

    c. Jacksonian

    d. lateral

23. The wheezing and the breathlessness of an asthma patient are due to the small airways in the _____ narrowing.

    a. trachea

    b. nasal cavity

    c. bronchioles

    d. lungs

24. _____ is an acquired, abnormal response to a substance that does not normally cause a reaction.

    a. Alkalosis

    b. Seizure

    c. Type I diabetes mellitus

    d. Allergy

25. _____ is a severe, life-threatening allergic reaction.

    a. Hyperventilation

    b. Hypoglycemia

    c. Anaphylactic shock

    d. Congestive heart failure

26. _____ is the loss of carbon dioxide from the blood, causing alkalosis.

    a. Hyperglycemia

    b. Hyperventilation

    c. Hypoglycemia

    d. Hemiplegia

27. _____ is the more severe form of diabetes mellitus and occurs between the ages of 10 and 16.

    a. Type I

    b. Type II

    c. Epilepsy

    d. Hypoglycemia

28. _____ is the result of the pancreas not producing sufficient insulin.

    a. A seizure

    b. Hyperventilation

    c. Diabetes

    d. Angina

29. Too little glucose in the bloodstream causes a person to experience

    a. hypoglycemia.

    b. hyperglycemia.

    c. seizures.

    d. allergies.

30. _____ is commonly called hardening of the arteries.

    a. Myocardial infarction

    b. Arteriosclerosis

    c. Cerebrovascular accident (CVA)

    d. Congestive heart failure

31. _____ is a condition in which patient symptoms include pain from pressure, swelling, and severe responses to heat.

    a. Avulsed tooth

    b. Abscessed tooth

    c. Broken prosthesis

    d. Soft tissue injury

32. _____ is a condition commonly known as a dry socket.

    a. Avulsed tooth

    b. Abscessed tooth

    c. Alveolitis

    d. Fistula

33. The dental assistant is responsible for observing signs and symptoms of the patient and trying to prevent syncope. Which of the following is not a preventive method or technique?

    a. Talking to the patient

    b. Assuring the patient everything is normal

    c. Keeping needles out of sight

    d. Dental assistant leaves the room after patient complains of dizziness

34. The patient may complain and demonstrate early signs of syncope. Which is not an early sign of syncope?

    a. Feeling flushed

    b. Having an upset stomach

    c. Choking

    d. Pale skin color

35. To maintain proficiency in emergency management, the dental assistant needs formal training every _____.

    a. year

    b. 2 years

    c. 5 years

    d. 6 years

36. If the emergency kit contains controlled substances, it _____ be kept locked up.

    a. may

    b. must

    c. is never to

    d. should

37. What is the name of the device that is used to measure the oxygen saturation in a patient's blood?

a. Sphygmomanometer   b. Pulse oximeter

c. Automated external defibrillator   d. Electrodes

38. The condition in which the body is deprived of its oxygen supply is called

a. hypoxia.   b. hypoglycemia.

c. erythema.   d. ischemia.

39. What is the device called that is used to record the electrical activity of the heart?

a. Capnograph   b. Radiograph

c. Electrocardiograph   d. Sonograph

40. Anticonvulsant drugs may cause which of the following dental conditions?

a. Gingival recession   b. Gingival swelling

c. Gingival hypoplasia   d. Gingival hyperplasia

Matching

Asthma may be caused by an allergy to a substance. Match the term with the definition.

Term

1. ___D___ Allergy
2. ___C___ Antibodies
3. ___E___ Antigens
4. ___A___ Hypersensitivity
5. ___B___ Allergens

Definition

a. Body overreacts
b. Antigen triggers allergic reaction
c. Also called immunoglobulins
d. Exaggerated reaction of immune system to offending agent
e. Foreign bodies

A number of other allergic reactions may take place in the dental office. Match the condition with its response.

Condition

6. ___C___ Dermatitis
7. ___D___ Edema
8. ___E___ Erythema
9. ___A___ Urticaria
10. ___B___ Angioedema

Response

a. Large urticaria (hives)
b. Hives may occur on skin surface
c. A skin reaction
d. Swelling
e. Redness

Epilepsy manifests in the form of varying types of seizures. Knowing the characteristics of each may help determine when a colleague or patient is having a seizure and how to respond to it. The following is a list of types of epilepsy and seizure disorders. Match the term with its characteristics.

Disorder

11. ___D___ Grand mal seizure
12. ___B___ Petit mal seizure
13. ___C___ Jacksonian epilepsy
14. ___A___ Status epilepticus

Characteristics

a. Continuous seizures
b. Person retains consciousness, also known as a simple partial seizure
c. Momentary loss of consciousness, also known as an absence seizure
d. Most common seizure, lasts 2 to 5 minutes

Stroke is a leading cause of disability and death for Americans. Match the term with its condition.

Term	Condition
15. _____ D _____ Cerebral infarction	a. Rupture of a blood vessel
16. _____ C _____ Cerebral embolism	b. Weakness, numbness, or paralysis on one side
17. _____ a _____ Cerebral hemorrhage	c. Blood clot
18. _____ b _____ Hemiplegia	d. Stroke-like symptoms that disappear in 24 hours
19. _____ e _____ Transient ischemic attacks	e. Sudden onset caused by blood loss to brain

Critical Thinking

1. Even though the number of emergencies is not great in a dental office, the dental assistant must always be observant of the patient and be prepared to deal with emergencies. What observations would the dental assistant be making while patients are escorted from the waiting room to the treatment room?

2. Advancements in medical care have allowed treatments that were not available in the past. List some of these treatments that dental patients may have had that could present complications during dental treatment.

3. Explain why the American Heart Association changed the "ABCs of CPR" to the "CABs of CPR."

4. Anxious or fearful patients are common in dental offices. How are symptoms for hyperventilation and syncope different? Are they treated differently?

CASE STUDY 1

Rose has arrived at the dental office for an extraction. When the dental assistant escorts Rose from the waiting room to the treatment room, the assistant asks how she is doing. Rose responds, "I am a little nervous about this appointment. My hands feel a little clammy."

1. What are signs of vasodepressor syncope?

2. Explain the "fight or flight syndrome."

3. What can the dental assistant do if the patient shows signs of fainting?

4. What preventive measures can the dental assistant take to limit the anxiety?

5. List treatments administered to assist patients in recovering from signs of fainting.

CASE STUDY 2

The patient is being treated for a loose temporary crown. The crown is loose but very much attached to the remaining tooth. An instrument used to lift the crown off pops the crown up and it flips to the back of the patient's throat. The patient immediately coughs, spits, gags, and leans forward, while having difficulty breathing.

1. State the symptoms of a universal distress signal.

2. Describe the dental team's actions in response to a universal distress signal.

3. Name other items causing FBAO.

CASE STUDY 3

About halfway through a long, scheduled dental treatment, Barbara becomes agitated and restless, and has difficulty breathing. The dental team halts the treatment and asks Barbara whether she is okay. Barbara states that she needs her inhaler to deal with asthma symptoms, and she has forgotten it.

1. What can cause asthma?

2. What are the most common allergens responsible for asthma?

3. Are asthma attacks more frequent at particular times?

4. After use of a bronchodilator, how quickly should the patient improve?

SKILL COMPETENCY ASSESSMENT

16-1 Administration of Oxygen

Student's Name _____ Date _____

Instructor's Name _____

Skill: Identification of the oxygen system used. Tanks are stored upright and secure and are green. The oxygen inhalation equipment must be readily available for use at all times.

Performance Objective: The student will follow a routine procedure that meets guidelines and protocol for locating oxygen equipment and know how to administer oxygen during an emergency. In some instances, the dental assistant may routinely administer oxygen in conjunction with the nitrous oxide gas under supervision of the dentist.

	Self-Evaluation	Student Evaluation	Possible Points	Instructor Evaluation	Comments
Equipment and Supplies 1. Oxygen tank with gauge at top or gauge in the dental treatment area.			2		
2. Oxygen mask and tubing.			2		
Competency Steps (follow aseptic procedures) 1. Position the patient comfortably in a supine or Trendelenburg position.			2		
2. Explain the procedure to the patient and reassure the patient that everything is being taken care of (if an emergency should occur).			3		
3. Place the oxygen mask over the patient's nose and drape the tubing on either side of the face (adjust to fit securely over the nose).			3		
4. Start the flow of oxygen immediately. It should flow at 2 to 4 liters per minute.			3		
5. Instruct the patient to breathe through the nose and keep the mouth closed.			3		

	Self-Evaluation	Student Evaluation	Possible Points	Instructor Evaluation	Comments
6. Continue to calm the patient by talking softly in reassuring tones.			2		

TOTAL POINTS POSSIBLE   20

TOTAL POINTS POSSIBLE—2nd attempt   18

TOTAL POINTS EARNED   _____

Points assigned reflect importance of step to meeting objective: Important = 1, Essential = 2, Critical = 3. Students will lose 2 points for repeated attempts. Failure results if any of the critical steps are omitted or performed incorrectly. If using a 100-point scale, determine score by dividing points earned by total points possible and multiplying the results by 100.

SCORE: _____

SKILL COMPETENCY ASSESSMENT

16-2 CPR for an Adult, One Rescuer

Student's Name _____ Date _____

Instructor's Name _____

Skill: To perform cardiopulmonary resuscitation on a patient who is not breathing and has no pulse.

Performance Objective: The student properly performs CPR in an emergency on the non-responsive patient.

	Self-Evaluation	Student Evaluation	Possible Points	Instructor Evaluation	Comments
Equipment and Supplies 1. Resuscitation mouth piece, mask, or barrier device			2		
2. Gloves			2		
Competency Steps (*follow aseptic procedures*) 1. Assess patient condition and look for breathing.			3		
2. Direct someone to call 9–1-1 or call yourself if alone.			3		
3. Wash hands and put on gloves if possible.			2		
4. Check for pulse at carotid artery.			3		
5. If no pulse, begin chest compressions ($\times$ 30).			3		
6. Position patient's head and give two rescue breaths using mask.			2		
7. Continue for 4 cycles and recheck pulse.			2		
TOTAL POINTS POSSIBLE			22		
TOTAL POINTS POSSIBLE—2nd attempt			20		
TOTAL POINTS EARNED			_____		

Points assigned reflect importance of step to meeting objective: Important = 1, Essential = 2, Critical = 3. Students will lose 2 points for repeated attempts. Failure results if any of the critical steps are omitted or performed incorrectly. If using a 100-point scale, determine score by dividing points earned by total points possible and multiplying the results by 100.

SCORE: _____

SKILL COMPETENCY ASSESSMENT

16-3 Rescue Breathing for Adults

Student's Name _____ Date _____

Instructor's Name _____

Skill: Identifying the patient's consciousness or unconscious state. Call for help, or have someone call for emergency services.

Performance Objective: The student will follow a routine procedure that meets the guidelines and protocol to assess the patient's condition. If an emergency occurs, the dental assistant must be prepared to respond to a patient who ceases breathing and/or to assist the dentist in rescue breathing for a patient.

	Self-Evaluation	Student Evaluation	Possible Points	Instructor Evaluation	Comments
Equipment and Supplies 1. Resuscitation mouthpiece.			3		
2. Gloves (latex or vinyl—optional)			3		
Competency Steps (*follow aseptic procedures*) 1. Determine if the patient is responding. Ask "Are you okay?"			3		
2. If patient gives no response: a. Have someone call emergency services. b. If alone, call quickly and return to the patient.			3 3		
3. Wash hands (if possible). Place on gloves.			3		
4. If patient is not breathing, tilt back the head, lift the chin, position the resuscitation mouthpiece, and close the nose by pinching it together.			3		
5. Give two slow breaths. a. Watch the chest gently rise while breaths are being given. b. Turn the face to the side and listen. c. Watch for air to return.			3 2 2 2		

	Self-Evaluation	Student Evaluation	Possible Points	Instructor Evaluation	Comments
6. Check the pulse: a. Carotid artery, side closest to you. b. Use the forefinger and middle finger to palpate the pulse.			3 3		
7. If the pulse is present but the patient is not breathing:					
a. Give one slow breath every 5 seconds.			2		
b. Continue Step A for one minute (12 times).			2		
8. Recheck the pulse and breathing after each 12 breaths or each minute.			3		
9. Continue rescue breathing for as long as the pulse remains. a. If the pulse ceases, begin CPR. b. If the pulse remains, continue rescue breathing until breathing is restored or until someone else arrives and takes over.			3 3 3		
10. Dispose of the resuscitation mouthpiece in a biohazard container.			3		
11. Remove gloves and wash hands.			3		
12. Document activities in the patient's chart.			3		

TOTAL POINTS POSSIBLE 61

TOTAL POINTS POSSIBLE—2nd attempt 59

TOTAL POINTS EARNED _____

Points assigned reflect importance of step to meeting objective: Important = 1, Essential = 2, Critical = 3. Students will lose 2 points for repeated attempts. Failure results if any of the critical steps are omitted or performed incorrectly. If using a 100-point scale, determine score by dividing points earned by total points possible and multiplying the results by 100.

SCORE: _____

SKILL COMPETENCY ASSESSMENT

16-4 Operating an Automated External Defibrillation (AED) Unit

Student's Name _____ Date _____

Instructor's Name _____

Skill: When a site has an automated defibrillator, the chances of survival for patients who experience cardiac arrest increase. The dental assistant should be familiar with the proper use of the defibrillator.

Performance Objective: The student will follow a routine procedure that meets guidelines and protocol to assess the patient's condition. If an emergency occurs, the dental assistant must be prepared to respond to a patient who is unconscious, not breathing, and has no pulse. The defibrillator equipment may be available in the facility for emergencies and will have a voice system that will indicate when and where to place the electrodes.

	Self-Evaluation	Student Evaluation	Possible Points	Instructor Evaluation	Comments
Equipment and Supplies 1. Gloves (latex or vinyl—optional)			3		
2. Automated external defibrillation (AED) unit			3		
Competency Steps (*follow aseptic procedures*) If there is no pulse, follow the CABs of CPR. Perform CPR until the defibrillator is attached. 1. Press "Analyze" on the defibrillation unit.			3 3 3		
2. Follow each step as the unit instructs.			3		
3. Attach the AED to patient as indicated by instructions on lid of unit.			3		

	Self-Evaluation	Student Evaluation	Possible Points	Instructor Evaluation	Comments
4. State loudly, "Everybody clear of patient."			3		
a. Verify that everyone is clear of patient.			2		
b. Press analysis control switch on AED.			2		
c. Assessment takes 10 to 20 seconds.			2		
d. Everyone should remain clear during this time.			2		
5. If device indicates that a shock is not advised, resume CPR.			3		
6. Once the unit begins charging, a synthesized voice message or light indicator indicates it is charging. Assume that ventricular fibrillation (VF/VT) is present. The AED will indicate the need to deliver shock.			3		
7. Verify that everyone is clear of unit. The AED delivers shocks without additional actions from the operator. It may indicate "Shock now."			2		
8. Give three consecutive shocks.			3		
9. Check the patient's pulse.			3		
10. If no pulse is present, assess the vital signs, support airway, and breathing.			2		
11. If no pulse is present, give CPR for one minute.			2		
12. Check the pulse. If it is not present, press "Analyze" on the AED.			2		
13. Defibrillate up to three times.			2		

	Self-Evaluation	Student Evaluation	Possible Points	Instructor Evaluation	Comments
14. If VF persists after nine shocks, repeat sets of three stacked shocks with one minute of CPR between each set until the "No shock indicated" message is received on the AED or until the patient revives.			3		

TOTAL POINTS POSSIBLE   57

TOTAL POINTS POSSIBLE—2nd attempt   55

TOTAL POINTS EARNED   _____

Points assigned reflect importance of step to meeting objective: Important = 1, Essential = 2, Critical = 3. Students will lose 2 points for repeated attempts. Failure results if any of the critical steps are omitted or performed incorrectly. If using a 100-pomt scale, determine score by dividing points earned by total points possible and multiplying the results by 100.

SCORE: _____

SKILL COMPETENCY ASSESSMENT

16-5 Heimlich Maneuver (Subdiaphragmatic Thrusts) for a Conscious Adult

Student's Name _____ Date _____

Instructor's Name _____

Skill: The person may begin choking and clutch throat with hands. The rescuer can ask, "Are you choking?" If the patient cannot expel the foreign body, the Heimlich maneuver is performed.

Performance Objective: The student will follow a routine procedure that meets guidelines and protocol to assess the patient's condition. If an adult is conscious and has a blocked airway, the rescuer can talk to him or her and perform the Heimlich maneuver to open up the blocked airway.

	Self-Evaluation	Student Evaluation	Possible Points	Instructor Evaluation	Comments
Equipment and Supplies No equipment required.					
Competency Steps (*follow aseptic procedures*) 1. Verify that the patient is choking. Ask, "Are you choking?"			3		
2. If the patient is standing, tell him or her what the procedure is going to be, position yourself behind the patient, and proceed to wrap your arms around patient's abdomen.			3		
3. Place thumb side of fisted hand against middle of abdomen, just above umbilicus.			3		
4. Grasp hands together, keeping one hand fisted and other wrapped on top of it.			3		
5. Give quick, upward thrusts with hands against abdomen.			3		
6. Repeat procedure until patient expels object or until patient becomes unconscious.			3		

	Self-Evaluation	Student Evaluation	Possible Points	Instructor Evaluation	Comments
7. Wash hands.			2		
8. Document the procedure.			3		

TOTAL POINTS POSSIBLE   23

TOTAL POINTS POSSIBLE—2nd attempt   21

TOTAL POINTS EARNED   _____

Points assigned reflect importance of step to meeting objective: Important = 1, Essential = 2, Critical = 3. Students will lose 2 points for repeated attempts. Failure results if any of the critical steps are omitted or performed incorrectly. If using a 100-pomt scale, determine score by dividing points earned by total points possible and multiplying the results by 100.

SCORE: _____

SKILL COMPETENCY ASSESSMENT

16-6 Adult with Airway Obstruction

Student's Name _____ Date _____

Instructor's Name _____

Skill: If the patient becomes unconscious, position the patient on the floor and immediately activate emergency medical services (EMS).

Performance Objective: The student will follow a routine procedure that meets guidelines and protocol to assess the patient's condition. If an adult is unconscious and has a blocked airway, the rescuer performs abdominal thrusts to open the blocked airway.

	Self-Evaluation	Student Evaluation	Possible Points	Instructor Evaluation	Comments
Equipment and Supplies 1. Gloves			3		
2. Resuscitation device			3		
Competency Steps (*follow aseptic procedures*) 1. If the person is unconscious, activate EMS immediately.			3		
2. Lay the person on his or her back.			3		
3. Perform the tongue-jaw lift followed by finger sweep to remove the object.			3		
4. Open the airway: a. Place the resuscitation device. b. Try to ventilate. c. If the airway is still obstructed, reposition the patient's head and try to ventilate again.			3 3 3 3		
5. Place the heel of the hand against the person's abdomen.			3		

	Self-Evaluation	Student Evaluation	Possible Points	Instructor Evaluation	Comments
6. Kneel astride patient's thighs. Give up to five abdominal thrusts in a motion toward diaphragm.			3		
7. Repeat Steps 3 through 6 until effective or help arrives.			3		

TOTAL POINTS POSSIBLE   36

TOTAL POINTS POSSIBLE—2nd attempt   34

TOTAL POINTS EARNED   _____

Points assigned reflect importance of step to meeting objective: Important = 1, Essential = 2, Critical = 3. Students will lose 2 points for repeated attempts. Failure results if any of the critical steps are omitted or performed incorrectly. If using a 100-point scale, determine score by dividing points earned by total points possible and multiplying the results by 100.

SCORE: _____

SKILL COMPETENCY ASSESSMENT

16-7 Treatment of a Patient with Syncope

Student's Name _____ Date _____

Instructor's Name _____

Skill: To properly handle and treat the patient presenting with syncope.

Performance Objective: The student will demonstrate the proper technique for dealing with a syncopal patient.

	Self-Evaluation	Student Evaluation	Possible Points	Instructor Evaluation	Comments
Equipment and Supplies					
1. Oxygen tank with gauge at top or gauge in the dental treatment area			3		
2. Oxygen mask and tubing			3		
3. Spirits of ammonia			1		
Competency Steps (*follow aseptic procedures*)					
1. Position the patient in Trendelenberg position.			2		
2. Establish that the airway is open. If it is not, perform the head tilt, chin lift.			2		
3. Assess for breathing.			2		
4. Administer oxygen.			1		
5. If the patient is not revived within the first 15 seconds, remove the oxygen mask and pass ammonia-soaked gauze under patient's nose for 1 to 2 seconds.			2		
6. Full revival should occur within 1–2 minutes.			2		

	Self-Evaluation	Student Evaluation	Possible Points	Instructor Evaluation	Comments
7. If the patient still does not revive, begin procedures for CPR.			3		
8. Postpone dental treatment and call for patient transport.			2		

TOTAL POINTS POSSIBLE   21

TOTAL POINTS POSSIBLE—2nd attempt   19

TOTAL POINTS EARNED   _____

Points assigned reflect importance of step to meeting objective: Important = 1, Essential = 2, Critical = 3. Students will lose 2 points for repeated attempts. Failure results if any of the critical steps are omitted or performed incorrectly. If using a 100-pomt scale, determine score by dividing points earned by total points possible and multiplying by 100.

SCORE: _____

Clinical Dental Procedures

CHAPTER **17**

Introduction to the Dental Office and Basic Chairside Assisting

SPECIFIC INSTRUCTIONAL OBJECTIVES

The student should strive to meet the following objectives and demonstrate an understanding of the facts and principles presented in this chapter:

1. Describe the design of a dental office, explaining the purpose of each area.
2. Describe the equipment and function of the equipment in each area.
3. Describe the daily routine to open and close the dental office.
4. Explain the basic concepts of chairside assisting.
5. Identify the activity zones and classifications of motion.
6. Describe the necessary steps to prepare the treatment room.
7. Explain the necessary steps to seat the patient for treatment.
8. Describe the ergonomics of the operator and the assistant at chairside.
9. Describe the necessary steps to dismiss the patient after treatment is finished.
10. Identify the special needs of certain patients.

SUMMARY

It is important for the dental assistant to understand the various dental office designs and how each area relates to patient care. Each dentist lays out his or her office to meet the needs of the practice. The assistant learns the function of each area in the dental office and the equipment that is used in this area. Responsibilities and the job description of the dental assistant are discussed in relation to preparing for the patient and seating and then dismissing the patient. Concepts of assisting are described including assisting for a left- or right-handed dentist. Dental health professionals go to great lengths to ensure patient and employee safety and an ergonomic work environment.

Examining the needs of various special needs patients gives the dental assistant the information to plan and prepare for these patients to eliminate problems and make their experience a positive one.

202

© 2013 Cengage Learning. All Rights Reserved. May not be scanned, copied or duplicated, or posted to a publicly accessible website, in whole or in part

EXERCISES AND ACTIVITIES

True or False

1. The sterilization area of the dental office should be near the treatment room.
   a. True
   b. False

2. Dental treatment rooms are also called operatories.
   a. True
   b. False

3. A reclined position with the nose and knees on the same plane may be called a supine position.
   a. True
   b. False

4. The air-water syringe is used to remove saliva and fluids from the patient's mouth.
   a. True
   b. False

5. The operating light is used to set light-cured materials.
   a. True
   b. False

6. Hands-free communication systems are becoming increasingly more popular in dental offices.
   a. True
   b. False

7. The transfer zone for right-handed operators is at the 7 to 12 o'clock position.
   a. True
   b. False

8. Motion that involves the finger, wrist, and elbow is considered a Class III motion.
   a. True
   b. False

9. Ergonomics is very important for dental team members.
   a. True
   b. False

10. If a patient is hearing impaired, the dental assistant must maintain a position in which the patient can see the dental assistant's lips.
    a. True
    b. False

Multiple Choice

1. Which of the following rooms should have their decor changed as often as needed to keep the atmosphere friendly and positive for patients as they enter the dental office?
   a. Restroom
   b. Dentist's private office
   c. Reception room
   d. Sterilizing area

2. Which of the following may be included in the dental business office?

   1. Appointment scheduling
   2. Filing system
   3. Toothbrush center
   4. Computer terminals
   5. Patient records

      a. 1, 2, 3, 5   c. 1, 3, 4, 5
      b. 1, 2, 3, 4   d. 1, 2, 4, 5

3. The assistant should arrive early to open the office and prepare for the day's schedule. Which of the following is not a part of opening the office?

   a. Turn on the master switches, lights, dental units, vacuum system, and air compressor.
   b. Turn off the water supply to the manual processing tanks.
   c. Change into appropriate clinical clothing and follow OSHA guidelines.
   d. Turn on the communication systems.

4. The _____ should be well ventilated because of chemical fumes and exhaust from the equipment.

   a. reception area   c. treatment room
   b. business area   d. sterilizing room

5. Dental stools for staff should be made available that provide for which of the following requirements?

   a. Fixed back rest for vertical adjustment   c. Fixed back rest to support lumbar region
   b. Good support, comfort   d. Thin seat

6. One characteristic of good assistant positioning is

   a. good visibility 4 to 6 inches above the operator.
   b. that the front edge of the assistant stool is even with the patient's elbow.
   c. that the assistant's feet are touching the floor.
   d. that the assistant is positioned on the stool so that weight is on outside edge of seat.

7. The special needs patient is defined as a

   a. child patient.   c. hearing-impaired patient.
   b. pregnant patient.   d. All of the above

8. The sterilization room area should accomplish and provide the following:

   1. Good air circulation
   2. Sink
   3. Vibrator
   4. Instrument ultrasonic equipment
   5. Vacuum former
   6. Sterilizers

      a. 1, 2, 4, 5   c. 1, 2, 4, 6
      b. 2, 3, 5, 6   d. 1, 2, 3, 5

9. The reception room is to be kept tidy by the dental staff. What tasks are required to maintain this look?

   a. Dust and vacuum   c. Magazines are current
   b. Reading materials and chairs are straightened at end of day   d. All of the above

10. In the dental office design plan, this room must provide occupational safety from ionizing radiation.

    a. Patient education room
    c. Radiography room
    b. X-ray processing room
    d. Dental office laboratory

11. The dental office laboratory is a separate area in the office design. The laboratory may contain the all of the following *except* the

    a. vibrator.
    c. patient filing system.
    b. vacuum former.
    d. dental lathe.

12. In selecting a dental unit, _____ is not considered one of the basic modes of delivery.

    a. rear delivery
    c. side delivery
    b. mobile cart
    d. front delivery

13. The assistant's cart is usually set up with the following instrumentation except for the

    a. air-water syringe.
    c. three handpieces.
    b. HVE.
    d. saliva ejector.

14. The air-water syringe provides which of the following?

    a. Combination of air and water
    c. Water
    b. Air
    d. All of the above

15. The ultrasonic unit is used to remove

    a. caries.
    c. hard deposits.
    b. restorations.
    d. temporaries.

Matching

Match each classification of motion with its proper definition.

Classification

1. _c_ Class I
2. _e_ Class II
3. _a_ Class III
4. _b_ Class IV
5. _d_ Class V

Definition

a. Involves finger, wrist, and elbow movement
b. Involves movement of the entire arm and shoulder
c. Involves only finger movement
d. Involves movement of the arm and twisting of the body
e. Involves movement of the fingers and wrist

Match the room to an office by its design and function.

Room

6. _d_ Reception desk
7. _c_ Business office
8. _a_ Sterilizing area
9. _b_ X-ray processing room

Function

a. Near treatment room, has good air circulation to protect from the chemical fumes that may be exhausted.
b. Small room near the treatment rooms. Equipment would include a manual processing tank, drying racks, and a safelight.
c. Area or space where patients can pay bills and schedule appointments. This area may also be used for private conversations with patients.
d. Adjacent to the reception area. Greeting area for the patient and place where telephone calls are received.

Match the following activity zones for a right-handed operator with clock positions.

Zone	Clock Position
10. _c_ Operating	a. 12–2 o'clock
11. _d_ Assistant	b. 4–7 o'clock
12. _a_ Static/rear delivery	c. 7–12 o'clock
13. _b_ Transfer	d. 2–4 o'clock

 Critical Thinking

1. For the dental assistant, ergonomics is key for comfort and the ability to perform duties effectively and efficiently. List the ways in which the chairside dental assistant can ensure proper positioning.

2. Positioning around the patient must be efficient and effective. Describe the five activity zones for a left-handed operator and the activities performed in each zone.

3. Identify and explain classifications of motion involving Classes I, II, and III.

 CASE STUDY 1

The dental receptionist makes an appointment for a patient who speaks no English. The patient brought a friend to assist in this initial appointment process.

1. What recommendations can the receptionist make to the patient when he or she comes for the dental exam?

2. What steps will the dental staff take to make the patient aware that they are making every effort to understand the patient and will assist the patient in any way they can?

CASE STUDY 2

A dental assistant is interviewing for an opening for a chairside assistant position. During the interview a tour of the operatories was provided. There were various observations made about the dental unit, work practices with the equipment, and the ergonomics of accessing the equipment.

1. Name the types of dental units that could be available.

2. Name the types of carts that most units contain.

3. How are operator lights attached or mounted? Who do the lights need to be accessible to? What types of lighting help to improve operations? What are the control switches on lights for and what parts of lights need to be covered with barriers?

CASE STUDY 3

Understanding a new work environment would include the personalized adaptation of both the operator and assistant stools. State the basic ergonomic requirements for each type of stool.

1. Operator stool

2. Assistant stool

CASE STUDY 4

The dentist's vision and expectations are reflected in the office design, which should always consider the patients that the dentist serves. The appearance of the dental office makes a statement about the dentist, the dental staff, and the quality of dental care. The reception room, reception desk, and business office are basic components of the office design.

1. What general features should the reception room offer and how does it affect the patient?

2. Describe the reception desk area and how it is expected to serve the patient.

3. Describe the business area and its function.

SKILL COMPETENCY ASSESSMENT

17-1 Daily Routine to Open the Office

Student's Name _____ Date _____

Instructor's Name _____

Skill: With the amount of equipment operated in the dental office, a routine schedule needs to be in place to ensure proper control. Usually the office is cleaned professionally, but the assistant should periodically check the overall appearance of the office.

Performance Objective: These tasks are performed by the assistant each morning. The assistant arrives at the office early to open the office and to prepare for the day's schedule.

	Self-Evaluation	Student Evaluation	Possible Points	Instructor Evaluation	Comments
Competency Steps					
1. Turn on master switches to the lights, each dental unit, the vacuum system, and the air compressor.			3		
2. Check the reception room.					
a. Turn on the lights.			2		
b. Straighten the magazines.			2		
c. Straighten the children's area.			2		
d. Unlock the patient's door to the office.			3		
3. Turn on the communication system.			3		
a. Check the answering machine or answering system.			3		
b. Start the computers.			3		
c. Unlock files.			2		
d. Organize the business area.			2		
4. Post copies of patient schedules in designated areas throughout the office.			2		
5. Turn on all equipment in the x-ray processing area.			2		
a. Change water in the processing tanks.			3		
b. Replenish solutions, if necessary.			3		
6. Change into appropriate clinical clothing following OSHA guidelines.			3		

	Self-Evaluation	Student Evaluation	Possible Points	Instructor Evaluation	Comments
7. Review the daily patient schedule.			2		
8. Prepare treatment room for the first patient.			3		
a. Check supplies.			2		
b. Place barriers, fill water reservoirs.			3		
c. Review patient records.			3		
d. Prepare appropriate trays and lab work for first patient.			3		
9. Turn on any sterilizing equipment.			2		
a. Check solution levels.			3		
b. Prepare new ultrasonic solutions.			3		
c. Prepare new disinfectant solutions.			3		
d. Complete overnight sterilization procedures.			3		
10. Replenish supplies needed for the day.			3		

TOTAL POINTS POSSIBLE   71

TOTAL POINTS POSSIBLE—2nd attempt   69

TOTAL POINTS EARNED   _____

Points assigned reflect importance of step to meeting objective: Important = 1, Essential = 2, Critical = 3. Students will lose 2 points for repeated attempts. Failure results if any of the critical steps are omitted or performed incorrectly. If using a 100-point scale, determine score by dividing points earned by total points possible and multiplying the results by 100.

SCORE: _____

SKILL COMPETENCY ASSESSMENT

17-2 Daily Routine to Close the Office

Student's Name _____ Date _____

Instructor's Name _____

Skill: As with the opening routine, dental assistants usually share the responsibilities of closing the office.

Performance Objective: These tasks are performed by the assistant at the end of the day. The office evening routine includes closing the office for the evening and preparing for the next day. Each office has its own specific details.

	Self-Evaluation	Student Evaluation	Possible Points	Instructor Evaluation	Comments
Competency Steps					
1. Clean treatment rooms.			3		
a. Conduct in-depth cleaning of the dental chair and unit.			2		
b. Flush handpieces.			3		
c. Flush air-water syringes.			3		
d. Run solutions through evacuation hoses.			3		
e. Clean traps/filters.			3		
f. Maintain water reservoirs.			2		
2. Position the dental chair for evening housekeeping.			2		
3. Turn off all master switches.			3		
4. Process, mount, and file any x-rays.			3		
a. Follow manufacturer's instructions to shut down automatic processors.			3		
b. Turn off the water supply to manual processing tanks.			3		
5. Wipe counters and turn off the safety light.			3		
6. Sterilize all instruments.			3		
a. Set up trays for next day.			3		
b. Empty ultrasonic solutions.			3		
c. Turn off all equipment.			3		
d. Restock supplies.			2		

	Self-Evaluation	Student Evaluation	Possible Points	Instructor Evaluation	Comments
7. Make sure that all laboratory cases have been sent to the lab and that early morning cases have been received.			3		
8. Confirm and complete the appointment schedule for the next day.			3		
a. Complete insurance forms and responsibilities.			3		
b. Complete daily bookkeeping responsibilities.			3		
c. Pull charts for the next day.			3		
9. Turn off business office equipment.			3		
a. Turn on the answering machine or service.			3		
b. Lock patient and business office files.			2		
10. Straighten the reception room. For office security, lock all doors and windows.			3		
11. Change from uniform to street clothes, following OSHA guidelines.			3		
12. Turn off machines in the staff lounge and clean tables and counters.			2		

TOTAL POINTS POSSIBLE   81

TOTAL POINTS POSSIBLE—2nd attempt   79

TOTAL POINTS EARNED   _____

Points assigned reflect importance of step to meeting objective: Important = 1, Essential = 2, Critical = 3. Students will lose 2 points for repeated attempts. Failure results if any of the critical steps are omitted or performed incorrectly. If using a 100-pomt scale, determine score by dividing points earned by total points possible and multiplying the results by 100.

SCORE: ____

SKILL COMPETENCY ASSESSMENT

17-3 Seating the Dental Patient

Student's Name _____ Date _____

Instructor's Name _____

Skill: Greet the patient in the reception area and escort the patient to the treatment room. Prepare the patient for the dental treatment.

Performance Objective: The student will review the patient's medical and dental records, clean and prepare the treatment room with appropriate barriers, ready the tray setup, and remove any possible obstacles from the patient's pathway.

	Self-Evaluation	Student Evaluation	Possible Points	Instructor Evaluation	Comments
Equipment and Supplies					
1. Patient's medical and dental records (updated)			1		
2. Basic setup: mouth mirror, explorer, and cotton pliers			1		
3. Saliva ejector, evacuator (HVE), and air-water syringe tip			1		
4. Cotton rolls, cotton-tip applicator, and gauze sponges			1		
5. Lip lubricant			1		
6. Patient napkin and napkin clip			1		
7. Tissue			1		
8. Protective eyewear			1		
Competency Steps (*follow aseptic procedures*)					
1. Greet and escort the patient to the treatment room. Show the patient where to place personal items. You may offer mouth rinse.			3		
2. Seat the patient in the dental chair. Have the patient sit all the way back in the chair. Offer the patient tissue to remove lipstick and offer lubricant for the lips.			3		

	Self-Evaluation	Student Evaluation	Possible Points	Instructor Evaluation	Comments
3. Place the napkin on the patient and give the patient protective eyewear.			2		
4. Review the patient's health history for any changes since the last visit. Check whether the patient has any questions. Provide a brief explanation/confirmation of treatment to be performed at this appointment. Place x-rays on the view box.			4		
5. Position the patient for treatment, adjust the headrest until the patient's head is well supported and the patient is comfortable, and adjust the dental light for the appropriate arch.			4		
6. Position the operator's stool and the rheostat.			3		
7. Position the assistant's stool. Put on the mask and protective eyewear, and then wash hands and don gloves before being seated chairside.			3		
8. Position the tray setup. Prepare the saliva ejector, evacuator tip, air-water (three-way) syringe tip, and dental handpieces.			3		

TOTAL POINTS POSSIBLE   33

TOTAL POINTS POSSIBLE—2nd attempt   31

TOTAL POINTS EARNED   _____

Points assigned reflect importance of step to meeting objective: Important = 1, Essential = 2, Critical = 3. Students will lose 2 points for repeated attempts. Failure results if any of the critical steps are omitted or performed incorrectly. If using a 100-point scale, determine score by dividing points earned by total points possible and multiplying the results by 100.

SCORE: _____

SKILL COMPETENCY ASSESSMENT

17-4 Dismissing the Dental Patient

Student's Name _____ Date _____

Instructor's Name _____

Skill: After the treatment is completed, the patient is escorted from the treatment room to the reception area.

Performance Objective: The student will remove gloves, wash hands, and review the patient's dental treatment with the dentist. Documentation will be made on the patient's chart or input to the computer terminal by the assistant. The patient's chart and x-rays are gathered, the patient's personal items are returned, any obstacles are removed from the patient's pathway, and the patient is escorted to the reception area.

	Self-Evaluation	Student Evaluation	Possible Points	Instructor Evaluation	Comments
Equipment and Supplies					
1. Patient's medical and dental records			1		
2. Basic three: mouth mirror, explorer, and cotton pliers			1		
3. Saliva ejector, evacuator (HVE), and air-water syringe tip			1		
4. Cotton rolls, cotton tip applicator, and gauze sponges			1		
5. Lip lubricant			1		
6. Tissue			1		
7. Safety glasses			1		
Competency Steps					
1. When operator is finished with procedure, assistant rinses and evacuates the patient's mouth thoroughly. The dental light is positioned out of the patient's way.			3		

	Self-Evaluation	Student Evaluation	Possible Points	Instructor Evaluation	Comments
2. Remove any debris from the patient's face. (Patient can also look in mirror before leaving the treatment area.)			2		
3. Patient napkin (bib) is removed and placed over the used materials on the tray setup. Safety glasses are removed.			3		
4. Remove evacuator (HVE) tip, saliva ejector, and air-water syringe tip.			2		
5. Operator's stool and rheostat moved out of way of patient.			3		
6. Procedure documented in the patient chart or in the computer terminal (gloves must be removed and hands washed). Patient's chart and x-rays are gathered.			3		
7. Postoperative instructions are given to patient.			2		
8. Patient's personal items are returned and patient is escorted to reception area.			1		

TOTAL POINTS POSSIBLE   26

TOTAL POINTS POSSIBLE—2nd attempt   24

TOTAL POINTS EARNED   _____

Points assigned reflect importance of step to meeting objective: Important = 1, Essential = 2, Critical = 3. Student will lose 2 points for repeated attempts. Failure results if any of the critical steps are omitted or performed incorrectly. If using a 100-point scale, determine score by dividing points earned by total points possible and multiplying the results by 100.

SCORE: _____

CHAPTER 18

Basic Chairside Instruments and Tray Systems

SPECIFIC INSTRUCTIONAL OBJECTIVES

The student should strive to meet the following objectives and demonstrate an understanding of the facts and principles presented in this chapter:

1. Identify the parts of an instrument.
2. Describe how instruments are identified.
3. Identify the categories and functions of dental burs.
4. Describe the types and functions of abrasives.
5. Describe the various handpieces and attachments.
6. Describe the types of tray systems and color-coding systems.

SUMMARY

The basic instruments used in general dental procedures include common cutting and noncutting instruments. Instruments are generally categorized as hand instruments and rotary instruments. Each procedure requires special instruments to accomplish specific tasks. The assistant is responsible for keeping the instruments sterilized, organized, and in working condition.

EXERCISES AND ACTIVITIES

Multiple Choice

1. The _____ is *not* part of the dental hand instrument.
   a. flute
   b. handle
   c. shank
   d. working end

2. The _____ is the part of the instrument that connects the handle to the working end.

   a. handle
   b. shank

   c. blade
   d. bevel

3. The working end of the instrument may be a

   a. point.
   b. blade.

   c. nib.
   d. All of the above

4. Which part of the instrument actually performs the instrument's specific function?

   a. Handle
   b. Shank

   c. Working end
   d. Flute

5. (The) _____ formula was developed to standardize the exact size and angulation of an instrument.

   a. manufacturer's number
   b. Black's

   c. first number
   d. second number

6. Which of the following is *not* a cutting instrument?

   a. Chisel
   b. Excavator

   c. Carrier
   d. Angle former

7. Which of the following is *not* an example of a noncutting instrument?

   a. Carver
   b. Carrier

   c. File
   d. Hoe

8. Which of the following is *not* included in Black's three-number formula?

   a. The first number is the width of the blade.

   c. The second number represents the degree of the angle of the cutting edge to the blade.

   b. The second number is the measurement of the length of the blade.

   d. The third number provides measurement of the angle of the blade to the long axis of the handle.

9. _____ are used to assist in the design of the cavity preparation.

   a. Amalgam carriers
   b. Carvers

   c. Amalgam condensers
   d. Hand cutting instruments

10. _____ are used to shape and plane the enamel and dentin walls of the cavity preparation.

   a. Hoes
   b. Hatchets

   c. Chisels
   d. Angle formers

11. _____ are paired left and right and are used in a downward motion to refine the cavity walls.

   a. Excavators
   b. Hatchets

   c. Hoes
   d. Chisels

12. The _____ is used in a pulling motion to smooth and shape the floor of the cavity preparation.

   a. gingival margin trimmer
   b. hatchet

   c. hoe
   d. chisel

13. The _____, which is similar to the hatchet in regard to the position of the blade to the handle, is used to bevel the gingival margin wall of the cavity preparation.

   a. hatchet
   b. gingival margin trimmer

   c. hoe
   d. chisel

14. The _____ is used in a downward pushing motion to form and define point angles and to sharpen line angles.

   a. gingival margin trimmer

   b. angle former

   c. hatchet

   d. chisel

15. The _____, which is used to remove carious material, has a cutting edge that is rounded all the way around the periphery of the blade.

   a. gingival margin trimmer

   b. carrier

   c. excavator

   d. carver

16. The _____ examination setup instruments are common to all tray setups.

   a. composite

   b. plastic

   c. basic

   d. amalgam

17. Which of the following is *not* one of the basic examination setup instruments?

   a. Excavator

   b. Mouth mirror

   c. Explorer

   d. Cotton pliers

18. Which is *not* a type of mouth mirror?

   a. Concave

   b. Convex

   c. Front

   d. Plane

19. The operator uses a mirror that is called _____ to view areas of the mouth not visible with direct vision.

   a. retraction of light

   b. transillumination

   c. indirect vision

   d. direct vision

20. Known as _____, the mirror is used to direct the light to reflect and detect fractures in a tooth.

   a. retraction

   b. transillumination

   c. indirect vision

   d. direct vision

21. Which instrument's working end is a thin, sharp point of flexible steel?

   a. Excavator

   b. Cotton pliers

   c. Explorer

   d. Plastic instrument

22. _____ are used to transport and manipulate various materials. They are available with either locking or nonlocking handles.

   a. Explorers

   b. Excavators

   c. Cotton pliers

   d. Probes

23. The working end of the _____ consists of a rounded or blunted blade that is marked in millimeters.

   a. explorer

   b. probe

   c. plastic

   d. carver

24. The amalgam _____ is designed to carry and dispense amalgam into the cavity preparation.

   a. condenser

   b. carrier

   c. carver

   d. burnisher

25. _____ are used to remove excess restorative material and to carve tooth anatomy in the restoration before the material hardens.

   a. Condensers

   b. Carriers

   c. Carvers

   d. Burnishers

26. _____ knives are used to trim excess filling material.
    a. Carver
    b. Finishing
    c. File
    d. Burnisher

27. _____ spatulas are used to mix composite resin materials.
    a. Cement
    b. Laboratory
    c. Plastic
    d. Surgical

28. Which of the following is *not* a use or characteristic of the crown and collar scissors?
    a. Trim matrix bands
    b. Cut retraction cord
    c. Trim amalgam
    d. Straight blade

29. The _____ of the bur is inserted into the handpiece.
    a. neck
    b. head
    c. diamond
    d. shank

30. The _____ of the bur is the working end of the bur.
    a. neck
    b. head
    c. diamond
    d. shank

31. Cutting burs have _____ cutting blades or surfaces.
    a. 8
    b. 4
    c. 14
    d. 10

32. There are _____ basic cutting bur shapes.
    a. 3
    b. 6
    c. 9
    d. 12

33. _____ burs or stones are used for rapidly reducing tooth structure during cavity preparation, polishing and finishing composite restorations, and occlusal adjustment.
    a. Surgical
    b. Finishing
    c. Laboratory
    d. Diamond

34. _____ are nonbladed instruments used to finish and polish restorations.
    a. Abrasives
    b. Diamonds
    c. Mandrels
    d. Finishing burs

35. Which of the following instruments have abrasive material that may be made of garnet, diamond, and quartz?
    a. Cutting burs
    b. Fissure burs
    c. Discs
    d. Finishing burs

36. _____ discs are used for rapid cutting and have diamond particles bonded to both sides of steel discs.
    a. Sandpaper
    b. Diamond
    c. Carborundum
    d. Separating

37. The _____ end of the handpiece is where burs, stones, and attachments are held.
    a. connection
    b. working
    c. rheostat
    d. shank

38. Which of the following will reduce frictional heat from the use of the high-speed handpiece?
    a. Air
    b. Water
    c. Air-water spray
    d. All of the above

39. The _____ holds the shank portion of the bur in place.

    a. head

    b. chuck

    c. handle

    d. neck

40. What will activate and control the speed of the handpiece?

    a. Power source

    b. Fiber-optic light source

    c. Friction

    d. Rheostat

41. The low-speed handpiece is often called the

    a. contra-angle.

    b. right angle.

    c. straight handpiece.

    d. latch type.

42. At the dental unit, the low-speed handpiece will not

    a. polish teeth.

    b. remove soft carious material.

    c. polish appliances.

    d. define cavity walls.

43. Which of the following cannot be sterilized?

    a. Burs

    b. Handpieces

    c. Sandpaper discs

    d. Rotary instruments

44. High-speed handpieces operate at _____ rpm.

    a. 400,000

    b. 30,000

    c. 100,000

    d. 250,000

45. A _____ tray system provides an efficient means of transporting instruments.

    a. positioning

    b. preset

    c. rubberized

    d. color-coded

46. The _____ chisel is used for Class III or IV cavity preparation.

    a. gingival marginal trimmer (GMT)

    b. binangle

    c. Wedelstaedt

    d. contra-angle

47. The dental handpiece is not used for

    a. removing dental decay.

    b. polishing teeth.

    c. polishing and finishing restorations.

    d. probing.

48. Identify this instrument:

© Cengage Learning 2013

    a. Enamel hatchet

    b. Straight chisel

    c. Gingival marginal trimmer

    d. Excavator

49. Identify this instrument:

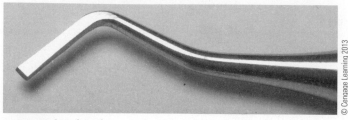

a. Straight chisel

b. Gingival marginal trimmer

c. Enamel hatchet

d. Carver

50. Identify this bur:

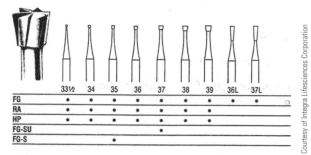

a. Pear

b. Inverted cone

c. End cutting

d. Round

51. Identify this bur:

a. Wheel

b. Inverted cone

c. Tapered fissure cross-cut

d. Tapered fissure straight

Matching

Hand cutting instruments are used to assist in the design of the cavity preparation. Match the instrument with its use.

Instrument

1. ___C___ Hatchet

2. ___A___ Hoe

3. ___D___ Gingival

4. ___C___ Angle former

5. ___B___ Chisel

Use

a. Used in pulling motion to shape floor of cavity preparation

b. Shape and plane enamel/dentin walls of cavity preparation

c. Used in downward motion to form/define point angles margin trimmer

d. Bevel gingival margin wall of cavity preparation

e. Used in downward motion to refine cavity walls

Instruments are classified by function to describe a specific use. Match each noncutting instrument with its respective use.

Instrument

6. _B_ Amalgam carriers

7. _E_ Amalgam gun

8. _A_ Amalgam condensers

9. _C_ Carvers

10. _D_ Explorer

Use

a. Sometimes called pluggers

b. Carry and dispense amalgam into cavity preparations

c. Carve tooth anatomy in restorations

d. Detect any irregularity

e. Has spring action and is single ended and made of plastic

Dental burs are rotary instruments. Match each part of the bur with its respective description.

Bur

11. _B_ Shank

12. _C_ Neck

13. _A_ Head

Description

a. Working end of bur

b. Inserted into handpiece

c. Tapered connection of shank to the head

Identify each bur name with its respective function.

Bur Name

14. _C_ Round

15. _D_ Inverted cone

16. _A_ Plain fissure straight

17. _E_ Tapered fissure cross-cut

18. _B_ Diamond

Function

a. Forms cavity walls of preparation

b. Used for rapid reduction of tooth structure

c. Used to open the cavity and remove caries

d. Makes undercuts and removes caries

e. Forms divergent walls of the cavity preparation

Critical Thinking

1. The dental assistant should examine all instruments carefully. Name common examinations and evaluations of instruments.

2. What are the risks that occur when instruments that come out of sterilization are not dried before being stored?

3. Rotary instruments are used with a dental handpiece. At chairside, how are these instruments (burs) used?

4. How are rotary instruments such as laboratory burs used?

5. Abrasives are nonbladed instruments. Name some categories of abrasive materials and how they would be used in the finishing process.

CASE STUDY 1

The dental assistant is responsible for keeping instruments sterilized and in working condition. All dental instruments must be properly cared for, maintained, and sterilized to ensure that the instruments will last a long time, function as designed, and are used safely.

1. When should instruments be cleaned?

2. Describe proper instrument cleaning.

3. How are hinged instruments cared for?

4. How are instruments prepared for sterilization?

CASE STUDY 2

At chairside, rotary instruments such as cutting burs are used. Burs are specified by shape, function, and number. The dentists often will ask for a bur by its number. As these burs are used for specific functions, the number can alert the dental assistant to the activity taking place within the tooth structure.

1. Describe the function of the round bur and provide a 1–6 number range of these burs, beginning with the smallest number.

2. Describe the function of the inverted cone bur and provide a 1–4 number range of these burs. What would the "L" indicate?

3. Describe the function of the plain fissure straight bur and provide a 1–3 number range of these burs. Compare the plain fissure straight and cross-cut burs.

4. Describe the function of the tapered fissure straight bur and provide a 1–5 number range of these burs.

CASE STUDY 3

The dentist selects the instruments that she or he feels the most confident and comfortable using. The dental assistant's role is to be able to recognize, identify, and describe these instruments with confidence.

1. Describe the binangle chisel and where in the tooth preparation it would be used. (Be able to photo recognize the correct instrument.)

2. Describe the enamel hatchet and where in the tooth preparation it would be used. (Be able to photo recognize the correct instrument.)

3. Describe the mesial marginal trimmer and where in the tooth preparation it would be used. (Be able to photo recognize the correct instrument.)

4. Describe the distal marginal trimmer and where in the tooth preparation it would be used. (Be able to photo recognize the correct instrument.)

CHAPTER 19

Instrument Transfer and Maintaining the Operating Field

The student should strive to meet the following objectives and demonstrate an understanding of the facts and principles presented in this chapter:

1. Describe the transfer zone.

2. Define a fulcrum and tactile sensation.

3. Describe the grasps, positions, and transfer of instruments for a procedure.

4. List the eight rules for instrument transfer.

5. Understand instrument transfer modification.

6. Describe and demonstrate how to maintain the oral cavity.

7. Explain the equipment used in the treatment of the oral cavity.

8. Describe techniques for moisture control and isolation.

9. Explain techniques for dental assistants performing expanded functions.

SUMMARY

Four-handed, sit-down dentistry has changed the role of the dental assistant. Working right at the chair with the dentist or dental hygienist, the assistant has become an important aspect of performing dental procedures on patients. Transferring instruments and evacuation are skills the dental assistant will use every day with every patient. Learning how to correctly perform these tasks and understanding what needs to be done during a procedure will enable the dental assistant to be a great asset to the operator and a comfort to the patient.

EXERCISES AND ACTIVITIES

True or False

1. A smooth transfer of instruments and materials occurs when the assistant is able to anticipate the operator's needs.
   a. **True**
   b. False

2. The assistant passes and receives instruments with the right hand when working with a right-handed dentist.
   a. True
   b. **False**

3. Using one hand for instrument transfer frees the other hand for evacuation.
   a. **True**
   b. False

4. The reverse palm-thumb grasp is sometimes called the thumb-to-nose grasp. (Op) Text
   a. **True**
   b. False

5. The way an instrument is grasped also dictates how it is exchanged.
   a. **True**
   b. False

6. The pen grasp is used to hold instruments that have straight shanks.
   a. True
   b. **False**

7. The modified pen grasp provides more control and strength in some procedures.
   a. **True**
   b. False

8. The only tool needed to maintain moisture control in the oral cavity is the saliva ejector.
   a. True
   b. **False**

9. The dental assistant doesn't transfer dental materials to the dentist.
   a. True
   b. **False**

10. With angled-shank instruments, the primary working end should be placed away from the assistant on the tray.
    a. **True**
    b. False

Multiple Choice

1. Proper instrument transfer is accomplished when which of the following is maintained?
   a. The operator's view remains on the oral cavity.
   b. Safety and comfort are maintained for the patient.
   c. Stress and fatigue for the operator and the assistant are reduced.
   d. **All of the above.**

2. Selecting the correct instrument grasp allows

    a. the operator control of the instrument.

    b. greater tactile sensation for the operator.

    c. reduced fatigue for the operator.

    d. All of the above.

3. The ability to maintain the operating field is a critical skill for the dental assistant to obtain. Which of the following skills are essential to oral evacuation tip placement?

    1. The fingers always rest on the occlusal surface.

    2. The evacuator tip is placed approximately one tooth distal to the tooth being worked on.

    3. The bevel of the tip is held parallel to the buccal or lingual surface of the teeth.

    4. The bevel of the tip is parallel to the apex surface of the teeth.

    5. The opening should be even with the occlusal surface.

    6. The primary working end should always be placed toward the cheek.

    a. 1, 5, 6

    b. 2, 3, 5

    c. 2, 3, 6

    d. 1, 3, 5

4. Name the grasp type used when the instrument is held between the pad of the thumb and the pad of the index finger, with the side of the middle finger on the opposite side of the thumb.

    a. Reverse palm-thumb

    b. Palm

    c. Pen

    d. Thumb-to-nose

5. The _____ grasp is used to hold instruments that have angled shanks.

    a. thumb-to-nose

    b. modified pen

    c. pen

    d. palm

6. The two-handed transfer is used for which of the following instruments?

    a. Surgical forceps

    b. Air-water syringe

    c. Dental handpiece

    d. All of the above

7. The instrument grasp shown below is called the _____ grasp.

    a. reverse palm-thumb

    b. modified pen

    c. palm-thumb

    d. pen

© Cengage Learning 2013

8. At the beginning of a procedure, the dental assistant places the _____ in the right hand and the _____ in the left hand and when the dentist puts his or her hands in position, the dental assistant passes both instruments simultaneously.

    a. cotton pliers, explorer

    b. scissors, explorer

    c. explorer, mouth mirror

    d. mouth mirror, explorer

9. The operator receives the air-water syringe by the

(a) handle.

c. tip.

b. hose.

d. The operator never needs to use the air-water syringe.

10. Which device provides a clear, dry field; isolation; and light all at the same time?

a. Air-water syringe

c. Obturation unit

b. High-speed handpiece

(d) Isolite System

Matching

Match the term with the best description.

1. ___d___ Transfer zone

2. ___a___ Fulcrum

3. ___b___ Tactile sensation

4. ___c___ Transfer hand

a. A point of rest on which the fingers are stabilized and can pivot.

b. The feeling sensed by touch. The pressure of the instrument exchanged in an instrument transfer.

c. The hand that delivers and receives instruments.

d. Where the assistant brings the instrument to the operator (area just below the patient nose and chin).

Match each grasp type with its best definition.

5. ___b___ Pen grasp

6. ___c___ Palm grasp

7. ___d___ Reverse palm-thumb

8. ___a___ Modified pen

a. Provides more control in some procedures

b. Grasped in the same manner as a pen or pencil

c. Used with surgical pliers

d. Used to hold the evacuation tip in patient's mouth

The one-handed transfer is the most common instrument transfer. Following are the three steps for the instrument transfer. Match each transfer step with its description.

9. ___b___ Approach

10. ___c___ Retrieval

11. ___a___ Delivery

a. Rotate hand toward the operator and place the instrument in the operator's fingers.

b. Lift the instrument from the tray, holding it near the non-working end.

c. Extend the little finger and close around the handle of the instrument.

Critical Thinking

1. Various techniques and methods of moisture control/isolation are identified in this chapter. Keeping the field dry during a procedure is critical in most procedures.

   a. Describe the use of cotton rolls.

   b. Explain how cotton rolls are placed.

   c. Describe where cotton rolls are placed.

   d. Describe methods of removing cotton rolls.

2. At the beginning of a procedure, the operator needs the mirror and the explorer to examine the area to be treated.

   a. Describe the mirror and explorer transfer.

   b. Would this be a one-handed or two-handed transfer?

3. There are times when the instrument transfer must be modified.

   a. Indicate whether the operator should leave the fulcrum position.

   b. Name some of these modifications.

CASE STUDY 1

Miriam has a large quantity of saliva flow. During her dental procedure the dental assistant used various methods to keep the field of operation dry.

1. Name some of the methods of moisture control and isolation.

2. Describe how each of these methods would improve a dry field.

CASE STUDY 2

Each dentist you work with may have her or his own personalized method of instrument exchange and transfer. In four-handed, sit-down dentistry, the assistant must gain confidence and skill to properly pass and receive instruments from the operator.

1. What does efficient instrument transfer permit the operator to accomplish or maintain?

2. Describe a smooth transfer of instruments and materials.

3. Name the four outcomes of proper instrument transfer.

CASE STUDY 3

A smooth transfer of instruments and materials occurs when the assistant is able to anticipate the operator's needs.

1. Describe the role of the transfer hand.

2. Describe a one-handed versus a two-handed transfer.

3. Describe a signal that will alert the dental assistant to an instrument transfer exchange.

SKILL COMPETENCY ASSESSMENT

19-1 One-Handed Instrument Transfer

Student's Name _____ Date _____

Instructor's Name _____

Skill: The one-handed transfer is the most common transfer. The assistant picks up the next instrument to be transferred with one hand, and with that same hand receives the instrument the operator is finished using, then rotates the new instrument into the operator's hand.

Performance Objective: The student will demonstrate the exchange of dental instruments safely and efficiently with the working end delivered in the position of use.

	Self-Evaluation	Student Evaluation	Possible Points	Instructor Evaluation	Comments
Equipment and Supplies 1. Basic setup: mouth mirror, explorer, and cotton pliers			3		
2. Spoon excavator (for pen or modified pen grasp)			2		
3. Straight chisel, forceps, or elevators (for palm grasp)			2		
Competency Steps (*follow aseptic procedures*) *Approach* 1. Lift the instrument from the tray using the thumb, index finger, and second finger. Hold the instrument near the nonworking end.			3		
2. Turn the palm upward into passing position, rotating the nib toward the correct arch.			3		
3. Move toward operator's hand.			2		
Retrieval 4. Extend the little finger and close it around the handle of the instrument that the operator is holding.			3		

	Self-Evaluation	Student Evaluation	Possible Points	Instructor Evaluation	Comments
5. Lift the instrument out of the operator's hand.			3		
6. Pull this instrument toward the assistant's palm and wrist.			3		
Delivery 7. Rotate the hand toward the operator and place the new instrument in the operator's fingers.			3		
8. Once the operator has the new instrument, rotate the old instrument to the delivery position for use again or return it to the tray.			3		

TOTAL POINTS POSSIBLE   30

TOTAL POINTS POSSIBLE—2nd attempt   28

TOTAL POINTS EARNED   _____

Points assigned reflect importance of step to meeting objective: Important = 1, Essential = 2, Critical = 3. Students will lose 2 points for repeated attempts. Failure results if any of the critical steps are omitted or performed incorrectly. If using a 100-point scale, determine score by dividing points earned by total points possible and multiplying the results by 100.

SCORE: _____

SKILL COMPETENCY ASSESSMENT

19-2 Oral Evacuation for Specific Tip Placements

Student's Name _____ Date _____

Instructor's Name _____

Skill: To maintain the oral cavity to keep the area clear and clean for the operator and for patient comfort.

Performance Objective: The student will demonstrate the various oral evacuation tip placements for each quadrant when assisting a right-handed operator.

	Self-Evaluation	Student Evaluation	Possible Points	Instructor Evaluation	Comments
Equipment and Supplies 1. Basic setup: mouth mirror, cotton pliers, and explorer			1		
2. HVE tip and air-water syringe tip			1		
3. Cotton rolls			1		
4. Dental handpiece			1		
Competency Steps (*follow aseptic procedures*) 1. Carefully place the evacuator tip in the patient's mouth (avoid bumping the teeth, lips, or gingiva).			3		
2. Place the evacuator tip in the mouth and position it before the operator positions the handpiece or instrument.			2		
3. Place the evacuation tip approximately one tooth distal to the tooth being worked on.			2		
4. Hold the bevel of the evacuator tip parallel to the assigned surface (buccal or lingual).			2		

	Self-Evaluation	Student Evaluation	Possible Points	Instructor Evaluation	Comments
5. Hold the middle of the evacuator tip opening even with the occlusal surface.			1		
6. Hold the evacuator tip still while the handpiece or instruments are being used or exchanged.			2		
7. Whenever possible, the evacuator tip should not rest on gingival tissue but rather on a cotton roll.			4		
8. Demonstrate areas of the mouth to avoid to prevent the patient's gagging reflex.			2		
9. Keep the evacuator tip away from the mucosal tissue.			2		

TOTAL POINTS POSSIBLE   24

TOTAL POINTS POSSIBLE—2nd attempt   22

TOTAL POINTS EARNED   _____

Points assigned reflect importance of step to meeting objective: Important = 1, Essential = 2, Critical = 3. Students will lose 2 points for repeated attempts. Failure results if any of the critical steps are omitted or performed incorrectly. If using a 100-point scale, determine score by dividing points earned by total points possible and multiplying the results by 100.

SCORE: _____

CHAPTER 20

Anesthesia and Sedation

SPECIFIC INSTRUCTIONAL OBJECTIVES

The student should strive to meet the following objectives and demonstrate an understanding of the facts and principles presented in this chapter:

1. Describe methods used to manage the pain and anxiety associated with dental procedures.

2. Explain various topical anesthetics and their placements.

3. Describe types of local anesthetics.

4. Identify the injection sites for the maxillary and mandibular arches.

5. Describe the equipment and materials needed to administer local anesthetic.

6. List the steps for preparing for the administration of local anesthetic.

7. Identify supplemental techniques to administer anesthetics.

8. Discuss the role of nitrous oxide in the care of the dental patient.

9. Demonstrate the ability to assist in the administration of nitrous oxide.

SUMMARY

Because most procedures require some form of anesthesia, the dentist may select one or a combination of methods to control pain, depending on the patient and the procedure. The dental assistant is responsible for preparing, safely transferring, and caring for the anesthetic syringe and accessories. During this time, the assistant must be aware of the various topical solutions, the application sites, how to apply the topical anesthetic, and possible patient reactions. In addition, the assistant follows the dentist's directions for the administration of sedation and monitoring requirements.

EXERCISES AND ACTIVITIES

Multiple Choice

1. When a(n) _____ anesthetic is administered, the patient becomes unconscious.

    a. local

    b. topical

    c. general

    d. infiltration

2. The patient may experience _____ after conscious sedation.

    a. a headache

    b. nausea

    c. brief periods of amnesia

    d. All of the above

3. An oral sedation like benzodiazepine can be used as a sedative hypnotic to keep the patient

    a. drowsy.

    b. relaxed.

    c. a and b.

    d. None of the above

4. If benzodiazepine is used as an anti-anxiety drug, the patient will be

    a. relaxed.

    b. drowsy.

    c. a and b.

    d. None of the above

5. _____ reactions are symptoms due to an overdose of anesthetic solution.

    a. Allergic

    b. Toxic

    c. Paresthesia

    d. Topical

6. Local anesthetics used for injections are available in _____ form.

    a. topical

    b. gas

    c. liquid

    d. gel

7. Which of the following is not an amide compound found in local anesthetic solutions?

    a. Lidocaine

    b. Mepivacaine

    c. Prilocaine

    d. Procaine

8. _____ -duration solutions last longer than 90 minutes and contain a vasoconstrictor.

    a. Intermediate

    b. Long

    c. Short

    d. All of the above

9. The most common vasoconstrictor used in dentistry is

    a. oxygen.

    b. nitrous oxide sedation.

    c. epinephrine.

    d. distilled water.

10. Which of the following is not among the most common vasoconstrictor ratios?

    a. 1:20,000

    b. 1:50,000

    c. 1:10,000

    d. 1:100,000

11. _____ is the sensation of feeling numb.

    a. Hemorrhage

    b. Paresthesia

    c. Impulse

    d. Allergy

12. The injection method that places anesthetic solution in tissue near the small terminal nerve branches for absorption is (a)

    a. computerized.

    b. local infiltration.

    c. field block.

    d. nerve block.

13. The injection method that deposits anesthetic near larger terminal nerve branches is (a)

    a. nerve block.
    b. computerized.
    c. local.
    d. field block.

14. The injection method that deposits anesthetic solutions near a main nerve trunk is (a)

    a. field block.
    b. computerized.
    c. electronic.
    d. nerve block.

15. The _____ part of the syringe is cleaned with a brush and checked for sharpness before sterilizing.

    a. barrel
    b. piston rod
    c. threaded end
    d. harpoon

16. Which injection would use a long needle?

    a. Infiltration
    b. Incisive
    c. Mental
    d. Infraorbital

17. Inhalation anesthesia is administered through the

    a. face mask.
    b. laryngeal mask airway.
    c. endotracheal tube.
    d. All of the above.

18. The _____ is the slanted tip of the needle.

    a. lumen
    b. gauge
    c. bevel
    d. shank

19. All of the following are common for adults *except*

    a. general anesthesia.
    b. inhalation anesthesia.
    c. intramuscular sedation.
    d. intravenous conscious sedation.

20. The _____ cylinder contains the anesthetic solution.

    a. computer
    b. cartridge
    c. electronic
    d. topical

21. The syringe end of the needle penetrates the anesthetic solution at the

    a. aluminum cap.
    b. rubber plunger.
    c. piston rod.
    d. diaphragm.

22. Which of the following conditions indicate that the anesthetic cartridge should be discarded?

    a. Large bubbles
    b. Extruded plunger
    c. Corrosion
    d. All of the above

23. The injection that places local anesthetic directly into the cancellous bone is (the)

    a. periodontal ligament.
    b. intrapulpal.
    c. electronic.
    d. intraosseous.

24. Benefits from use of nitrous oxide sedation include the following:

    a. Provides relaxation and relieves apprehension.
    b. Makes time pass quickly.
    c. Allows patient to be comfortable while receiving treatment.
    d. All of the above.

25. Which of the following is a contraindication for the use of nitrous oxide sedation?

    a. Patient is unable to breathe through the nose.
    b. Patient fears dental treatment.
    c. Patient has very a sensitive gag reflex.
    d. Patient has a heart condition and will benefit from oxygen.

26. The _____ meter adjusts the gas flow through the unit.

    a. reservoir
    b. flow

    c. nosepiece
    d. mask

27. The nitrous oxide gas cylinder color is

    a. white.
    b. blue.

    c. green.
    d. orange.

28. The concentration of solution for a topical anesthetic is _____ than that used for local anesthetics.

    a. higher
    b. lower

29. The _____ needle is used for injections that require little penetration of the soft tissue, such as infiltration.

    a. long
    b. short

30. The _____ needle is used for mandibular nerve block injections.

    a. short
    b. long

31. Nitrous oxide sedation will _____ the pain threshold without the loss of consciousness.

    a. lower
    b. raise

Matching

Match the injection site with the teeth most affected.

Injection	Effect
1. __d__ Infiltration	a. A mandibular quadrant
2. __c__ Middle superior alveolar	b. Mandibular premolars, canines
3. __a__ Inferior alveolar nerve	c. Maxillary premolars in one quadrant
4. __b__ Mental nerve block	d. Individual teeth

The type of syringe most commonly used for dental procedures is the aspirating syringe. Recommended by the ADA, it is designed to allow the operator to check the position of the needle before depositing the anesthetic solution. Match the part with its function.

Part	Function
5. __d__ Thumb ring	a. Holds the cartridge
6. __e__ Plunger	b. Barbed tip end that engages the cartridge
7. __b__ Harpoon	c. Where the needle attaches to the syringe
8. __c__ Threaded end	d. Allows the operator to aspirate; should not come loose
9. __a__ Barrel	e. Located inside the syringe; the rod applies force

Critical Thinking

1. Benzodiazepine is a commonly prescribed drug for oral sedation of dental patients. The drug can be prescribed in several ways. Name these prescribed ways and how the patient benefits from each.

2. Needlesticks can occur during transfer of the syringe or during the recap procedure. List the procedure to follow when a needlestick occurs.

3. Anesthetic administration is to be charted carefully and in detail. The dental assistant may be directed by the dentist (with supervision) to do the charting. List the steps that the charting would include.

CASE STUDY 1

Brooke has completed a comprehensive dental exam. During the consultation and treatment planning, Brooke expressed the anxiety she has when going to the dental office. She was unsure how she would handle the several visits required for the planned treatment.

1. Name an anti-anxiety type of sedation.

2. If a drug is prescribed, what effects will the patient feel?

3. When would this medication be taken?

CASE STUDY 2

In charting anesthetic administration for Laura, the following chart notations are made: R-PSANB. Define each symbol.

1. R.

2. PSANB. Define the injection.

3. Where is the location for this injection?

4. Which teeth or tissues are affected?

CASE STUDY 3

Most dental procedures require some form of anesthesia. One of the dental assistant's major responsibilities is the care and handling of the equipment to prepare for local anesthetic.

1. What equipment is needed to administer local anesthetic?

2. What should the thumb ring be checked for?

3. Describe needle lengths.

4. Explain two ADA cartridge colors and their respective concentrations, with or without epinephrine.

SKILL COMPETENCY ASSESSMENT

20-1 Preparing the Anesthetic Syringe

Student's Name _____ Date _____

Instructor's Name _____

Skill: Routine steps should be followed for all patients in the management of pain and anxiety. The dental assistant must be aware of anesthetic solutions, techniques, application sites, and possible patient reactions.

Performance Objective: The student will follow a routine procedure that meets the regulations and the protocol set forth by the dentist and regulatory agencies, keeping in mind that assistant duties vary from state to state. The dental assistant prepares the syringe out of the view of the patient. (The dentist then places the topical anesthetic, or if the dental assistant is working in an expanded functions state and has requisite training, the assistant places the topical anesthetic, and then loads the syringe.)

	Self-Evaluation	Student Evaluation	Possible Points	Instructor Evaluation	Comments
Equipment and Supplies					
1. Sterile syringe			2		
2. Selected disposable needle			2		
3. Selected anesthetic cartridge, needlestick protector			3		
4. 2 × 2 gauze sponge moistened with 91% isopropyl alcohol or 70% ethyl alcohol			1		
This procedure is described for a right-handed person. **Competency Steps** 1. Following aseptic procedures, select disposable needle and the anesthetic that the dentist has specified for this procedure.			3		
2. Remove the sterile syringe from the autoclave bag. Inspect the syringe to be sure that it is ready for use. Tighten the thumb bar or ring.			2		
3. Hold the syringe in the left hand and use the thumb ring to fully retract the piston rod.			3		

	Self-Evaluation	Student Evaluation	Possible Points	Instructor Evaluation	Comments
4. With the piston rod retracted, place the cartridge in the barrel of the syringe. Once the cartridge is in place, release the piston rod (rubber stopper toward piston).			3		
5. With moderate pressure, push the piston rod into the rubber stopper until it is fully engaged.			3		
6. Remove the protective plastic cap from the syringe end of the needle, and then screw or press the needle onto the syringe hub. The needle must be secure but not too tight. Needle guards are often placed on the protective cap.			3		
7. If the needle is placed before placing the cartridge, take precautions. Name two.			2		
8. Carefully remove the protective cover from the needle. Holding the syringe, expel a few drops to ensure that the syringe is properly working.			3		
9. Replace the cap and place on the tray, ready for use.			2		

TOTAL POINTS POSSIBLE   32

TOTAL POINTS POSSIBLE—2nd attempt   30

TOTAL POINTS EARNED   _____

Points assigned reflect importance of step to meeting objective: Important = 1, Essential = 2, Critical = 3. Students will lose 2 points for repeated attempts. Failure results if any of the critical steps are omitted or performed incorrectly. If using a 100-point scale, determine score by dividing points earned by total points possible and multiplying the results by 100.

SCORE: _____

SKILL COMPETENCY ASSESSMENT

20-2 Assisting with the Administration of Topical and Local Anesthetics

Student's Name _____ Date _____

Instructor's Name _____

Skill: The dental assistant will observe safety precautions at all times during this procedure. The patient is informed of the procedure but not alerted to such words as "pain," "shot," and so on.

Performance Objective: The student will follow a routine procedure that meets the regulations and protocol set forth by the dentist and regulatory agencies, keeping in mind that assistant duties vary from state to state. The dental assistant checks with the dentist for instructions on the type of anesthetic and needle for the procedure. Following those instructions, the assistant will prepare the equipment and material on the procedure tray setup.

   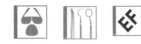

	Self-Evaluation	Student Evaluation	Possible Points	Instructor Evaluation	Comments
Equipment and Supplies					
1. Patient's medical dental history and chart.			2		
2. Basic setup: mouth mirror, explorer, and cotton pliers			2		
3. Air-water syringe tip and evacuator tip (HVE)			2		
4. Cotton rolls, cotton-tip applicator, and 2 × 2 gauze sponges			2		
5. Topical anesthetic			1		
6. Aspirating syringe			2		
7. Anesthetic cartridge			2		
8. Selection of needles			2		
Competency Steps (*follow aseptic procedures*) ***Topical Anesthetic*** 1. After seating the patient, review and update the patient's medical dental history.			2		
2. Explain the procedure and prepare the patient for topical application.			2		

	Self-Evaluation	Student Evaluation	Possible Points	Instructor Evaluation	Comments
3. Follow aseptic procedures; place a small amount of topical anesthetic on the cotton-tip applicator.			1		
4. Dry the oral mucosa with a sterile 2 × 2 gauze sponge. Keep the tissue retracted.			2		
5. Place topical anesthetic on the injection site and leave for designated time.			3		
Local Anesthetic Application 6. While waiting for the topical anesthesia to take effect, assemble the syringe, cartridge, and needle as prescribed by the dentist.			3		
7. When the operator indicates, take the cotton-tip applicator and prepare to pass the syringe.			2		
8. Check the needle bevel so that it is directed toward the alveolar bone, and then loosely replace the protective cap on the needle.			3		
9. Pass the syringe below the patient's chin, placing the thumb ring over the dentist's thumb. Once the dentist grasps the syringe at the finger rest and takes the syringe, remove the protective guard.			3		
10. During the injection, watch the patient for any adverse signs or reaction.			3		
11. The injection is completed and the operator recaps the syringe by sliding the needle into the protective guard. If a second injection is given, remove the cartridge, insert a new one, test the syringe by expelling a few drops, check the bevel, and position the needle for the dentist to retrieve.			2		

	Self-Evaluation	Student Evaluation	Possible Points	Instructor Evaluation	Comments
12. Place the recapped syringe on the tray out of the way but nearby in case more anesthetic is needed.			2		
13. Rinse the patient's mouth with the air-water syringe and evacuate to remove water, saliva, and the taste of anesthetic solution.			2		
Unloading Anesthetic Syringe 1. After the procedure is completed and the patient is dismissed, don utility gloves to clean up, and disassemble the syringe and prepare it for sterilization.			2		
2. Retract the piston to release the harpoon from the cartridge.			2		
3. Remove the cartridge from the syringe.			2		
4. Carefully remove the needle with the protective cap in place. Carefully unscrew the needle (do not unscrew the needle adapter). Discard the needle in the sharps container.			3		
5. Prepare the syringe for sterilization.			2		

TOTAL POINTS POSSIBLE   56

TOTAL POINTS POSSIBLE—2nd attempt   54

TOTAL POINTS EARNED   _____

Points assigned reflect importance of step to meeting objective: Important = 1, Essential = 2, Critical = 3. Students will lose 2 points for repeated attempts. Failure results if any of the critical steps are omitted or performed incorrectly. If using a 100-point scale, determine score by dividing points earned by total points possible and multiplying the results by 100.

SCORE: _____

SKILL COMPETENCY ASSESSMENT

20-3 Administration and Monitoring of Nitrous Oxide Sedation

Student's Name _____ Date _____

Instructor's Name _____

Skill: The dental assistant will observe safety precautions at all times during this procedure. The patient is informed of the procedure and will be able to talk and follow directions during the relaxed state. The assistant monitors the patient as directed.

Performance Objective: The student will follow a routine procedure that meets regulations and protocol set forth by the dentist and regulatory agencies. The dental assistant checks with the dentist for instructions on the type of anesthetic. Check the tubing that is connected to the tank of nitrous oxide and oxygen, check breathing tubes and mask, and check the reservoir bag for leakage. Replace the oxygen and nitrous tanks as directed. Monitor or administer sedation equipment as directed.

	Self-Evaluation	Student Evaluation	Possible Points	Instructor Evaluation	Comments
Equipment and Supplies 1. Nitrous oxide unit with controls and gauge			2		
2. Tanks of nitrous oxide and oxygen			2		
3. Sterile nitrous oxide nosepieces for patient			2		
Competency Steps (*follow aseptic procedures*) ***Preparation*** 1. Check all equipment and verify that it is working properly.			2		
2. Check that gas levels are adequate.			2		
Administration 3. Seat the patient and place in supine position.			1		
4. The dentist or assistant explains to the patient the effects, sensation, and potential hazards of nitrous oxide.			2		
5. The patient gives informed consent and allows for administration to continue.			3		

	Self-Evaluation	Student Evaluation	Possible Points	Instructor Evaluation	Comments
6. Attach a sterile nitrous oxide scavenger mask to the tubing.			2		
7. Place a nosepiece mask over the nose of the patient, ensuring a proper fit with tubing draped to each side.			3		
8. Instruct the patient to breathe slowly through the nose.			3		
9. The dentist or assistant begins the flow of oxygen (5+ liters per minute) and nitrous oxide. (Some offices provide a flow of oxygen for one minute before nitrous oxide is begun.)			3		
10. The dentist or assistant will sit with the patient to monitor any effects as the nitrous oxide is administered. a. Make adjustments for comfort level of sedation. b. Watch for Guedel's signs, Stage 1. Talk with the patient and ask how the patient is feeling.			3 3		
11. The dentist or assistant will watch the patient's chest rise and fall during breathing.			3		
12. The local anesthetic solution is administered within a few minutes of nitrous oxide application. If the patient is comfortable, the procedure can continue.			2		
Recovery 13. When the dental procedure is near completion, turn off the nitrous oxide.			2		
14. The patient will breathe oxygen for a minimum of 5 minutes or until all signs of nitrous oxide sedation have disappeared.			2		
15. Remove nosepiece from the patient's nose.			2		

	Self-Evaluation	Student Evaluation	Possible Points	Instructor Evaluation	Comments
16. Turn off the oxygen at the unit; the flow meter for the nitrous oxide and oxygen will read zero.			3		
17. Seat the patient upright and ask how the patient feels.			2		
18. Ask the patient to stay seated for a minute or two until the head clears.			1		
19. Dismiss the patient when the patient feels all right.			2		
20. Complete all documentation on the patient's chart, including notation about administration of the nitrous oxide.			2		
21. Give the patient the nosepiece to use later or dispose of.			2		
22. Disinfect the tubing.			2		

TOTAL POINTS POSSIBLE   58

TOTAL POINTS POSSIBLE—2nd attempt   56

TOTAL POINTS EARNED   _____

Points assigned reflect importance of step to meeting objective: Important = 1, Essential = 2, Critical = 3. Students will lose 2 points for repeated attempts. Failure results if any of the critical steps are omitted or performed incorrectly. If using a 100-point scale, determine score by dividing points earned by total points possible and multiplying the results by 100.

SCORE: _____

Dental Radiography

CHAPTER 21

Introduction to Dental Radiography and Equipment

SPECIFIC INSTRUCTIONAL OBJECTIVES

The student should strive to meet the following objectives and demonstrate an understanding of the facts and principles presented in this chapter:

1. Explain the history of radiation and the use of the Hittorf-Crookes and Coolidge tubes.

2. List the properties of radiation and explain the biological effects of radiation exposure.

3. Identify the components of a dental x-ray unit and explain the function of each component.

4. Describe the safety precautions when using radiation.

5. Explain how an x-ray is produced.

6. Describe the composition, sizes, types, and storage of dental x-ray film.

SUMMARY

Dental assistants must understand the physics and biological effects of ionization radiation, use their understanding during every radiographic exposure, understand the ALARA principle, and use the lead apron with cervical collar for the patient's safety every time an x-ray is taken. The assistant must label and store patient x-rays properly to prevent loss and thereby avoid the need for x-rays being retaken.

EXERCISES AND ACTIVITIES

Multiple Choice

1. _____ was the professor of physics who discovered x-rays.

   a. Kells

   b. Roentgen

   c. Walkoff

   d. Rollins

2. _____ took the first intraoral radiograph.

   a. Walkoff

   b. Roentgen

   c. Kells

   d. Rollins

3. _____ developed the bisecting technique.

   a. Rober

   b. McCormack

   c. Fitzgerald

   d. Coolidge

4. _____ developed the paralleling technique.

   a. Fitzgerald

   b. Coolidge

   c. Rober

   d. McCormack

5. The open-ended tube, commonly known as the cone, is called the

   a. position indicator device (PID).

   b. maximum permissible dose (MPD).

   c. radiation absorbed dose (rad).

   d. roentgen equivalent man (rem).

6. In addition to x-rays, other forms of electromagnetic energy include

   a. radio waves.

   b. television waves.

   c. visible light.

   d. All of the above.

7. _____ is the process by which atoms change into negatively or positively charged ions during radiation.

   a. Impulse

   b. Milliamperage

   c. Kilovoltage

   d. Ionization

8. Which of the following is *not* a characteristic of short, hard wavelengths?

   a. High frequency

   b. Low energy

   c. High penetrating power

   d. All of the above

9. _____ radiation is the central beam that comes from the x-ray tubehead.

   a. Leakage

   b. Primary

   c. Scatter

   d. Secondary

10. _____ radiation forms when the primary x-ray strikes or contacts any type of matter (solid, liquid, or gas).

    a. Leakage

    b. Primary

    c. Scatter

    d. Secondary

11. _____ radiation deflects from its path as it strikes matter.

    a. Leakage

    b. Primary

    c. Scatter

    d. Secondary

12. _____ radiation is a form of radiation that escapes in all directions from the tube or tubehead.

    a. Leakage

    b. Primary

    c. Scatter

    d. Secondary

13. A_____ equals the amount of radiation that will ionize one cubic centimeter of air.

    a. rad

    b. roentgen

    c. rem

    d. GY

14. The _____ is an abbreviation for the radiation dose to which body tissues are exposed, which is measured in terms of its estimated biological effects.

    a. Sv

    b. R

    c. GY

    d. mr

15. The period between the radiation exposure and the development of biological effects is called the _____ period.

    a. radiosensitive

    b. sievert

    c. latent

    d. RBE

16. Circuit boards and controls are located in the _____ of the dental x-ray unit.

    a. milliamperage

    b. kilovoltage

    c. electronic timer

    d. control panel

17. The most common setting(s) for the kilovoltage is (are)

    a. 30.

    b. 70 to 90.

    c. 10 to 15.

    d. 30 to 59.

18. The most common settings for the milliamperage are

    a. 10 to 15.

    b. 30 to 50.

    c. 70 to 90.

    d. 20 to 40.

19. During the _____ process, current passes through the cathode filament and heats it to an extremely high temperature.

    a. bisecting technique

    b. thermionic emission

    c. blurred image

    d. cross-section technique

20. Electromagnetic radiation with short wavelengths with high frequency equals _____ energy.

    a. less

    b. more

    c. magnetic

    d. kinetic

21. D-speed film is called

    a. Ektaspeed.

    b. Ultraspeed.

    c. low speed.

    d. hyper speed.

22. Recommendations by the International Commission on Radiological Protection recommend the following occupational exposure dose limits:

    a. 50 rems

    b. 2 rems

    c. 10 mA

    d. 7 mA

23. The orthopantomograph unit took the first acceptable _____ radiographs.

    a. PID

    b. intraoral

    c. panoramic

    d. Both a. and b.

24. The _____ group of cells can be affected by radiation.

    a. somatic

    b. genetic

    c. Both a. and b.

    d. None of the above

25. _____ cells, which divide rapidly, are radiosensitive cells.

    a. Anode

    b. Basal

    c. Cathode

    d. Thermionic

26. Some cells are more radiosensitive than others. Identify the most radiosensitive tissues and organs.

    1. Salivary glands

    2. Lymphoid

    3. Kidney

    4. Reproductive cells

    5. Intestinal epithelium

    6. Muscle

    7. Bone marrow

    8. Nerves

        a. 1, 3, 6, 8

        b. 1, 2, 3, 5

        c. 2, 4, 6, 8

        d. 2, 4, 5, 7

27. Using InSight film instead of D-type film reduces the time that the patient is exposed to radiation by up to _____ %.

    a. 20

    b. 50

    c. 60

    d. 10

28. _____ film is the highest-speed dental film and allows for the greatest reduction in radiation exposure for the patient.

    a. D-speed, Ultraspeed

    b. F-speed, InSight

    c. A-speed

    d. G-speed

29. _____ is the degree of darkness on an x-ray.

    a. Density

    b. Contrast

    c. Obscureness

    d. Opacity

30. What characteristic of a wavelength categorizes its electromagnetic energy?

    a. Frequency

    b. Peak

    c. Length

    d. Ionization

Matching

Match each type of radiation with the best definition.

Type

1. _____ Primary

2. _____ Secondary

3. _____ Scatter

4. _____ Leakage

Definition

a. Escapes in all directions

b. Formed when primary x-ray strikes the patient or contacts matter

c. Central beam that comes from the x-ray tubehead

d. Deflected from its path as it strikes matter

Match each x-ray tube component with its respective function.

Component	Function
5. _____ Cathode	a. Directs the flow of x-rays; made of a tungsten target
6. _____ Anode	b. Solid metal; made of aluminum
7. _____ Filter	c. Lead plate
8. _____ Central beam	d. Negative side where electrons will originate
9. _____ Collimator	e. Hard x-rays with short wavelengths

Dental intraoral film packets range in size according to radiographic exposures. Match each film size with its respective use.

Film Size	Use
10. _____ No. 0	a. Long bite-wing film
11. _____ No. 1	b. Adult
12. _____ No. 2	c. Occlusal film
13. _____ No. 3	d. Narrow anterior film
14. _____ No. 4	e. Child

 Critical Thinking

1. Knowing the composition of the intraoral film packet is necessary in order to identify its contents during film exposure and processing. Name the film packet contents.

2. The dental assistant has the responsibility to know and understand intraoral dental x-ray film types. The dentist may use one of three choices based on film speed and exposure benefits. Name the three choices normally found in the dental office, their speed differentials, and which involves the least radiation exposure for the patient.

3. Assume that a patient is to have an 18 film series (full mouth). Two methods of exposure include using a long, round PID or using a rectangular PID. Explain both methods, and identify which benefits the patient the most in terms of reduced radiation exposure.

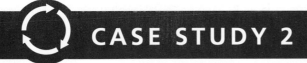

CASE STUDY 1

In the course of the day, the dental assistant has exposed films on adults and children and for special requests. Each of these assignments required choosing a particular film type.

1. A full mouth series was required for an adult. What intraoral film size would typically be used?

2. In this adult case, there is severe crowding in the anterior. What size film might be necessary?

3. The dental hygienist has requested an adult set of bite-wings but wants only two films. The area to be covered by a No. 2 film would not be adequate. What size would be used?

4. The child patient is being checked for progress in the mixed dentition. The dentist has ordered one film of the upper and lower. The film should cover canine to canine. What film type and number would be required?

CASE STUDY 2

Sue, an adult patient, has complained of a toothache. The dentist prescribes a periapical of tooth #3. When the dental assistant takes the intraoral film, it will be a periapical exposure of a maxillary first molar.

1. Explain what happens when the control panel is turned on.

2. Name the measurement unit for electrical current on the control panel. What is the relationship between amount of electrical current and radiation?

3. Define and describe kilovoltage.

4. Describe the electronic timer on a dental x-ray unit.

5. List any variation between child and adult mAs.

CASE STUDY 3

Holly is being examined to determine the diagnosis for recurrent caries. The doctor prescribes x-rays. Holly expresses her concerns about radiation and its effects. The dentist and the dental assistant understand that Holly needs assurance about the effects of dental x-rays compared to other radiation sources.

1. Define ALARA.

2. List means of protecting patients who are pregnant from radiation.

3. List tissues that are radiosensitive in the dental region.

4. Define MPD.

5. Name two major categories of exposure to daily radiation.

6. Explain the latent period and "long-term effects."

CHAPTER 22

Production and Evaluation of Dental Radiographs

SPECIFIC INSTRUCTIONAL OBJECTIVES

The student should strive to meet the following objectives and demonstrate an understanding of the facts and principles presented in this chapter:

1. Describe a diagnostic-quality x-ray.

2. Identify the means of producing quality radiographs.

3. List the types of film exposures.

4. Explain the bisecting principle and technique.

5. Explain the paralleling principle and techniques including a full-mouth radiographic survey and bite-wing series.

6. Describe special radiographs on various patients, including occlusal, pediatric, edentulous, and endodontic radiographs, and special needs/compromised patients.

7. Describe manual film-processing equipment and technique.

8. List and explain the composition of processing solutions.

9. Describe automatic processing equipment and explain the technique.

10. Explain and demonstrate how to mount dental x-rays.

11. List common radiographic errors that occur during exposure and processing of x-ray films.

12. Explain how to duplicate dental radiographs.

13. Describe the storage of final radiographs and legal implications concerning dental radiographs.

14. List standardized procedures and state policies that dental offices follow to ensure quality radiographs.

SUMMARY

The dentist uses both intraoral films placed in the patient's mouth for exposure, and extraoral films placed outside the patient's mouth to produce quality radiographs used in diagnosing dental conditions. Simply, a quality radiograph facilitates accurate diagnosis.

The two techniques used to expose radiographs are bisecting and paralleling. Both techniques are described in this chapter, but the paralleling technique and equipment required for this technique are demonstrated in each area of the mouth for adults and children.

Once the radiographs have been exposed, they must be processed. Manual and automatic processing equipment and techniques are described and compared. Chemical components of the developing and fixing solutions are listed, and the role they play in converting the latent image into a visible permanent radiograph is discussed.

Radiographs are then mounted for viewing. There are various types of dental x-ray mounts to choose from, and helpful hints to determine the order the x-rays are mounted, especially when learning, are addressed.

Common radiographic errors during processing and exposing x-rays are listed and examples provided. Careful attention to positioning during x-ray exposure and detailed step-by-step procedures for processing can assist in the elimination of errors.

Patient radiographs are needed for many reasons. For instance, insurance companies require copies of the patient's x-rays to determine insurance coverage, and other dental offices require a copy of the patient's x-rays for their own diagnoses. Radiographs can be duplicated so that the original radiographs never have to leave the office. The special film and equipment needed for this process are discussed. Dental offices are required to properly store final radiographs to prevent losses, and thereby avoid the need for x-rays to be retaken.

EXERCISES AND ACTIVITIES

Multiple Choice

1. Which intraoral technique for film exposures does the American Association of Dental Schools and the American Academy of Oral and Maxillofacial Radiology recommend?

    a. Paralleling

    b. Bisecting

    c. Horizontal

    d. Occlusal

2. The _____ radiograph pictures the entire tooth and surrounding area.

    a. bite-wing

    b. occlusal

    c. periapical

    d. edentulous

3. The _____ radiograph pictures the crown, the interproximal spaces, and the crest area of the alveolar bone of both the maxillary and the mandibular teeth.

    a. bite-wing

    b. occlusal

    c. periapical

    d. edentulous

4. A clear film would indicate _____ exposure.

    a. double

    b. no

    c. under

    d. over

5. When the image on the film is light and a herringbone/tire track pattern is visible, this operator error was the result of

    a. the film being placed backward in the mouth.

    b. double exposures.

    c. underexposed film.

    d. overexposed film.

6. With the _____ technique for exposing occlusal radiographs, the central ray is directed perpendicular to the bisecting plane.

   a. cross-section
   b. topographic
   c. Both a. and b.
   d. None of the above

7. Which vertical angulation error is caused by too little angulation?

   a. Elongation
   b. Foreshortening
   c. Both a. and b.
   d. None of the above

8. _____ occurs when the cone is angled toward the mesial or the distal surfaces instead of the interproximal area.

   a. Cone cutting
   b. Overlapping
   c. Foreshortening
   d. Elongation

9. Given that most of these processors are compact and some have daylight loader units, which processing method reduces processing time?

   a. Automatic
   b. Manual
   c. Both a. and b.
   d. None of the above

10. Which processing solution chemically reduces the exposed area of the emulsion, making images visible to the naked eye?

    a. Developer
    b. Fixer
    c. Both a. and b.
    d. None of the above

11. Which processing solution removes the unexposed and undeveloped crystals from the film emulsion?

    a. Developer
    b. Fixer
    c. Water
    d. None of the above

12. The paralleling technique is the most commonly used because it

    a. is accurate.
    b. produces excellent diagnostic-quality radiographs.
    c. results in less exposure to patient's head and neck.
    d. All of the above

13. In an endodontic procedure, the _____ technique is preferred because it reduces distortion.

    a. bisecting
    b. paralleling
    c. bite-wing
    d. occlusal

14. Which of the following areas should be covered on an endodontic film?

    a. Cover entire length of the tooth
    b. Cover surrounding area at apex
    c. Central ray to be perpendicular to the tooth
    d. All of the above

15. The paralleling technique is uncomfortable for some adults and small children if the patient has a

    a. small mouth.
    b. sensitive mouth.
    c. low palatal vault.
    d. All of the above

16. Which of the following actions may help prevent gagging for those patients who have a sensitive gag reflex?

    a. Try to persuade the patient to breathe through the nose.
    b. Try to get the patient to think of something else.
    c. Work quickly while talking to the patient.
    d. All of the above

17. The process in which solutions combine with oxygen is called

    a. oxidation.

    b. duplication.

    c. reticulation.

    d. trituration.

18. Name the chemical that shrinks and hardens the emulsion gelatin.

    a. Sodium sulfite

    b. Acetic acid

    c. Potassium alum

    d. Potassium bromide

19. What is an image called that is found on a developed x-ray film but is not a part of the normal anatomy and pathology?

    a. Artifact

    b. Fogged

    c. Reticulation

    d. Distortion

20. What method can be used to evaluate the dark room for light leaks?

    a. Taking multiple exposures of a step wedge

    b. A coin test

    c. A spin top test

    d. Exposure of a dosimeter

Matching

The direction of the central rays creates vertical angulation, which will work with most patients. Match the area with the vertical angulation.

Area

1. _____ Incisor/lateral

2. _____ Cuspids

3. _____ Bicuspids (premolars)

4. _____ Molars

Angulation

a. Maxillary +45, mandibular –20

b. Maxillary +20, mandibular –5

c. Maxillary +40, mandibular –15

d. Maxillary +30, mandibular –10

LABELING

Identify the following radiographs as bite-wing, occlusal, or periapical.

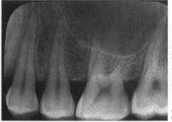

A

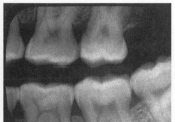

B

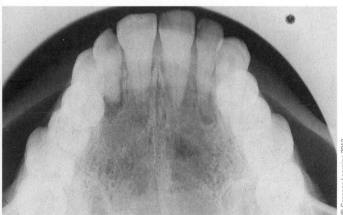

C

A._____

B._____

C._____

Label the arches on the cross-section occlusal radiographs.

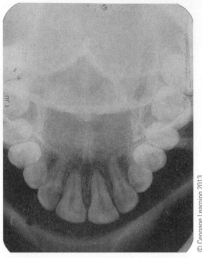

D

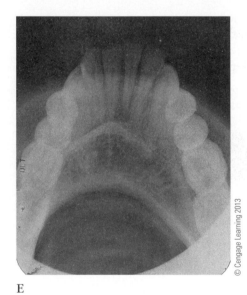

E

D._____

E._____

Critical Thinking

1. Taking radiographs is part of a routine dental exam. How frequently are bite-wing x-rays taken? What specific features are detected in these x-rays?

2. There are two methods used to mount a full series of x-rays. State the name of each method and explain the difference between the two.

3. Correct positioning is necessary for quality films. When using the paralleling technique, film positioning is done by first placing the film correctly in the holder and then rechecking the film once it is in the patient's mouth. Explain the proper positioning of the film in the holder.

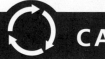 **CASE STUDY 1**

During Vernon's 12-month dental exam, the dentist prescribes routine bite-wings. Taken correctly, bite-wing x-rays can be used for diagnosing various teeth and structure conditions.

1. Enumerate what bite-wing radiographs picture.

2. Bite-wing radiographs are also known as _____.

3. Where are bite-wings taken?

4. A bite-wing will cover the _____.

5. Bite-wings are used for detecting/examining _____.

6. Describe the differences between horizontal and vertical positioning.

CASE STUDY 2

At 7-year-old Scott's routine dental exam, the dentist observed new decay and loose teeth. The dentist prescribes a full-mouth series of radiographs to help in determining Scott's present dental health.

1. What will a full-mouth series detect?

2. Will the number of films taken for Scott be the same as for an adult?

3. Is radiation exposure time the same for children and adults?

4. What observations of a child's mouth should be made before placing the films?

CASE STUDY 3

Dental assistant Ella has taken her first full-mouth series of radiographs. The films are dry and she begins to mount them.

1. What equipment and supplies are required for mounting radiographs?

2. What information is necessary for labeling the mount, and will it be entered in pen or in pencil?

3. What direction should the dot on the film face? What is this called?

4. What mounting technique is used in most dental offices and is recommended by the ADA?

5. In mounting a full-mouth set of radiographs, dividing them into three groups is recommended. Name the three groups.

6. After all radiographs are mounted, performing a quick check is advisable. Name the observations made during this quick check.

SKILL COMPETENCY ASSESSMENT

22-1 Radiography Infection Control

Student's Name _____ Date _____

Instructor's Name _____

Skill: Routine steps should be followed for all treatment areas to maintain absolute clinical asepsis. The patient is informed about the procedure.

Performance Objective: The student will follow a routine procedure that meets the regulations and protocol set forth by the dentist and regulatory agencies, keeping in mind that assistant duties vary from state to state. The dental assistant checks with the dentist for instructions on the type of radiographs needed for diagnosis, prepares the patient and area, takes the radiographs, and processes and mounts the films for viewing according to infection control protocol.

	Self-Evaluation	Student Evaluation	Possible Points	Instructor Evaluation	Comments
Equipment and Supplies					
1. Barriers for the x-ray room			2		
2. X-ray film of proper size			2		
3. Rinn XCP materials (assembled for use) or other paralleling technique aids			2		
4. Film barriers (optional)			1		
5. Lead apron with thyroid collar			3		
6. Container for exposed film			2		
Competency Steps (follow aseptic procedures)					
1. Wash and dry hands.			2		
2. Place appropriate barriers on the dental chair, film, and x-ray equipment.			2		
3. Prepare the equipment and supplies needed for the procedure: sterile Rinn XCP instruments, tissue or a paper towel, and cup or container with patient's name.			3		

	Self-Evaluation	Student Evaluation	Possible Points	Instructor Evaluation	Comments
4. After the patient is seated and positioned (lead apron), glasses and a mask may be worn. Wash and dry hands. Don treatment gloves.			3		
5. After x-rays are exposed and removed from the patient's mouth, wipe them off and place them in a cup/container or on a covered surface.			3		
6. When all x-ray exposures are complete, remove the lead apron from the patient, following aseptic protocol (methods include removing with contaminated gloves on and disinfecting apron, or removing contaminated gloves and placing on overgloves and removing apron).			2		
7. After the patient is dismissed, remove and dispose of all barriers.			2		
8. Any areas that were not covered with a barrier must be disinfected, including the x-ray film.			3		

TOTAL POINTS POSSIBLE   32

TOTAL POINTS POSSIBLE—2nd attempt   30

TOTAL POINTS EARNED   _____

Points assigned reflect importance of step to meeting objective: Important = 1, Essential = 2, Critical = 3. Students will lose 2 points for repeated attempts. Failure results if any of the critical steps are omitted or performed incorrectly. If using a 100-point scale, determine score by dividing points earned by total points possible and multiplying the results by 100.

SCORE: _____

SKILL COMPETENCY ASSESSMENT

22-2 Full-Mouth X-Ray Exposure with Paralleling Technique

Student's Name _____ Date _____

Instructor's Name _____

Skill: Routine steps should be followed for all treatment areas to maintain absolute clinical asepsis. The patient is informed about the procedure, which will include film placement and exposure for the central incisors in each arch and one-half of the maxillary arch and one-half of the mandibular arch. The same technique would be used to expose the opposite arches.

Performance Objective: The dental assistant will follow a routine procedure that meets the regulations and protocol set forth by the dentist and regulatory agencies, keeping in mind that assistant duties vary from state to state. The dental assistant checks with the dentist for the request that a full-mouth set of radiographs be taken; prepares the equipment (Rinn XCP instruments), area, and patient; takes the radiographs; and processes and mounts the films for viewing according to infection control protocol.

	Self-Evaluation	Student Evaluation	Possible Points	Instructor Evaluation	Comments
Equipment and Supplies					
1. Barriers for the x-ray room and equipment			2		
2. X-ray film (appropriate size and number of films)			2		
3. X-ray film barriers (optional)			1		
4. Cotton rolls (optional)			1		
5. Rinn XCP materials (assembled for use) or other paralleling technique aids			2		
6. Lead apron with thyroid collar			3		
7. Container for exposed film			2		
8. Paper towel or tissue			1		
Competency Steps **(follow aseptic procedures)** 1. Review the patient's chart.			3		
2. Wash and dry hands.			2		
3. Place appropriate barriers on the dental chair, film, and x-ray equipment.			2		

	Self-Evaluation	Student Evaluation	Possible Points	Instructor Evaluation	Comments
4. Prepare the equipment and supplies needed for the procedure, including sterile Rinn XCP instruments, tissue or paper towel, and a cup or container with the patient's name.			3		
5. Turn the x-ray machine on and check mA, kV, and exposure time.			3		
6. Seat and position the patient upright.			2		
7. Have the patient remove any facial jewelry, earrings, eyeglasses, and detachable appliances that may interfere with the exposing process.			2		
8. Place a lead apron with a thyroid collar on the patient.			3		
9. After the patient is prepared, wash and dry hands and don latex treatment gloves.			3		

TOTAL POINTS POSSIBLE   37

TOTAL POINTS POSSIBLE—2nd attempt   35

TOTAL POINTS EARNED   _____

Points assigned reflect importance of step to meeting objective: Important = 1, Essential = 2, Critical = 3-Students will lose 2 points for repeated attempts. Failure results if any of the critical steps are omitted or performed incorrectly. If using a 100-point scale, determine score by dividing points earned by total points possible and multiplying the results by 100.

SCORE: _____

SKILL COMPETENCY ASSESSMENT

22-3 Exposing Occlusal Radiographs

Student's Name _____ Date _____

Instructor's Name _____

Skill: Routine steps should be followed for all treatment areas to maintain absolute clinical asepsis. The patient is informed about the procedure. This procedure will include technique selection determined by the view that the dentist needs for diagnosis (topographic or cross-sectional).

Performance Objective: The dental assistant will follow a routine procedure that meets the regulations and protocol set forth by the dentist and regulatory agencies, keeping in mind that assistant duties vary from state to state. The dental assistant checks with the dentist for the request of technique selection to be taken; prepares the equipment and supplies, area, and patient; takes the radiographs; and processes and mounts the films for viewing according to infection control protocol.

	Self-Evaluation	Student Evaluation	Possible Points	Instructor Evaluation	Comments
Equipment and Supplies					
1. Barriers for the x-ray room			2		
2. Occlusal film (2 for children and 4 for adults)			2		
3. Lead apron with thyroid collar			3		
4. Container or barrier for exposed film			2		
Competency Steps **(follow aseptic procedures)** 1. Wash and dry hands.			2		
2. Place appropriate barriers.			2		
3. Prepare the film, tissue or paper towel, and cup or container with the patient's identification.			2		
4. Seat the patient upright and place the lead apron on the patient.			3		
5. Wash and dry hands and don treatment gloves.			2		

	Self-Evaluation	Student Evaluation	Possible Points	Instructor Evaluation	Comments
Topographic Technique					
6. For a maxillary view, position the patient so that the maxillary arch is parallel to the floor. Positioning is similar to that used for the bisecting technique.			3		
7. Place film in the mouth with the smooth/plain side toward the cone.			3		
8. Have the patient close on the film, leaving about a 2-mm edge beyond the incisors.			2		
9. Move the cone to a vertical angulation of +65 degrees to +75 degrees.			2		
10. Direct the cone over the bridge of the nose, with the lower edge of the cone covering the incisors.			2		
11. For a mandibular view using the topographic technique, tilt the patient's head backward.			2		
12. Place the smooth side of the film on the occlusal surfaces of the teeth with the central incisors at the front edge of the film.			2		
13. Have the patient close gently on the film.			1		
14. Vertical angulation will vary with each patient from −45 degrees to −55 degrees.			1		
15. Center the cone over the film, directing the central ray at the middle and tip of the chin.			2		
Cross-Section Technique					
1. **For a maxillary view** using this technique, the patient should be upright, with the head tilted slightly backward.			2		
2. Film placement is the same as that for topographic technique. The cone is positioned over the top of the patient's head with the central ray directed perpendicular to the film.			2		

	Self-Evaluation	Student Evaluation	Possible Points	Instructor Evaluation	Comments
3. Be sure that the cone covers the maxillary area to be exposed.			2		
4. **For a mandibular view,** the patient's head should be tilted backward.			2		
5. Film placement is the same as with the topographic technique.			2		
6. The cone is positioned under the patient's chin with the central ray directed perpendicular to the film. The patient may have to lift the chin to position the cone.			2		

TOTAL POINTS POSSIBLE   52

TOTAL POINTS POSSIBLE—2nd attempt   50

TOTAL POINTS EARNED   _____

Points assigned reflect importance of step to meeting objective: Important = 1, Essential = 2, Critical = 3. Students will lose 2 points for repeated attempts. Failure results if any of the critical steps are omitted or performed incorrectly. If using a 100-point scale, determine score by dividing points earned by total points possible and multiplying the results by 100.

SCORE: _____

SKILL COMPETENCY ASSESSMENT

22-4 Full-Mouth Pediatric X-Ray Exposure

Student's Name _____ Date _____

Instructor's Name _____

Skill: Routine steps should be followed for all treatment areas to maintain absolute clinical asepsis. The patient is informed of the procedure. This procedure includes technique selection that is determined by the dentist's needs for diagnosis. Evaluate the child's cooperation and behavior. Work quickly and confidently.

Performance Objective: The dental assistant will follow a routine procedure that meets the regulations and protocol set forth by the dentist and regulatory agencies. The dental assistant checks with the dentist for the request of a full-mouth set of radiographs to be taken and identifies the eight films; prepares the equipment (Rinn XCP instruments), area, and patient; takes the radiographs; and processes and mounts the films for viewing according to infection control protocol.

	Self-Evaluation	Student Evaluation	Possible Points	Instructor Evaluation	Comments
Equipment and Supplies					
1. Barriers for the x-ray room and equipment			2		
2. X-ray film, six size 0 films and two size 2 films			2		
3. X-ray film barriers (optional)			1		
4. Cotton rolls (optional)			1		
5. Rinn XCP materials (assembled for use) or other paralleling technique aids			2		
6. Lead apron with thyroid collar			3		
7. Container or barrier for exposed film			2		
8. Paper towel or tissue			1		
Competency Steps (follow aseptic procedures)					
1. Review the patient's chart.			3		
2. Wash and dry hands.			2		
3. Place appropriate barriers on dental chair, film, and x-ray equipment.			2		

	Self-Evaluation	Student Evaluation	Possible Points	Instructor Evaluation	Comments
4. For children, prepare film 2.			2		
5. Assemble sterile Rinn XCP instruments, and prepare tissue or paper towel and a cup or container with patient's name.			2		
6. Turn on the x-ray machine and check mA, kV, and exposure time.			3		
7. Seat and position the patient upright.			2		
8. Place a lead apron with a thyroid collar on the patient.			3		
9. After the patient is prepared, wash and dry hands and don latex treatment gloves.			2		
10. Tell the patient about the procedure.			2		
Exposing Occlusal Radiographs Maxillary Occlusal Film/Topographic Technique 1. **For a maxillary view,** position the patient so that the maxillary arch is parallel to the floor. Positioning is similar to that used for the bisecting technique.			3		
2. Place film in the mouth with the smooth/plain side toward the cone.			3		
3. Have the patient close on the film, leaving about a 2-mm edge beyond the incisors.			2		
4. Move the cone to a vertical angulation of +65 to +75 degrees.			2		
5. Direct the cone over the bridge of the nose, with the lower edge of the cone covering the incisors.			2		

	Self-Evaluation	Student Evaluation	Possible Points	Instructor Evaluation	Comments
Mandibular Occlusal X-Ray/Topographic Technique					
1. For a mandibular view, using the topographic technique, tilt the patient's head backward until the mandibular arch is parallel to the floor.			.2		
2. Place the smooth side of the film on the occlusal surfaces of the teeth, with central incisors at the front edge of the film.			2		
3. Have the patient close gently on the film.			1		
4. Vertical angulation will vary with each patient from −40 degrees to −55 degrees.			1		
5. Center the cone over the film, directing the central ray at the middle and tip of the chin.			2		
Deciduous Bite-Wings Technique					
1. Position the tab or positioning ring on the film.			2		
2. Center the film with the smooth side of the film toward the ring or tab.			2		
3. Position the film, covering the deciduous first and second molars with the front edge of the film to the middle of the cuspid.			3		
4. Holding the tab, place the film near the lingual surface of the teeth in the patient's mouth, positioning the film to cover the mandibular deciduous molars.			3		
5. While holding the tab in place, have the patient close and slowly rotate the fingers out of the way.			2		

	Self-Evaluation	Student Evaluation	Possible Points	Instructor Evaluation	Comments
6. When using a positioning instrument, place the bite-wing holder into the patient's mouth, away from the lingual surface of the teeth. The film should cover the deciduous molars and be parallel to them. Have the patient close slowly on the bite-wing holder and hold it in place.			3		
7. Begin cone positioning for premolar bite-wings with vertical angulation set at 0.			3		
Positioning for Maxillary Deciduous Molars 1. For the maxillary deciduous molars, tilt the film/film holder, place it in the patient's mouth, and position it away from the lingual surfaces toward the middle of the palate.			3		
2. Place the anterior edge of the film behind the middle of the cuspid to cover the area of the two molars.			3		
3. Holding the film in place, have the patient close slowly on the bite-block. Holding the metal rod, slide the positioning ring toward the patient's face.			2		
4. Bringing the tube head toward the ring, place open cone evenly around ring. Note the angle of the film/film holder, positioned so the central ray will pass through the contact point of the first and second deciduous molars.			2		
5. Center the bite-block on the deciduous molars. The distal of the cuspid is seen and the first and second deciduous molars have the contact between them open.			2		

	Self-Evaluation	Student Evaluation	Possible Points	Instructor Evaluation	Comments
Positioning for the Mandibular Deciduous Molars 1. Tilt the mandibular deciduous molars film/film holder, place in the patient's mouth, gently positioning between the lingual surfaces of the teeth and tongue.			2		
2. The anterior edge of the film will be at the middle of the cuspid to ensure the film will cover the area of the two deciduous molars.			2		
3. Have the patient close on the bite-block.			2		
4. Place the film in the space between the tongue and the mandibular arch.			2		
5. The film, teeth, and plane of the open end of the cone are all parallel. The first and second deciduous molars are seen on the film with the contact point open.			2		

TOTAL POINTS POSSIBLE   97

TOTAL POINTS POSSIBLE—2nd attempt   95

TOTAL POINTS EARNED   _____

Points assigned reflect importance of step to meeting objective: Important = 1, Essential = 2, Critical = 3. Students will lose 2 points for repeated attempts. Failure results if any of the critical steps are omitted or performed incorrectly. If using a 100-point scale, determine score by dividing points earned by total points possible and multiplying the results by 100.

SCORE: _____

SKILL COMPETENCY ASSESSMENT

22-5 Processing Radiographs Using a Manual Tank

Student's Name _____ Date _____

Instructor's Name _____

Skill: Routine steps should be followed for all treatment areas to maintain absolute clinical asepsis. The dental assistant prepares the equipment, supplies, and area, and takes the exposed radiographs to the darkroom to process. The processing area is to be well ventilated and to exclude all white light.

Performance Objective: The dental assistant will follow a routine procedure that meets the regulations and protocol set forth by the dentist and regulatory agencies, keeping in mind that assistant duties vary from state to state. The dental assistant will process (develop, fix, and wash) the dental x-rays according to infection control protocol.

	Self-Evaluation	Student Evaluation	Possible Points	Instructor Evaluation	Comments
Equipment and Supplies					
1. Barriers for darkroom counter			2		
2. Exposed radiographs			2		
3. X-ray rack			1		
4. Processing tank			1		
5. Safety light			1		
6. Timer			1		
7. Thermometer			1		
8. Pencil			1		
9. Electric film dryer			1		
Competency Steps (follow aseptic procedures)					
1. Wash and dry hands (gloves must be worn if x-rays are contaminated).			2		
2. Place barriers on a clean surface in the darkroom.			2		
3. With a thermometer, check the temperature of the developer (check the processing chart for the corresponding temperature and time).			2		

	Self-Evaluation	Student Evaluation	Possible Points	Instructor Evaluation	Comments
4. Check the quantity of processing solutions and replenish if necessary.			2		
5. If performing the first processing of the morning or afternoon, stir the developer and fixer. Stir with corresponding rods to match solutions—do not interchange.			3		
6. Check that x-ray rack clips are working.			2		
7. Label the x-ray rack in pencil with the patient's name, date of exposure, and number of x-rays taken.			3		
8. Turn on safety lights; turn off white lights.			3		
9. Remove films from wrappers and place on x-ray racks. Maintain absolute asepsis.			2		
10. Check each film to ensure it is attached securely and placed parallel to adjacent film and not touching it.			2		
11. Place in the developer tank, agitating the rack to eliminate bubbles on the emulsion surface.			2		
12. Place the tank cover on the processing tank. If the temperature is at 70°F in the developer, set the timer for 4 minutes. Clean the area and dispose of barriers and wrappers.			2		
13. When the timer goes off, remove the x-ray rack from the developer, letting the excess solution drip into the developer before placing the rack in running water. Let it rinse for 30 seconds.			2		

	Self-Evaluation	Student Evaluation	Possible Points	Instructor Evaluation	Comments
14. Remove the x-ray rack from rinsing, letting excess water drip off, and then immerse the rack in the fixing solution for 8 minutes (a quick fix for the dentist can be 3 minutes, and then return the film for the remaining time).			3		
15. Replace the processing lid and set the timer for 8 minutes.			3		
16. When 8 minutes have lapsed, remove the x-ray rack of films from the fixer, and place in running water. The final wash takes 20 minutes.			2		
17. After 20 minutes, remove the rack of x-rays from the water and place in an x-ray dryer for an additional 15 to 20 minutes or until drying is complete.			2		
18. When x-rays are dry, remove from the rack and place in a labeled x-ray mount.			2		
TOTAL POINTS POSSIBLE			52		
TOTAL POINTS POSSIBLE—2nd attempt			50		
TOTAL POINTS EARNED			_____		

Points assigned reflect importance of step to meeting objective: Important = 1, Essential = 2, Critical = 3. Students will lose 2 points for repeated attempts. Failure results if any of the critical steps are omitted or performed incorrectly. If using a 100-point scale, determine score by dividing points earned by total points possible and multiplying the results by 100.

SCORE: _____

SKILL COMPETENCY ASSESSMENT

22-6 Processing Radiographs Using an Automatic Processor

Student's Name _____ Date _____

Instructor's Name _____

Skill: Routine steps should be followed for all treatment areas to maintain absolute clinical asepsis. The dental assistant prepares the equipment, supplies, and area, and takes the exposed radiographs to the automatic processor to process.

Performance Objective: The dental assistant will follow a routine procedure that meets the regulations and protocol set forth by the dentist and regulatory agencies, keeping in mind that assistant duties vary from state to state. The dental assistant will process (develop, fix, wash, and dry) the dental x-rays according to infection control protocol.

	Self-Evaluation	Student Evaluation	Possible Points	Instructor Evaluation	Comments
Equipment and Supplies 1. Exposed radiographs			2		
2. Automatic x-ray processor with day loader			2		
Competency Steps *(follow aseptic procedures)* 1. Turn on the automatic x-ray processor at the beginning of each day.			2		
2. Wash and dry hands.			2		
3. Place exposed radiographs in the daylight loader with two additional containers/cups.			2		
4. Don gloves and position gloved hands through the sleeves of the loader.			2		
5. Remove each radiograph from its packet, placing the film in an uncontaminated container. Do not touch (contaminate) film while removing the packet.			3		
6. Place empty packets in the other container.			2		

	Self-Evaluation	Student Evaluation	Possible Points	Instructor Evaluation	Comments
7. After all x-rays are unwrapped, remove gloves and place them in the contaminated container with the empty packets.			2		
8. With clean hands, feed the un-wrapped films into machine slowly. Start on one side of the processor and rotate to the other. Repeat. If using a film holder, place all films in a holder and re-lease for processing. Continue until all films are processed. Maintain absolute asepsis.			3		
9. Remove processed films from the outlet area and place in a labeled x-ray mount.			2		

TOTAL POINTS POSSIBLE   24

TOTAL POINTS POSSIBLE—2nd attempt   22

TOTAL POINTS EARNED   _____

Points assigned reflect importance of step to meeting objective: Important = 1, Essential = 2, Critical = 3.Students will lose 2 points for repeated attempts. Failure results if any of the critical steps are omitted or performed incorrectly. If using a 100-point scale, determine score by dividing points earned by total points possible and multiplying the results by 100.

SCORE: _____

SKILL COMPETENCY ASSESSMENT

22-7 Mounting Radiographs

Student's Name _____ Date _____

Instructor's Name _____

Skill: The dental assistant prepares the equipment, supplies, and area. It may take several practice sessions, but soon the operator will be able to quickly identify any incorrectly mounted x-rays and place them correctly.

Performance Objective: This procedure is performed by the dental assistant. A viewbox may or may not be used when mounting the radiographs. The American Dental Association recommends that dental offices use labial mounting.

	Self-Evaluation	Student Evaluation	Possible Points	Instructor Evaluation	Comments
Equipment and Supplies					
1. Radiographs			3		
2. Lighted viewbox			2		
3. X-ray mount (full, 18 x-ray mount)			2		
4. Clean, dry surface			2		
Competency Steps *(follow aseptic procedures)*					
1. Wash and dry hands.			1		
2. Label the x-ray mount with the patient's name and the date of exposure (in pencil).			3		
3. Turn on the light in the x-ray viewbox (optional).			1		
4. Place radiographs on a clean surface, all dots outward (convex) to view.			3		
5. Categorize all x-rays into three groups: bite-wings (four in number), anteriors (six in number), and posteriors (eight in number).			2		
6. Place the bite-wing x-rays in the mount, dots convex, molars toward the outside, bicuspids toward the inside, x-rays mounted according to the curve of the Spee.			2		

	Self-Evaluation	Student Evaluation	Possible Points	Instructor Evaluation	Comments
7. Place the anterior x-rays with the maxillary on the upper, and the mandibular on the lower. Incisal edges closest to each other in mount and roots positioned as they grow. Centrals are placed in middle and cuspids on the outer sides. Maxillary centrals are much larger than mandibular ones.			2		
8. Place remaining posterior x-rays, molars toward the outside and bicuspids toward the inside. Maxillary molars have three roots, while mandibular have two roots. Biting surfaces are more closely positioned.			2		
9. Review mounted x-rays to verify proper placement.			3		

TOTAL POINTS POSSIBLE   28

TOTAL POINTS POSSIBLE—2nd attempt   26

TOTAL POINTS EARNED   _____

Points assigned reflect importance of step to meeting objective: Important = 1, Essential = 2, Critical = 3. Students will lose 2 points for repeated attempts. Failure results if any of the critical steps are omitted or performed incorrectly. If using a 100-point scale, determine score by dividing points earned by total points possible and multiplying the results by 100.

SCORE: _____

SKILL COMPETENCY ASSESSMENT

22-8 Processing Duplicating Technique

Student's Name _____ Date _____

Instructor's Name _____

Skill: The dental assistant prepares the equipment, supplies, and area. Copies of x-rays can be made by a duplication process in the darkroom.

Performance Objective: The dental assistant will follow a routine procedure that meets the regulations and protocol set forth by the dentist and regulatory agencies, keeping in mind that assistant duties vary from state to state. The radiographs to be duplicated are taken to the darkroom by the dental assistant to duplicate.

	Self-Evaluation	Student Evaluation	Possible Points	Instructor Evaluation	Comments
Equipment and Supplies 1. Duplicating film and radiographs to be duplicated			2		
2. X-ray duplicating machine			2		
3. Automatic x-ray processor with daylight loader			2		
Competency Steps *(follow aseptic procedures)* 1. Place x-rays in the desired position on the duplicator, dot upward.			3		
2. If the machine has a viewing light, turn it on to assist in x-ray placement.			2		
3. Turn off viewing light under safety light conditions, and place duplicating film over the x-rays with the emulsion side facing downward and contacting the x-ray (the notch will be in the upper left corner).			3		
4. Cover the lid and latch tightly. Set the timer to 4 to 5 seconds (may vary by machine).			2		
5. Activate the machine to expose the film.			2		

	Self-Evaluation	Student Evaluation	Possible Points	Instructor Evaluation	Comments
6. When completed, remove duplicating film under safety light conditions and process the film.			2		

TOTAL POINTS POSSIBLE   20

TOTAL POINTS POSSIBLE—2nd attempt   18

TOTAL POINTS EARNED   _____

Points assigned reflect importance of step to meeting objective: Important = 1, Essential = 2, Critical = 3. Students will lose 2 points for repeated attempts. Failure results if any of the critical steps are omitted or performed incorrectly. If using a 100-point scale, determine score by dividing points earned by total points possible and multiplying the results by 100.

SCORE: _____

Extraoral and Digital Radiography

SPECIFIC INSTRUCTIONAL OBJECTIVES

The student should strive to meet the following objectives and demonstrate an understanding of the facts and principles presented in this chapter:

1. Identify extraoral films and describe exposing techniques.
2. Identify normal and abnormal radiographic landmarks.
3. Identify imaging systems used for dental purposes.
4. Describe digital radiography.
5. Identify the components of digital radiography.
6. Explain the procedure for using digital radiography.
7. Describe 3-D imaging systems.

SUMMARY

Manufacturers, dental team members, and patients are responsible for following safety precaution measures when using radiography equipment. Steps must be used to minimize risk to the patient and all dental personnel.

The dentist is responsible for having dental assistants properly credentialed and trained to expose and process radiographs. The dentist is also responsible for supervising dental assistants in these tasks. In 1981, the Consumer Patient Radiation Health and Safety Act was enacted. This federal law requires each state to inform the Secretary of Health and Human Services how compliance with the act is accomplished.

Dental assistants must be trained in aseptic techniques, radiation hygiene, and maintenance of quality assurance and safety, and they must obtain proper education in exposure and processing techniques. They must understand the physics and biological effects of ionizing radiation, utilize their understanding during every radiographic exposure, understand the ALARA principle, and use the lead apron with cervical collar for the patient's safety every time an x-ray is taken. The assistant must label and store patient x-rays properly to prevent loss and thereby avoid the need for x-rays to be retaken.

EXERCISES AND ACTIVITIES

Multiple Choice

1. Extraoral radiographs are used by the dentist to identify

   a. large areas of the skull on a single radiograph.

   b. both maxillary and mandibular areas at the same time.

   c. conditions or artifacts that are not otherwise diagnosed in other ways.

   d. All of the above

2. Panoramic radiographs may be taken of

   a. patients who have trismus.

   b. patients in wheelchairs.

   c. edentulous patients.

   d. All of the above

3. All of the following are extraoral radiographs except _____ radiographs.

   a. panoramic

   b. periapical

   c. cephalometric

   d. transcranial temporomandibular joint

4. All of the following may cause a ghost image *except*

   a. an earring.

   b. eyeglasses.

   c. caries.

   d. a facial piercing.

5. The cephalometric radiograph records

   a. sinuses.

   b. implant evaluation.

   c. TMJ assessment.

   d. All of the above

6. The cephalometric unit consists of all of the following *except* a

   a. bite-block.

   b. cephalostat.

   c. head-holding device.

   d. cassette holder.

7. The line from the tragus of the ear to the floor of the orbit is also called the

   a. midsagittal plane.

   b. lateral.

   c. transcranial.

   d. Frankfort plane.

8. Which dental specialist uses primarily cephalometric radiographs in practice?

   a. Endodontist

   b. Prosthodontist

   c. Periodontist

   d. Orthodontist

9. The radiographic principle of imaging one section or layer of the body while blurring images from other areas is called

   a. tomography.

   b. magnetic resonance imagery.

   c. paralleling.

   d. bisecting.

10. What positioning error has occurred when taking a panoramic radiograph if the anterior teeth appear blurred and the spine appears superimposed over the ramus areas of the mandible?

    a. Patient is positioned too far back.

    b. Patient's head is tilted downward.

    c. Patient's head is tilted upward.

    d. Patient is positioned too far forward.

11. What positioning error has occurred when taking a panoramic radiograph if a dark radiolucent area appears above the apices of the maxillary teeth?

    a. Patient is positioned too far back.

    b. Patient's tongue was not resting on the roof of the mouth.

    c. Patient's head is tilted upward.

    d. Patient is positioned too far forward.

12. When visualized on a radiograph, which term describes the dense compact bone that forms the tooth socket?

    a. Cementum

    b. Interradicular bone

    c. Cortical plate

    d. Lamina dura

13. When visualized on a radiograph, which term describes the compact edge of the cortical bone that shows as radiopaque between the teeth?

    a. Genial tubercle

    b. Mandibular canal

    c. Coronoid process

    d. Alveolar crest

14. When visualized on a radiograph, which term describes the process of the temporal bone that lies in the lower anterior section, just behind the ear?

    a. Mastoid

    b. Hamular

    c. Styloid

    d. Zygomatic

15. What imaging technique is mainly used to diagnose TMJ disease?

    a. Panoramic

    b. Computed tomography

    c. Ultrasonography

    d. Magnetic resonance imaging

16. Which type of imaging technique is storage phosphor imaging?

    a. Indirect digital imaging

    b. Tomography

    c. Magnetic resonance imaging

    d. Cephalometric imaging

17. _____ is the merging of multiple images that were taken at different times to reveal features that changed in any one of the images.

    a. Digitization

    b. Pixilation

    c. Digital subtraction

    d. Storage phosphor imaging

18. What type of imaging unit is Cone Beam Volumetric Imaging?

    a. Magnetic resonance imaging

    b. Computerized tomography

    c. Cephalometric imaging

    d. Three-dimensional imaging

19. What is the type of imaging most often used when planning an implant surgery?

    a. Panoramic imaging

    b. Computed tomography

    c. Magnetic resonance imaging

    d. Cephalometric imaging

20. When visualized on a radiograph, which term describes the radiolucent area on the lingual side of the mandible at the midline?

    a. Lamina dura

    b. Mental foramen

    c. Lingual foramen

    d. Mandibular foramen

Matching

Match each dental x-ray unit with the appropriate patient positioning.

Unit

1. _____ Cephalometric

2. _____ Panoramic

3. _____ Transcranial temporomandibular joint

Positioning

a. Patient holds cassette to side of head

b. Patient may sit or stand

c. Head reclines against cassette

Match each component of the panoramic unit with its function.

Component	Function
4. _____ Exposure controls	a. Flat, hard container that holds the film
5. _____ Head positioner	b. Collimator has narrow vertical slit
6. _____ X-ray tubehead	c. Outside the x-ray room; includes kV and mA
7. _____ Cassette holder	d. Chin rest, notched bit-block, forehead rest

LABELING

Using the following panoramic radiograph, identify the maxillary landmarks using abbreviations.

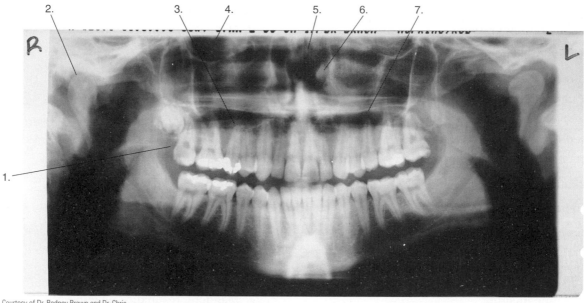

Courtesy of Dr. Rodney Brawn and Dr. Chris

1. _____

2. _____

3. _____

4. _____

5. _____

6. _____

7. _____

Using the following periapical radiograph, identify the parts of the tooth and surrounding structures using abbreviations.

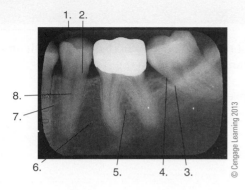

1. _____

2. _____

3. _____

4. _____

5. _____

6. _____

7. _____

8. _____

Critical Thinking

1. What causes a lead apron artifact in a panoramic radiograph?

2. Each manufacturer of digital radiography equipment will provide detailed instructions on preparation of the equipment and computer. Name two advantages and two disadvantages of digital radiography.

3. Describe the advantages of three-dimensional radiography.

CASE STUDY 1

Crisa is preparing for her first panoramic exposure. The patient is a retired woman who has some difficulty in walking. Crisa has checked with the dentist to verify the panoramic technique request.

1. In preparation for the exposure, what steps are performed to prepare the cassette?

2. How will the cassette be labeled?

3. Describe the aseptic procedure taken.

4. How is the panoramic machine prepared for the patient?

5. Explain the differences between the midsagittal plane and Frankfort plane positions.

CASE STUDY 2

Dental assistant Katie is preparing to interpret radiographs. Being familiar with the terminology used in radiographic interpretation and learning landmarks will make this step easier and more meaningful.

1. Define anatomical landmarks, radiopacity, and radiolucency.

2. Define each of the following: enamel, dentin, cementum, pulp chamber, pulp canals or root canals, periodontal ligament/space, lamina dura, cortical plate, interradicular bone, and interdental bone.

3. Enumerate the abbreviations for the eight mandibular landmarks; cross reference with the labeling of the panoramic and periapical radiograph.

4. Enumerate the abbreviation for the seven maxillary landmarks, cross reference with the labeling of the panoramic radiograph.

CASE STUDY 3

The dentist has purchased new equipment—a digital radiology computer—and the dental office team members are happy and anxious to share with their patients all of the equipment's useful features. Sue is the dental assistant responsible for preparing the equipment for the first patient.

1. Describe equipment preparation steps.

2. Describe patient preparation.

3. Enumerate steps involved in taking the exposure.

SKILL COMPETENCY ASSESSMENT

23-1 Exposing Panoramic Radiographs

Student's Name _____ Date _____

Instructor's Name _____

Skill: Routine steps should be followed for all treatment areas to maintain absolute clinical asepsis. The patient is informed about the procedure. This procedure will include technique selection determined by what the dentist needs for diagnosis.

Performance Objective: The dental assistant will follow a routine procedure that meets the regulations and protocol set forth by the dentist and regulatory agencies. The dental assistant checks with the dentist for the request of the technique to be performed and prepares the cassette, panoramic machine, and patient for exposure.

	Self-Evaluation	Student Evaluation	Possible Points	Instructor Evaluation	Comments
Equipment and Supplies					
1. Panoramic film			2		
2. Cassette			2		
3. Bite-block			2		
4. Barrier for the bite-block			2		
5. Lead apron without thyroid collar			3		
6. Panoramic machine			3		
Competency Steps ***Preparation for the Panoramic Radiographic Exposure*** 1. Under safety light conditions, load cassette in darkroom.			2		
2. Place panoramic film between cassette intensifying screens.			3		
3. Cassette must be firmly closed to prevent light leaks.			3		
4. Cassette is labeled left/right with patient name, date, and the dentist's name.			3		
5. Place cassette into the cassette holder of the panoramic machine.			2		

	Self-Evaluation	Student Evaluation	Possible Points	Instructor Evaluation	Comments
6. Prepare the bite-block. Place protective barrier on the bite-block (sterilization should occur between patients).			2		
7. Adjust the machine to patient's approximate height and set the kilovoltage and milliamperage according to manufacturer's guidelines.			3		
Prepare the Patient for Panoramic Exposure 8. Explain the procedure to the patient. Answer any questions.			2		
9. Ask patient to remove eyeglasses, earrings, tongue bars, facial piercing materials, hair pins/clips, necklaces, hearing aids, and partial/full dentures (anything that might interfere with exposure).			3		
10. Place and secure lead apron on patient (lead apron without collar). Apron is double-sided for front and back.			2		
11. Guide patient into position, whether sitting or standing. Ask patient to stand/sit as straight as possible, keeping vertebral column perfectly straight.			2		
12. Raise machine to the appropriate level so that the patient can easily bite on bite-block. Have the patient move forward until the upper and lower teeth are secured in the bite-block groove. If patient is edentulous, the alveolar ridges should be positioned over the grooves of the bite-block. Cotton rolls can assist in proper positioning.			3		
13- Turn the light on and adjust patient accordingly. Have midsagittal plane/Frankfort plane positioned.			2		
14. The midsagittal plane must be parallel with the floor. Divides the face in right and left halves.			2		

	Self-Evaluation	Student Evaluation	Possible Points	Instructor Evaluation	Comments
15. The Frankfort plane—an imaginary line from the middle of the ear to just below the eye socket across the bridge of nose— must be parallel to the floor.			2		
16. Before exposure, have the patient swallow, and then ask the patient to place the tongue at the roof of the mouth, and close lips around bite-block. Reassure the patient and instruct her or him to remain still during the exposure.			3		
17. After exposure is complete, guide the patient away from the panoramic machine and remove the apron.			2		
18. Remove the cassette and proceed with film processing.			2		

TOTAL POINTS POSSIBLE   57

TOTAL POINTS POSSIBLE—2nd attempt   55

TOTAL POINTS EARNED   ____

Points assigned reflect importance of step to meeting objective: Important = 1, Essential = 2, Critical = 3. Students will lose 2 points for repeated attempts. Failure results if any of the critical steps are omitted or performed incorrectly. If using a 100-point scale, determine score by dividing points earned by total points possible and multiplying the results by 100.

SCORE: _____

SKILL COMPETENCY ASSESSMENT

23-2 Digital Radiology Techniques

Student's Name _____ Date _____

Instructor's Name _____

Skill: Routine steps should be followed for all treatment areas to maintain absolute clinical asepsis. The patient is informed about the procedure, which includes technique selection determined by the dentist's needs for diagnosis. The steps comprise guidelines to follow during the general procedure of using digital radiology.

Performance Objective: The dental assistant will follow a routine procedure that meets the regulations and protocol set forth by the dentist and regulatory agencies. The dental assistant checks with the dentist for the technique request. All manufacturers of digital radiography systems provide detailed instructions on preparing the equipment and patient, taking the exposure, and using the computer. The dental assistant prepares the computer, which is activated to select the type of radiography to be exposed.

	Self-Evaluation	Student Evaluation	Possible Points	Instructor Evaluation	Comments
Equipment Preparation 1. Turn on computer, activate the computer screen, and select the type of radiography to be exposed.			3		
2. Enter patient's identification information and date.			2		
3. Select sterilized/disinfected sensor and place approved barrier over sensor.			2		
4. Place sensor into appropriate x-ray film holder.			2		
5. Prepare x-ray machine and adjust settings. (Follow manufacturer's instructions for settings.)			2		
Preparation of the Patient **(Patient is prepared in the same way as for traditional radiograph exposure.)**					
1. Seat patient so that the midsagittal plane is perpendicular to the floor.			3		
2. Adjust chair to comfortable level.			3		
3. Adjust headrest to position patient's head so that occlusal plane is parallel to floor.			2		

	Self-Evaluation	Student Evaluation	Possible Points	Instructor Evaluation	Comments
4. Place lead apron with thyroid collar on patient.			3		
5. Request that patient remove eyeglasses and any objects from the mouth that might interfere with the procedure.			2		
6. Quickly inspect the oral cavity for anything that could alter placement of the sensor.			2		
Taking the Exposure 1. Place the sensor in the patient's mouth and carefully move it into position for the exposure.			2		
2. Align the x-ray cone and PID; direct central rays in the same way as the x-ray film exposure technique.			2		
3. Using the keyboard or mouse, activate sensor exposure.			2		
4. Press the exposure button to expose sensor.			3		
Direct Digital Imaging System 5. Wait until image appears on the monitor and evaluate it. If the dentist determines that the image is of diagnostic quality, continue to next image to be exposed.			2		
6. If a positioning error occurs, do not remove the sensor from the patient's mouth; evaluate the error and correct the sensor position or realign the PID.					
7. If the image is satisfactory, remove the sensor or reposition it for additional exposures. Repeat until all exposures are acquired.			2		
Indirect Digital Imaging System 1. Remove the imaging plate from the patient's mouth.			1		
2. Remove the imaging plate from the film holder and remove the plastic barrier.			2		

	Self-Evaluation	Student Evaluation	Possible Points	Instructor Evaluation	Comments
3. Place the imaging plate into the dark container until all exposures are taken.			2		
4. After all exposures are taken, place imaging plates on the scanner and activate in a semi-dark room.			3		
5. Images begin appearing on the monitor. Evaluate for quality of diagnostic images. Retake any images that do not meet the dentist's needs. Erase the image from the plates and disinfect according to manufacturer's instructions.			3		
6. Replace barrier and retake any unacceptable exposure.			2		
After Exposure 1. Save images in patient file, and back up the file on the computer or supplemental storage system.			3		

TOTAL POINTS POSSIBLE   58

TOTAL POINTS POSSIBLE—2nd attempt   56

TOTAL POINTS EARNED   ____

Points assigned reflect the importance of the step in meeting the objective: Important = 1, Essential = 2, Critical = 3. Students will lose 2 points for repeated attempts. Failure results if any of the critical steps are omitted or performed incorrectly. If using a 100-point scale, determine score by dividing points earned by total points possible and multiplying the results by 100.

SCORE: _____

SECTION 7

Dental Specialties

CHAPTER 24

Endodontics

The student should strive to meet the following objectives and demonstrate an understanding of the facts and principles presented in this chapter:

1. Define endodontics and describe what an endodontist does.

2. Describe pulpal and periapical disease.

3. Identify diagnostic procedures.

4. Identify instruments used in endodontic procedures and describe their functions.

5. Identify materials used in endodontics and describe their functions.

6. Describe endodontic procedures and the responsibilities of the dental assistant.

7. Describe endodontic retreatment.

8. Explain surgical endodontic procedures and the instruments used.

SUMMARY

Endodontics comprises the diagnosis and treatment of pulp and periapical tissue diseases. Procedures include diagnosis, root canal treatment, and periapical surgery.

The endodontist is assisted by dental assistants who perform traditional assisting responsibilities in addition to expanded duties specific to endodontics as allowed by state dental practice acts.

Endodontic diagnosis includes patient medical and dental history; clinical examination, including pulp testing; and review of communication if the patient is sent from a referring dentist.

9590.

EXERCISES AND ACTIVITIES

Multiple Choice

1. Which of the following procedures is dealt with and included in the branch of dentistry called endodontics?

   a. Diagnosis

   b. Root canal treatment

   c. Periapical surgery

   d. All of the above

2. _____ is the process by which an agent encloses or grasps a toxic substance and makes it nontoxic.

   a. Zinc oxide-eugenol

   b. Sodium hypochlorite

   c. Chelation

   d. Ethyl chloride

3. An ultrasonic unit can be used during an endodontic procedure for all of the following *except*

   a. troughing around posts.

   b. opening calcified canals.

   c. as a spreader in the root canal procedure.

   d. Can be used for all of the above

4. A localized destruction of tissue and accumulation of exudate in the periapical region is called a _____ abscess

   a. fistula type

   b. periapical

   c. pulpitis

   d. necrosis

5. The endodontic bender is designed to bend all of the following *except*

   a. reamers.

   b. files.

   c. burs.

   d. pluggers.

6. Irritations of the pulp can be caused by

   a. heat.

   b. impact trauma.

   c. fractures.

   d. All of the above

7. Intracanal instruments that are made of fine metal wire with tiny, sharp projections along the instrument shaft are called

   a. barbed broaches.

   b. files.

   c. reamers.

   d. Gates-Glidden drills.

8. Which files are used only in a push-and-pull motion?

   a. K-type

   b. Hedström

   c. Reamer

   d. Broach

9. Which of the following are placed on reamers and files to mark the length of the root canal?

   a. Rubber stops

   b. File stops

   c. Endo stops

   d. All of the above

10. The instrument used to remove excess gutta percha is called a

    a. spreader.

    b. Glick 1.

    c. plugger.

    d. spoon.

11. Which of the following instruments has a long, twisted shank, has blades that are far apart, and is used in a twisting motion?

    a. File

    b. Broach

    c. Reamer

    d. Gates-Glidden drill

12. A thermoplastic material that is flexible at room temperature and is used to fill the canal is (a)

    a. rubber stop.
    b. file stop.

    c. gutta percha.
    d. marker.

13. _____ is(are) a material that comes in powder/liquid form, is(are) thick when mixed, is(are) used with obturating materials, and is(are) inserted in the canal.

    a. Gutta percha
    b. Sealer

    c. Paper points
    d. Marker

14. Which piece of equipment measures the distance to the apex of the tooth and displays the information on a digital readout?

    a. Vitality scanner
    b. Pulp tester

    c. Heating unit
    d. Apex finder

15. During which phase of endodontic treatment is the pulp canal restored by being filled and sealed permanently?

    a. Reversible pulpitis
    b. Pulpotomy

    c. Obturation
    d. Hemisection

16. The master cone material is (a)

    a. paper point.
    b. Lentulo spiral.

    c. calcium hydroxide.
    d. gutta percha.

17. In which procedure are the apex of the root and the infection surrounding the area surgically removed?

    a. Amputation
    b. Hemisection

    c. Pulpectomy
    d. Apicoectomy

18. The retrograde filling materials that can be placed in the prepared cavity include

    a. amalgam.
    b. composite.

    c. gutta percha.
    d. All of the above

19. Which of the following are characteristics of intracanal instruments?

    1. Precise diameters
    2. Precise lengths
    3. Made of stainless steel
    4. Made of nickel titanium alloy wire
    5. Gutta percha
    6. Flexible
    7. Fracture resistant
    8. Corrosion resistant
        a. 1, 2, 3, 4, 5, 6, 7, 8
        b. 1, 2, 3, 5, 8

        c. 1, 2, 3, 4, 6, 7, 8
        d. 1, 2, 5, 6, 7, 8

20. Which of the following steps are *not* part of general root canal therapy?

    1. Administer anesthetic
    2. Lay a surgical flap
    3. Isolate the area
    4. Amputate the root
    5. Gain access to the pulp
    6. Locate canals
        a. 1, 2, 3
        b. 2, 4

        c. 1, 3, 5
        d. 1, 3, 6

21. The following condition, occurring when the pulp is inflamed but able to heal when the irritant is removed, is called _____ pulpitis.

    a. irreversible

    b. reversible

    c. chronic

    d. None of the above

22. The following condition, occurring when inflammation continues until pulpal tissue cannot recover, is called _____ pulpitis.

    a. irreversible

    b. reversible

    c. temporary

    d. None of the above

23. The death of the pulpal cells, often the result of irreversible pulpitis, is called

    a. apical periodontitis.

    b. pulpal necrosis.

    c. pulpotomy.

    d. periapical abscess.

24. A(n) _____ consists of numerous cells of the inflammatory process of chronic apical periodontitis.

    a. granuloma

    b. osteomyelitis

    c. exudate

    d. cellulitis

25. The _____, a long, tapered endodontic instrument that is pointed on the ends, is used to adapt the gutta percha into the canal.

    a. plugger

    b. spreader

    c. reamer

    d. broach

26. The _____, a long, tapered endodontic instrument that is flat on the ends, is used to condense filling material.

    a. plugger

    b. spreader

    c. reamer

    d. broach

27. The endodontic handpiece is attached to a _____-speed handpiece.

    a. high

    b. low

    c. triple

    d. variable

28. The removal of all pulpal tissues, beginning in the coronal portion of the tooth and terminating short of the apex in the root canal of the tooth, is called a(n)

    a. pulpectomy.

    b. pulpotomy.

    c. apicoectomy.

    d. hemisection.

29. The removal of the pulp in the coronal portion of the tooth, leaving the pulp in the root canal intact and vital, is called a(n)

    a. pulpectomy.

    b. pulpotomy.

    c. apicoectomy.

    d. hemisection.

30. The surgical removal of one root and the overlying crown is called a(an)

    a. root amputation.

    b. hemisection.

    c. apicoectomy.

    d. pulpectomy.

31. Radiographs are a useful endodontic diagnostic tool. If inflammation has extended beyond the apex of the tooth, a radiograph will show a _____ area.

    a. radiopaque

    b. radiolucent

    c. Both a. and b.

    d. None of the above

32. Which of the following benefits is(are) provided by using a dental dam during an endodontic procedure?

    a. Improved operator visibility

    b. Tooth protected from saliva and solutions

    c. Aseptic field maintained

    d. All of the above used in endodontic treatment

33. What is the name of the instrument that provides magnification of the anatomical structures to allow greater precision in treatment?

    a. Endoscope

    b. Endodontic microscope

    c. Endodontic explorer

    d. Endodontic bender

34. What is the name of the system that warms the filling material and allows the dentist to backfill the canal?

    a. Endodontic reamer system

    b. Endodontic plugger system

    c. Endodontic irrigation system

    d. Endodontic obturation system

35. What is the name of the procedure in which the root canal apex in a necrotic tooth is treated?

    a. Apexogenesis

    b. Apicoectomy

    c. Apexification

    d. Apicotomy

Matching

Match the image of the instrument to the name of the instrument.

A. Endodontic pluggers

B. Finger spreader

C. Handled spreader

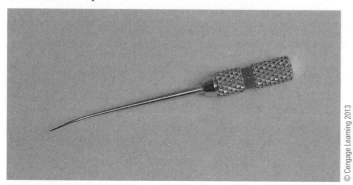

© Cengage Learning 2013

1. ____B____

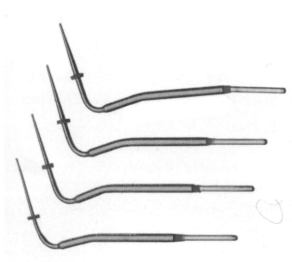

Courtesy of Sybron Endo

3. ____A____

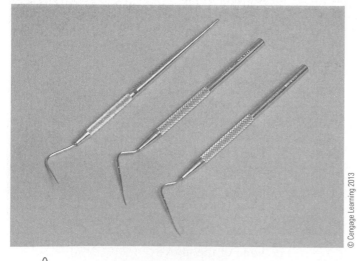

© Cengage Learning 2013

2. ____C____

Critical Thinking

1. Patient cases that require advanced knowledge of treatment are often referred to a specialist. What type of communication does the general dentist send along with the patient to the endodontist?

2. Dental assistants' efficiency depends on their knowledge of the instruments used during endodontic treatment. Name the hand instruments and their functions, and be able to visually identify these instruments.

3. The dental assistant must be able to demonstrate knowledge by anticipating what will be required during the initial endodontic treatment visit. Describe the three phases of this examination.

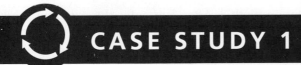

CASE STUDY 1

Ed has been referred to an endodontist by his general dentist, who determined that Ed's maxillary first molar will need a root canal. This is Ed's first appointment with the endodontist and he hopes that the procedure will be explained.

1. List the extraoral tissues to be evaluated.

2. Describe how the intraoral soft tissues are to be evaluated.

3. List other parts of the clinical examination that will aid in the final diagnosis.

4. List the general steps in root canal treatment.

CASE STUDY 2

The dental assistant's efficiency is enhanced by being familiar with the instrumentation of endodontics. Being knowledgeable and skilled in instrument recognition and identification will lead to quick delivery of the items needed by the endodontist.

1. Define intracanal instrumentation.

2. Describe each of the following: barbed broaches, files, and reamers.

3. Describe the use of the rotary or engine instruments.

4. List the names of the hand instruments that may be used and their functions.

5. Name the endodontic materials that may be used.

CASE STUDY 3

Ed was not so lucky in his first endodontic treatment on tooth 3. After 3 months, the pain and aching in this tooth have still not receded. He contacted the dentist about what should or could be done to relieve the pain. A referral back to the endodontist was the next step.

1. Enumerate three possible causes for retreatment.

2. Describe the treatment option of reopening the tooth.

3. List the steps for accomplishing retreatment.

4. If the problem is at the apex, what treatment will likely be recommended?

SKILL COMPETENCY ASSESSMENT

24-1 Electronic Pulp Testing

Student's Name _____ Date _____

Instructor's Name _____

Skill: Routine steps should be followed for all treatment areas to maintain absolute clinical asepsis. The patient is informed about the procedure. The dental assistant performs traditional assisting responsibilities in addition to expanded duties specific to endodontics allowed by each state Dental Practice Act.

Performance Objective: The student will follow a routine procedure that meets the regulations and protocol set forth by the dentist and regulatory agencies, keeping in mind that assistant duties vary from state to state. The electronic pulp tester indicates whether the tooth is vital or nonvital. The current creates an electrical stimulus to the tooth, and responses to the stimulus are compared to determine the pulp vitality.

	Self-Evaluation	Student Evaluation	Possible Points	Instructor Evaluation	Comments
Equipment and Supplies 1. Basic setup: mouth mirror, explorer, and cotton pliers			3		
2. Electronic pulp tester			3		
3. Conducting medium, such as toothpaste			2		
Competency Steps *(follow aseptic procedures)* Follow these steps to electronically test the pulp. (Test control tooth first.)					
1. Place a small amount of toothpaste on the tip of the electrode.			2		
2. Dry the tooth before using the electrode.			3		
3. Ask the patient to signal when noticing a sensation, usually a tingling or hot feeling.			3		
4. Place the tip on the facial surface of the tooth and gradually increase the power. **Caution:** Do not place the electrode on a metal restoration, a wet surface, gingivae, or artificial crowns.			3		

	Self-Evaluation	Student Evaluation	Possible Points	Instructor Evaluation	Comments
5. If the patient feels any sensation, some degree of tooth vitality is indicated. If no sensation is felt, the pulp may be necrotic.			3		

TOTAL POINTS POSSIBLE   22

TOTAL POINTS POSSIBLE—2nd attempt   20

TOTAL POINTS EARNED   _____

Points assigned reflect importance of step to meeting objective: Important = 1, Essential = 2, Critical = 3. Students will lose 2 points for repeated attempts. Failure results if any of the critical steps are omitted or performed incorrectly. If using a 100-point scale, determine score by dividing points earned by total points possible and multiplying the results by 100.

SCORE: _____

SKILL COMPETENCY ASSESSMENT

24-2 Root Canal Treatment

Student's Name _____ Date _____

Instructor's Name _____

Skill: Routine steps should be followed for all treatment areas to maintain absolute clinical asepsis. The patient is informed about the procedure. The dental assistant performs traditional assisting responsibilities in addition to expanded duties specific to endodontics allowed by each state Dental Practice Act.

Performance Objective: The student will follow a routine procedure that meets the regulations and protocol set forth by the dentist and regulatory agencies, keeping in mind that assistant duties vary from state to state. The following sequence contains steps involved in a root canal treatment that requires two appointments. (Each office has a routine procedure that is carefully followed to ensure that all pertinent information is gathered for endodontic diagnosis and treatment.)

   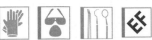

	Self-Evaluation	Student Evaluation	Possible Points	Instructor Evaluation	Comments
Equipment and Supplies					
1. Basic setup: mouth mirror, explorer, and cotton pliers			3		
2. Endodontic explorer and spoon excavator			2		
3. Locking cotton pliers			2		
4. Saliva ejector, evacuator tip (HVE), air-water syringe tip			3		
5. Cotton rolls, cotton pellets, and gauze sponges			3		
6. Anesthetic setup			3		
7. Dental dam setup			3		
8. High-speed handpiece and assortment of burs			3		
9. Low-speed handpiece			2		
10. Irrigating syringe and solution (sodium hypochlorite or hydrogen peroxide)			3		
11. Barbed broach, assorted reamers and files, and rubber stops			3		
12. Paper points (assortment)			2		

	Self-Evaluation	Student Evaluation	Possible Points	Instructor Evaluation	Comments
13. Temporization materials			2		
14. Permanent obturating materials (gutta percha or silver points and root canal sealer)			2		
15. Heat source			2		
16. Endodontic spreaders, pluggers, and Glick 1			3		
17. Articulating forceps and paper			2		
Competency Steps *(follow aseptic procedures)* **Administer Anesthetic** 1. Administer topical and local anesthetic.			2		
2. After the first appointment anesthetic may be unnecessary (to be indicated by the dentist).			2		
3. Prepare the syringe and assist during anesthetic administration.			3		
Isolate the Area 1. Prepare to isolate the tooth for treatment.			3		
2. Place the dental dam on the tooth being endodontically treated.			3		
3. After dental dam placement, wipe the area with disinfectant.			2		
4. State the benefits to the patient and/or the operator of the dental dam.			3		
Gain Access to the Pulp 1. The dentist uses a high-speed handpiece and bur to gain access to the pulp. The opening is through the crown to expose the pulp chamber.			2		
2. Evacuate and maintain good visibility for the dentist.			2		
3. Once the pulp is accessed, the dentist uses the endodontic explorer to locate main and accessory canals.			2		

	Self-Evaluation	Student Evaluation	Possible Points	Instructor Evaluation	Comments
Remove the Pulpal Tissues 1. The dentist will insert a barbed broach into the canal and withdraw pulpal tissue.			2		
2. Receive the barbed broach in a gauze sponge.			2		
Enlarge and Smooth the Root Canal 1. Using an x-ray, the dentist estimates the length of the root of the tooth. The assistant should record the length of the root on the patient's chart for reference.			2		
An apex finder may also be used. Use rubber stops to mark the length of the tooth on files/reamers.			1		
The dentist uses a series of small files to remove debris and enlarge canals (must be at least 25 file before Gates-Glidden burs can be used).			4		
As files enlarge the diameter of canal, the size of files and/or Gates burs increases.			2		
2. Prepare the stops on files and reamers. The dentist instructs the dental assistant to place rubber stops according to the measurement and precisely for each hand instrument. Keep the files and reamers in order and free of debris. (Duties vary depending on preferences of dentists; some dentists may want the assistant to sterilize reamers and files chairside, or they may request radiographs taken periodically.)			3		
Irrigate the Root Canal 1. Periodically, the canal is irrigated to remove debris. After the canal is flushed, it is dried with paper points.			2		
2. Prepare the irrigating solution in the disposable syringe and transfer to the operator. The operator flushes the solution into the canal, and the assistant evacuates the area. Then, transfer paper points in locking pliers to the operator. To dry the canal, measure 1 mm short of the apex. Receive the used saturated points in a gauze sponge.			3		

	Self-Evaluation	Student Evaluation	Possible Points	Instructor Evaluation	Comments
3. **Note:** The dentist may decide to place a temporary restoration and schedule another appointment with the patient in several days. Prepare the temporary restorative materials and either place the temporary or assist the dentist in placement. Remove the dental dam and dismiss the patient.			2		
Obturate the Root Canal 1. Obturation of the root canal is routinely performed at the second appointment. After seating the patient, remove the temporary and flush the canal.			2		
2. Radiographs are taken periodically throughout the procedure for the dentist to evaluate progress. Once the canal is adequately enlarged and free of disease, it is filled permanently.			2		
3. Materials and techniques for filling the canal may vary, but gutta percha materials are most common.			2		
4. The dentist selects a gutta percha point as the **master cone.** The cone is no more than 1 mm short of the prepared length. The dentist inserts the cone in the canal to check the fit. If the master cone is the correct length and fits snugly near the apex, the cone is removed and the root canal sealer is prepared.			2		
5. Root canal sealer is mixed and placed in the canal with a Lentulo spiral. The master cone is dipped into sealer and placed in the canal.			2		
6. A spreader is used to create space for additional accessory gutta percha cones. Dip each accessory gutta percha cone into the root canal sealer and pass it to the dentist for placement. Transfer spreader for use to create space for subsequent cones. This procedure is repeated until the canal is filled.			2		

	Self-Evaluation	Student Evaluation	Possible Points	Instructor Evaluation	Comments
7. Once the canal is filled, excess gutta percha in the crown of the tooth is removed with a hot Glick 1 or a heated plugger. The warm gutta percha is vertically condensed into the cervical portion.			2		
8. Hold a 2 × 2 piece of gauze to remove any excess gutta percha from the instruments.			2		
9. Take the final radiograph.			3		
10. The coronal portion of the tooth is sealed with a permanent restoration or a temporary restoration if a fixed prosthesis is the treatment of choice.			2		
11. Remove the dental dam and rinse the patient's mouth.			2		
12. The patient's occlusion is checked with articulating paper.			2		
13. Give the patient postoperative instructions and dismiss him or her.			2		

TOTAL POINTS POSSIBLE   117

TOTAL POINTS POSSIBLE—2nd attempt   115

TOTAL POINTS EARNED   _____

Points assigned reflect importance of step to meeting objective: Important = 1, Essential = 2, Critical = 3. Students will lose 2 points for repeated attempts. Failure results if any of the critical steps are omitted or performed incorrectly. If using a 100-point scale, determine score by dividing points earned by total points possible and multiplying the results by 100.

SCORE: _____

SKILL COMPETENCY ASSESSMENT

24-3 Apicoectomy

Student's Name _____ Date _____

Instructor's Name _____

Skill: The dental assistant prepares the equipment, supplies, and area. In this procedure, the apex of the root and infection surrounding the area is surgically removed.

Performance Objective: The dental assistant will follow a routine procedure that meets the regulations and protocol set forth by the dentist and regulatory agencies. Situations arise in which surgical endodontic treatment is needed to save the involved tooth from extraction. This procedure is performed by the dentist, who is assisted by the dental assistant.

	Self-Evaluation	Student Evaluation	Possible Points	Instructor Evaluation	Comments
Equipment and Supplies					
1. Basic setup: mouth mirror, explorer, and cotton pliers			3		
2. Endodontic explorer and spoon excavator			2		
3. Locking cotton pliers			2		
4. Saliva ejector, surgical evacuator tip, and air-water syringe tip			3		
5. Cotton rolls and gauze sponges			2		
6. Anesthetic setup			3		
7. Scalpel and blades			2		
8. Periosteal elevator and tissue retractors			2		
9. High-speed, very small-headed handpiece and assortment of burs			3		
10. Surgical curettes			2		
11. Irrigating syringe and sterile saline solution			2		
12. Hemostat and surgical scissors			3		
13. Amalgam setup			3		
14. Suture setup			3		

	Self-Evaluation	Student Evaluation	Possible Points	Instructor Evaluation	Comments
Competency Steps *(follow aseptic procedures)* 1. Prepare anesthetic to be administered to patient.			2		
The Incision 1. The dentist makes a flap incision with the scalpel and lifts tissue from the bone with a periosteal elevator.					
2. The dental assistant retracts the tissue for the dentist throughout the procedure.			3		
3. Transfer instruments, keeping the site clear and clean using surgical evacuator and tissue retractors.			3		
4. The dentist uses the high-speed handpiece to gain access to the root apex through the bone.			3		
5. The dentist removes debris and infection from around the apex of root with a surgical curette.			2		
6. The dental assistant evacuates and removes debris from instruments with a gauze sponge.			3		
7. The dental assistant prepares the handpiece and the sterile saline irrigation syringe.			2		
8. The dentist uses the high-speed handpiece and burs to remove a section of the exposed root tip. The root tip is beveled for better access, and the area is rinsed with the sterile saline to prepare the root to receive the retrograde filling material.			3		
Retrograde Filling 9. The dentist places retrograde filling material in the prepared cavity. Amalgam is commonly used, but gutta percha, zinc oxide eugenol, and composite are also used.			3		
Closing 10. Flap replacement and suturing are the final steps. Return the flap to position and hold it in place. The dentist then sutures the flap in place.			3		

	Self-Evaluation	Student Evaluation	Possible Points	Instructor Evaluation	Comments
11. The dental assistant prepares the suture and assists during placement. Once the suturing procedure is complete, the patient is given postoperative instructions and a prescription for pain medication, and is dismissed.			3		

TOTAL POINTS POSSIBLE   67

TOTAL POINTS POSSIBLE—2nd attempt   65

TOTAL POINTS EARNED   _____

Points assigned reflect importance of step to meeting objective: Important = 1, Essential = 2, Critical = 3. Students will lose 2 points for repeated attempts. Failure results if any of the critical steps are omitted or performed incorrectly. If using a 100-point scale, determine score by dividing points earned by total points possible and multiplying the results by 100.

SCORE: _____

CHAPTER 25

Oral and Maxillofacial Surgery

SPECIFIC INSTRUCTIONAL OBJECTIVES

The student should strive to meet the following objectives and demonstrate an understanding of the facts and principles presented in this chapter:

1. Describe the scope of oral and maxillofacial surgery.

2. Identify the surgical instruments used in various types of surgery and describe their functions.

3. Explain the aseptic procedures followed in the oral surgeon's office.

4. Describe evaluation procedures for new patients.

5. Describe how to prepare the patient for surgical treatment.

6. Explain surgical procedures, including tray setups and assisting responsibilities.

7. List postoperative instructions given to patients.

8. List and describe cancer and oral abnormalities detection.

9. List and describe biopsy techniques.

10. Describe temporomandibular (TMJ) disease.

11. List and describe the types of dental implants and explain the surgical procedures for placing the implants.

12. Explain the oral surgeon's relationship with the hospital.

Advanced Chairside Functions

13. Explain the function of sutures and when they are placed.

14. List the equipment and supplies needed for suture removal.

15. Determine and identify the location and number of sutures and how to evaluate the healing process.

16. Identify the following suture patterns: simple, continuous simple, sling, continuous sling, horizontal, and vertical mattress.

17. List the basic criteria for suture removal.

18. Explain the steps of removal for identified suture patterns.

19. Explain postoperative patient care.

SUMMARY

The dental surgery team may vary according to the surgeon's goals for the practice. In addition to the oral and maxillofacial surgeon, the team usually consists of the receptionist, the business office staff, the dental assistants, and, in some offices, a nurse or an anesthesiologist.

The surgical dental assistant's responsibilities often vary depending on the size of the practice.

EXERCISES AND ACTIVITIES

True or False

1. Surgical aspirating tips are used to aspirate blood and debris from the surgical site.

   a. True
   b. False

2. Universal forceps can be used on any of the four quadrants.

   a. True
   b. False

3. Cheek and lip retractors are used to hold the patient's mouth open during surgical procedures.

   a. True
   b. False

4. Surgical scissors are used to shape and contour the alveolar bone after the teeth are extracted.

   a. True
   b. False

5. One of the most common procedures is the removal of impacted teeth, especially the third molars.

   a. True
   b. False

6. The VELscope uses a blue-spectrum light that causes the soft tissues to fluoresce, thus allowing the dentist to visualize tissue that may be diseased or traumatized.

   a. True
   b. False

7. An excisional biopsy is also known as a smear biopsy.

   a. True
   b. False

8. An MDI is a small metal cap that fits on a dental implant and keeps tissue and debris from getting into the implant.

   a. True
   b. False

9. Alveolitis is the irrigation of a joint.

   a. True

   b. False

10. The surgical removal of a disk that is deteriorated or damaged is called a discectomy.

    a. True

    b. False

Multiple Choice

1. Oral and maxillofacial surgery involves surgery for

   a. functional malformations.

   b. facial injuries.

   c. facial aesthetics.

   d. All of the above

2. The surgical dental assistant would perform all the following tasks *except*

   a. transfer instruments.

   b. administer local anesthetic.

   c. maintain the operating field during procedures.

   d. take vital signs.

3. Which of the following instruments has straight, short beaks and fine serrations with a groove down the center of each beak, and is available in various sizes?

   a. Hemostat

   b. Needle holder

   c. Surgical scissors

   d. Rongeurs

4. Which of the following instruments has long serrated or grooved beaks and working ends that can be straight or curved, and is used to retract tissue or grasp loose objects?

   a. Surgical scissors

   b. Needle holder

   c. Hemostat

   d. Rongeurs

5. Which of the following instruments has pointed beaks with straight or angled blades, and can cut sutures or trim soft tissue?

   a. Scalpel

   b. Hemostat

   c. Needle holder

   d. Surgical scissors

6. Which of the following instruments is available in beveled or bi-beveled sides, can be used alone if bone is soft, and removes or shapes the bone?

   a. Mallet

   b. File

   c. Rongeurs

   d. Chisel

7. Which of the following instruments is usually double ended, comes in a variety of sizes and shapes, and is used in a back-and-forth motion to smooth the edges of alveolar bone?

   a. Mallet

   b. File

   c. Rongeurs

   d. Chisel

8. When multiple teeth are removed, which instrument would be used to contour the remaining ridge of the alveolar bone and eliminate sharp edges?

   a. Surgical scissors

   b. File

   c. Rongeurs

   d. Chisel

9. Which hinged instrument is used to remove teeth from the alveolar bone?

   a. Apical elevator

   b. Periosteal elevator

   c. Extraction forceps

   d. Root tip pick

10. _____ is a contouring process in which sharp edges and points on the alveolar ridge are contoured and smoothed.

    a. Alveolitis

    b. Osseointegration

    c. Exodontia

    d. Alveoplasty

11. A nonsurgical procedure that involves the oral surgeon removing a layer of cells from the surface lesion and spreading the gathered cells on a glass slab is called a(n)

    a. incisional biopsy.

    b. excisional biopsy.

    c. dental implant.

    d. exfoliative cytology.

12. The most common complication following an extraction is

    a. luxation.

    b. alveoplasty.

    c. alveolitis.

    d. exfoliative cytology.

13. The process in which a dental implant becomes fused with the bone and tissue is called

    a. orthognathi.

    b. alveoplasty.

    c. osseointegration.

    d. a stint.

14. The two most common dental implants are subperiosteal and endosteal. Which of the following are characteristics of a subperiosteal implant?

    1. Placed in the bone

    2. Often placed for denture patients

    3. Replaces one tooth

    4. Most common on the mandibular

    5. Abutment posts are above the mucoperiosteum

    6. Requires a ridge width of at least 2 mm

    7. Alveolar bone has atrophied

    8. Requires one or two surgeries

    a. 1, 2, 3, 4, 5, 6

    b. 1, 2, 5, 6

    c. 2, 3, 5, 8

    d. 2, 4, 7, 8

15. Surgical scalpels are used to incise the soft tissue and are then disposed of in the

    a. regular waste.

    b. sharps container.

    c. biohazard container.

    d. None of the above

16. A _____ is a retraction device used to grasp the tissue securely.

    a. cheek and lip retractor

    b. tissue retractor

    c. forceps

    d. hemostat

17. A retractor that is spoon shaped or has a long blade, and is placed between the border of the tongue and the lingual surfaces of the teeth, is called a

    a. cheek and lip retractor.

    b. tongue retractor.

    c. mouth prop.

    d. forceps.

18. The _____ is composed of mucosa and periosteum.

    a. periosteum

    b. mucoperiosteum

    c. gingiva

    d. alveolus

19. The term "luxates" indicates which type of motion?

    a. Dislocation

    b. Back-and-forth rocking

    c. Sawing

    d. Up and down

20. The term "subluxates" indicates which type of motion?

    a. Dislocation

    b. Back-and-forth rocking

    c. Sawing

    d. Up and down

21. When the oral surgeon removes a small section of a lesion and includes a small border of normal tissue, this is called an _____ biopsy.

    a. excisional

    b. incisional

    c. exfoliative

    d. extraction

22. The specialist who performs cyst and tumor removal is the

    a. periodontist.

    b. pedodontist.

    c. oral and maxillofacial surgeon.

    d. prosthodontist.

23. One of the most common procedures the oral surgeon performs is a(n)

    a. composite restoration.

    b. amalgam restoration.

    c. fixed prosthetic.

    d. third molar extraction.

24. Typical responsibilities of a surgical dental assistant include preparing the scalpel blade. Which of the following is the blade size selected for surgical procedures?

    a. 15

    b. 14

    c. 5

    d. 10

25. Which of the following are types of surgical retractors?

    a. Tissue

    b. Tongue

    c. Cheek

    d. All of the above

26. When removing or replacing scalpel blades on the scalpel handle, which of the following are used?

    a. Cotton pliers

    b. Hemostat

    c. Blade protector

    d. All of the above

27. The receptionist and the business staff play an important part in the oral surgery office. Which of the following are duties of the office staff?

    a. Communications from the referring dentist

    b. Financial arrangements

    c. Insurance claims

    d. All of the above

28. Ways to debride the suture site include

    a. using light air.

    b. using warm water spray.

    c. Both a. and b.

    d. None of the above

29. It is important for the patient to follow preoperative oral surgery instructions. All of the following are preoperative instructions *except*:

    a. Do not consume alcoholic beverages 24 hours before surgery.

    b. Arrange transportation to and from the office on the day of surgery.

    c. Food and drink can be consumed with no restrictions.

    d. Notify the dentist if a cold, a sore throat, a fever, or another illness develops prior to surgery.

30. Which type of suture is the most widely used?

    a. Sling suture

    b. Simple suture

    c. Continuous simple suture

    d. Mattress suture

31. Surgery to relieve pain and restore range of motion by realigning or reconstructing a joint is called
    a. arthroplasty.
    b. articular eminence recontouring.
    c. arthrocentesis.
    d. arthroscopy.

32. What is the most common complication following a tooth extraction?
    a. Bleeding
    b. Swelling
    c. TMJ disease
    d. Alveolitis

33. What type of implant is surgically placed directly into the bone?
    a. Endosteal
    b. Transosteal
    c. Subperiosteal
    d. Periosteal

34. Which type of imaging technology can aid the surgeon in treating patients with severe trauma?
    a. Panoramic imaging
    b. Cephalometric imaging
    c. Magnetic resonance imaging
    d. 3-Dimensional cone beam imaging

35. Which of the following procedures might an expanded functions dental assistant perform?
    a. Remove sutures
    b. Perform a biopsy
    c. Take and record vital signs
    d. Stabilize the patient's head and mandible during surgery

Matching

Match the elevator type with its use.

Elevator

1. ____ Periosteal
2. ____ Elevator
3. ____ Apical
4. ____ Root tip picks

Use

a. Narrow blades that loosen root or bone fragments
b. Tease root tips or fragments, paired left/right
c. Detaches the periosteum or lifts the mucoperiosteum
d. Single ended, T-shaped handle, useful for varied tasks

Match the oral surgery instrument with the photo of the instrument.

Instrument   **Photo**

a. ___3___ Hemostat   1.

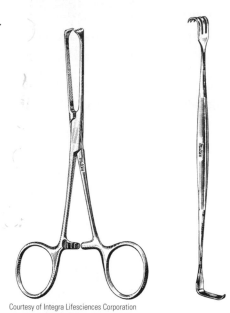

Courtesy of Integra Lifesciences Corporation

b. ___4___ Needle holder   2.

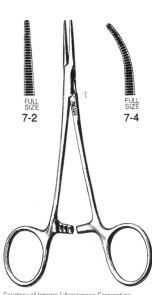

© Cengage Learning 2013

c. ___5___ Surgical curette   3.

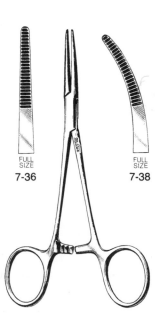

FULL SIZE 7-2   FULL SIZE 7-4   FULL SIZE 7-36   FULL SIZE 7-38

Courtesy of Integra Lifesciences Corporation

d. _2_ Surgical scissors

4.

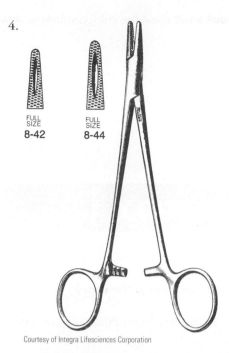

Courtesy of Integra Lifesciences Corporation

e. _1_ Tissue retractors

5.

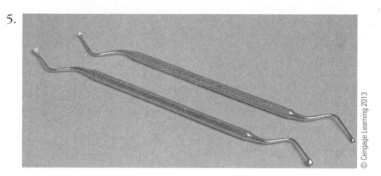

© Cengage Learning 2013

Critical Thinking

1. List four criteria for suture removal.

2. Surgical hand scrubbing has been updated. State what these changes are and state one major difference between general hand washing and surgical hand washing.

3. Describe how the scalpel is used and describe the common scalpel blades and their purposes.

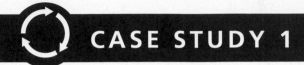

CASE STUDY 1

Donald has had an alveoplasty and the anesthesia is wearing off. He is glad that the dental team sent him home with postoperative instructions and a written appointment date. He was so groggy that he does not remember much of what they had told him at the office.

1. Describe how postoperative home-care instructions are provided.

2. List what to expect following an extraction.

3. List what to do following an extraction.

4. List five activities and substances that are to be avoided following an extraction.

5. If a patient still has questions, who should she or he contact?

6. State the differences, if there are any, between postoperative instructions for a general extraction and postoperative instructions for an implant procedure.

CASE STUDY 2

Dan's dental treatment included an uncomplicated extraction of a mandibular molar. However, a couple of days after the extraction, he called the office complaining of pain. When the dentist sees him and provides a thorough oral exam, the diagnosis is a dry socket.

1. Define dry socket by another name.

2. List the signs of a dry socket.

3. List the causes of a dry socket.

4. What procedural steps are part of treating a dry socket?

CASE STUDY 3

While a college student is studying during finals week, a throbbing pain begins in her jaw. The tissue over the last two molar teeth on the mandible is swollen. The student goes to the student health center and is referred to a dentist. She is in pain and cannot wait to go home to her local dentist. The nurse did indicate the possibility that the cause may be an infected third molar.

1. Are third molar teeth also known as wisdom teeth?

2. To what type of specialist would the general dentist refer patients for third molar extractions?

3. List factors determining the difficulty of a third molar removal.

4. What procedural steps does the dental assistant take as a part of the treatment?

SKILL COMPETENCY ASSESSMENT

25-1 Surgical Scrub

Student's Name _____ Date _____

Instructor's Name _____

Skill: Routine steps should be followed for all treatment areas to maintain absolute clinical asepsis. This procedure is performed by the dentist and the dental assistant before donning sterile gloves for a surgical procedure.

Performance Objective: The student will follow a routine procedure that meets the regulations and protocol set forth by the dentist and regulatory agencies, keeping in mind that assistant duties vary from state to state. However, for oral surgery, the surgical hand scrub is completed before donning sterile gloves.

	Self-Evaluation	Student Evaluation	Possible Points	Instructor Evaluation	Comments
Equipment and Supplies 1. Antimicrobial soap			2		
2. Sterile scrub brush or foam sponge			2		
3. Disposable sterile towels			2		
Competency Steps (*follow aseptic procedures*) 1. Remove watch and rings before the scrub.			2		
2. Use an antimicrobial soap, such as chlorhexidine gluconate.			2		
3. Wet the hands and forearms to the elbows with warm water.			3		
4. Dispense about 5 ml of soap into cupped hands and work into a lather.			2		
5. Beginning with the finger nails, scrub the fingers, hands, and forearms with a surgical scrub brush.			3		
6. Rinse thoroughly with warm water.			2		

	Self-Evaluation	Student Evaluation	Possible Points	Instructor Evaluation	Comments
7. Repeat the procedure with soap but without the scrub brush.			3		
8. Rinse with warm water, beginning at the fingertips and moving the hands and forearms through the water and up so that the water drains off the forearms last.			3		
9. Dry hands and arms thoroughly with disposable sterile towels.			2		
10. Don sterile surgical gloves.			2		
TOTAL POINTS POSSIBLE			30		
TOTAL POINTS POSSIBLE—2nd attempt			28		
TOTAL POINTS EARNED			_____		

Points assigned reflect importance of step to meeting objective: Important = 1, Essential = 2, Critical = 3. Students will lose 2 points for repeated attempts. Failure results if any of the critical steps are omitted or performed incorrectly. If using a 100-point scale, determine score by dividing points earned by total points possible and multiplying the results by 100.

SCORE: _____

SKILL COMPETENCY ASSESSMENT

25-2 Routine or Uncomplicated Extraction

Student's Name _____ Date _____

Instructor's Name _____

Skill: Routine steps should be followed for all treatment areas to maintain absolute clinical asepsis. The dental assistant must be prepared and thinking ahead to anticipate the dentist's needs.

Performance Objective: The student will follow a routine procedure that meets the regulations and protocol set forth by the dentist and regulatory agencies. The dental assistant assists the dentist throughout this procedure. (Assistant duties vary from state to state. Therefore, assistant performance may be evaluated by action, oral/written responses, and/or combined responses and action.)

	Self-Evaluation	Student Evaluation	Possible Points	Instructor Evaluation	Comments
Equipment and Supplies					
1. Mouth mirror and explorer			3		
2. Gauze sponges			2		
3. Surgical HVE tip			2		
4. University of Minnesota retractor for the tongue and cheek			2		
5. Local anesthetic setup			3		
6. Nitrous oxide setup (optional)			3		
7. Periosteal elevator			3		
8. Straight elevator			3		
9. Extraction forceps			3		
10. Surgical rongeurs			3		
11. Hemostat/needle holder			3		
12. Surgical curette			2		
13. Surgical scissors			3		
14. Suture setup			3		

	Self-Evaluation	Student Evaluation	Possible Points	Instructor Evaluation	Comments
Competency Steps (follow aseptic procedures) **Inspection** 1. Mount the patient's x-rays on the view box.			2		
2. Transfer the mirror and explorer to the dentist.			2		
3. Surgeon examines site of extraction.					
Anesthetic 1. Place topical anesthetic on the mucosa (or the assistant prepares the topical anesthetic and transfers it to the dentist).			3		
2. Prepare and pass the syringe to the dentist.					
3. Observe the patient.			3		
Procedure for Elevator (Identification and Use) 1. Pass the periosteal or a straight elevator and state its purpose and use.			3		
2. Receive the elevators.			2		
3. Have gauze ready to remove blood or debris from instruments.			2		
4. Maintain the operating field.			3		
5. Adjust the light.			2		
6. Retract tissues as directed.			3		
Forcep (Identification and Use) 1. Transfer forceps and elevators as needed by the dentist.			3		
2. Explain "luxates" and "subluxates."			2		
3. Keep instruments free of debris.			2		

	Self-Evaluation	Student Evaluation	Possible Points	Instructor Evaluation	Comments
4. Retract the patient's cheek or tongue.			3		
5. Observe the patient for signs of anxiety or syncope.			3		
Extraction Technique 1. Receive forceps with the extracted tooth in palm grasp.			3		
2. Transfer gauze to the dentist.			2		
3. Place the forceps and tooth on the tray for examination of fractured roots.			2		
Postextraction 1. Evacuate the alveolus (socket) with an HVE surgical tip. (The dentist examines the socket.)			2		
2. Pass the surgical curette. Dental assistant continues HVE suctioning.			2		
3. Hold gauze close to the patient's chin to remove debris from the curette.			2		
4. Remove debris from the curette until tooth and root fragments are removed (state why).			2		
5. Pass a folded, moistened gauze as a pressure pack.			2		
6. Instruct the patient to bite down on the gauze to apply pressure (state why).			2		
7. Ready suture materials as needed. Debride area with HVE tip. (Follow Steps 5 and 6 after suture placement.)			3		
8. Check and clean the patient's face.			2		
9. Return the patient to a sitting position.			2		

	Self-Evaluation	Student Evaluation	Possible Points	Instructor Evaluation	Comments
10. Allow a few minutes and then give postoperative instructions.			3		
11. Dismiss the patient.			2		

TOTAL POINTS POSSIBLE   107

TOTAL POINTS POSSIBLE—2nd attempt   105

TOTAL POINTS EARNED   _____

Points assigned reflect importance of step to meeting objective: Important = 1, Essential = 2, Critical = 3. Students will lose 2 points for repeated attempts. Failure results if any of the critical steps are omitted or performed incorrectly. If using a 100-point scale, determine score by dividing points earned by total points possible and multiplying the results by 100.

SCORE: _____

SKILL COMPETENCY ASSESSMENT

25-3 Multiple Extractions and Alveoplasty

Student's Name _____ Date _____

Instructor's Name _____

Skill: Routine steps should be followed for all treatment areas to maintain absolute clinical asepsis. Responsibilities of the dental assistant include evacuation and instrument transfer.

Performance Objective: The student will follow a routine procedure that meets the regulations and the protocol set forth by the dentist and regulatory agencies. The procedure is performed by the dentist, who is assisted by the dental assistant. This sterile procedure involves the removal of several teeth and contouring the bone. The dental assistant must be prepared and be thinking ahead of the dentist. (Assistant duties vary from state to state. Therefore, performance of the tasks below may be evaluated by performance, oral/written responses, and/or combined responses and action.)

	Self-Evaluation	Student Evaluation	Possible Points	Instructor Evaluation	Comments
Equipment and Supplies					
1. Basic setup: mouth mirror, explorer, and cotton pliers			3		
2. Gauze sponges			2		
3. Surgical HVE tip			2		
4. Luer-Lok syringe and sterile saline solution			2		
5. Retractor for the tongue and checks			3		
6. Local anesthetic			3		
7. Nitrous oxide setup (optional)			3		
8. Scalpel and blades			2		
9. Surgical rongeurs			2		
10. Hemostat and tissue retractors			2		
11. Periosteal elevator			3		
12. Straight elevator			3		
13. Extraction forceps (selected for site)			3		
14. Surgical curette			3		

	Self-Evaluation	Student Evaluation	Possible Points	Instructor Evaluation	Comments
15. Root tip picks			3		
16. Bone file			3		
17. Low-speed handpiece and surgical burs			3		
18. Suture setup			3		
Competency Steps **Inspection** 1. Assistant transfers mirror and explorer to the dentist. Teeth are examined for extraction.			2		
Anesthetic 1. Patient may request general anesthesia. Necessary materials are prepared.			3		
2. Intravenous sedation may be required for patient. Necessary materials are prepared.			3		
3. Assistant prepares materials necessary for local anesthetic.			3		
4. Assists in administration of the anesthetic.			3		
Procedure 1. The teeth are removed by the same technique described for routine extraction; root tips and debris are removed.			3		
Alveoplasty begins, one quadrant at a time 2. Assistant passes the scalpel (buccal to lingual, states purpose).			3		
3. Evacuates area as necessary. Maintains operating field. Flap of tissue reflected.			3		
4. Receives the scalpel.			3		
5. Transfers periosteal elevator (states purpose).			3		
6. Uses tissue forceps (states purpose).			3		

	Self-Evaluation	Student Evaluation	Possible Points	Instructor Evaluation	Comments
7. Maintains operating field.			3		
8. Transfers rongeurs (states purpose).			3		
9. Transfers low-speed handpiece with surgical burs.			3		
10. Keeps the rongeurs and burs free of debris.			3		
11. Intermittently uses the HVE and irrigation syringe with sterile saline solution, while final contouring is done with bone file.			3		
12. Maintains the operating field.			3		
13. Continues transfer of instruments as directed (final contouring, plastic stint try-in).			3		
14. Continues to maintain the surgical site, while the dentist continues to contour bone.			3		
15. Between placements, removes blood and debris from the stint. This area must be kept clean.			3		
Suturing 1. Prepares suture materials.			3		
2. Transfers suturing materials.			3		
3. Holds the flaps/tissue while dentist sutures.			3		
4. Prepares moist gauze pack and places over the surgical site or prepares the immediate denture for transfer.			4		
5. Transfers the immediate denture to the dentist.			4		
6. Patient is given recovery time.			2		
7. Postoperative instructions are given to the patient in oral and written forms.			4		

	Self-Evaluation	Student Evaluation	Possible Points	Instructor Evaluation	Comments
8. Patient is scheduled for a postoperative examination and suture removal.			3		

TOTAL POINTS POSSIBLE   133

TOTAL POINTS POSSIBLE—2nd attempt   131

TOTAL POINTS EARNED   _____

Points assigned reflect the importance of the step in meeting the objective: Important = 1, Essential = 2, Critical = 3. Students will lose 2 points for repeated attempts. Failure results if any of the critical steps are omitted or performed incorrectly. If using a 100-point scale, determine score by dividing points earned by total points possible and multiplying the results by 100.

SCORE: _____

SKILL COMPETENCY ASSESSMENT

25-4 Removal of Impacted Third Molars

Student's Name _____ Date _____

Instructor's Name _____

Skill: Routine steps should be followed for all treatment areas to maintain absolute clinical asepsis. This is a sterile procedure. The dental assistant transfers instruments and maintains the operating site.

Performance Objective: The student will follow a routine procedure that meets the regulations and protocol set forth by the dentist and regulatory agencies, keeping in mind that assistant duties vary from state to state. The procedure, removal of impacted third molars, is performed by the dentist. Because the teeth are impacted, the dentist will first have to expose the teeth by incising the tissue and removing the bone. The dental assistant must be prepared and be thinking ahead of the dentist. The assistant may be evaluated by action, verbal/written responses, and/or combined responses and actions.

	Self-Evaluation	Student Evaluation	Possible Points	Instructor Evaluation	Comments
Equipment and Supplies					
1. Basic setup: mouth mirror, explorer, and cotton pliers			3		
2. Gauze sponges			2		
3. Surgical HVE tip			3		
4. Irrigating syringe and sterile saline solution			3		
5. Retractor for the tongue and cheeks			3		
6. Local anesthetic setup			3		
7. Nitrous oxide setup (optional)			3		
8. Scalpel and blades			2		
9. Hemostat and tissue retractors			2		
10. Periosteal elevator			3		
11. Straight elevator			3		
12. Extraction forceps (if needed)			3		
13. Root tip picks			3		
14. Surgical curette			3		

	Self-Evaluation	Student Evaluation	Possible Points	Instructor Evaluation	Comments
15. Rongeurs			3		
16. Bone file			3		
17. Low-speed handpiece and surgical burs			3		
18. Surgical scissors			3		
19. Suture setup			3		
Competency Steps *(follow aseptic procedures)* **Anesthetic**					
1. The patient may request general anesthesia. Prepare the necessary materials.			3		
2. The patient may be required to have intravenous sedation. Prepare the necessary materials.			3		
3. Prepare the materials necessary for local anesthetic.			3		
4. Assist in the administration of the anesthetic.			3		
Procedure (when patient is adequately anesthetized) 1. Pass the scalpel (state the purpose).			3		
2. Maintain the operating field with a surgical HVE.			3		
3. Receive the scalpel.			3		
4. Pass the periosteal elevator. State its purpose. Evacuate.			3		
5. Use the tissue forceps. State its purpose.			3		
6. Receive the periosteal elevator and pass the handpiece and bur or the chisel and mallet. Dental assistant continues to evacuate as needed.			3		
7. Pass elevators and forceps as the operator needs them. State their purpose. Tooth may have to be sectioned.			3		

	Self-Evaluation	Student Evaluation	Possible Points	Instructor Evaluation	Comments
8. Keep the area clear with an HVE tip and periodically pass the dentist new gauze.			3		
9. Remove and examine the tooth to ensure that all of the tooth has been removed.			3		
10. Transfer instruments (curettes, rongeurs, bone file, or burs) and remove debris from the working ends with gauze.			3		
11. Prepare the irrigating syringe with sterile water.			3		
12. Evacuate the site thoroughly. Transfer instruments as needed and remove debris from instrument ends.			3		
Suturing 1. Prepare the suture materials (tissue flap is returned to normal position).			3		
2. Place the suture in the needle holder.			3		
3. Pass the suturing material.			3		
4. Retract the patient's cheeks while the oral surgeon sutures.			3		
5. Prepare the gauze pack (moist, folded, and ready) following suturing.			2		
6. Pass the gauze pack to the dentist.			2		
Postsurgery 1. Stay with the patient during recovery.			3		
2. Escort the patient when the patient is ready to leave. Patient should reschedule appointment in 5 to 7 days for suture removal.			3		
3. Ensure that the patient has necessary prescription(s).			3		

	Self-Evaluation	Student Evaluation	Possible Points	Instructor Evaluation	Comments
4. Give postoperative instructions orally and in writing (ice pack and prescription for pain). Patient scheduled to return in 6 to 7 days.			3		

TOTAL POINTS POSSIBLE   130

TOTAL POINTS POSSIBLE—2nd attempt   128

TOTAL POINTS EARNED   ____

Points assigned reflect importance of step to meeting objective: Important = 1, Essential = 2, Critical = 3. Students will lose 2 points for repeated attempts. Failure results if any of the critical steps are omitted or performed incorrectly. If using a 100-point scale, determine score by dividing points earned by total points possible and multiplying the results by 100.

SCORE: _____

SKILL COMPETENCY ASSESSMENT

25-5 Biopsy

Student's Name _____ Date _____

Instructor's Name _____

Skill: Routine steps should be followed for all treatment areas to maintain absolute clinical asepsis. This is a sterile procedure. The dental assistant readies all materials that are sent to the laboratory, as well as the tray setup.

Performance Objective: The student will follow a routine procedure that meets the regulations and protocol set forth by the dentist and regulatory agencies. The procedure is performed by the dentist, who is assisted by the dental assistant. The dental assistant must be prepared and be thinking ahead of the dentist. (Assistant duties vary from state to state. Therefore, assistant performance may be evaluated by action, verbal/written responses, and/or combined responses and action.)

	Self-Evaluation	Student Evaluation	Possible Points	Instructor Evaluation	Comments
Equipment and Supplies					
1. Mouth mirror			2		
2. Local anesthetic setup			3		
3. Retractors (tongue, cheek, and tissue)			3		
4. Gauze sponges			2		
5. Surgical HVE tip			3		
6. Scalpel and blades			3		
7. Tissue scissors and hemostat			3		
8. Small container with a preservative solution, such as formalin			3		
9. Suture setup			3		
Competency Steps (*follow aseptic procedures*) **Anesthetic**					
1. Prepare the materials necessary for local anesthetic.			3		
2. Assist in administration of the anesthetic.			3		

	Self-Evaluation	Student Evaluation	Possible Points	Instructor Evaluation	Comments
Procedure 1. Transfer the scalpel with the specific blade the surgeon prefers. State the purpose of the scalpel and blade.			3		
2. Maintain the operating field with a surgical HVE ready for use if necessary (State the related warning.)			3		
3. Receive the scalpel.			3		
4. Pass the tissue forceps. State its purpose.			3		
5. Retract the patient's cheeks and tongue.			3		
6. If needed, use gauze to control hemorrhage.			3		
7. Have the specimen container ready for the operator. State its purpose.			3		
8. Once the tissue biopsy has been placed, tightly cap the container.			3		
Suturing Biopsy Site Closed with Sutures 1. Prepare the suture materials while the dentist prepares the biopsy and information for the pathology laboratory.			3		
2. Place the suture in the needle forcep.			3		
3. Transfer the suture needle and thread on the forcep.			3		
4. Retract the patient's cheeks while the oral surgeon sutures.			3		
5. Transfer the suture scissors.			3		
Postsurgery 1. Dismiss the patient and reschedule in one week for suture removal and lab results.			3		

	Self-Evaluation	Student Evaluation	Possible Points	Instructor Evaluation	Comments
2. Give the patient postoperative instructions.			3		
3. Gather pertinent information on the biopsy.			3		
4. Prepare the biopsy container for pick-up by the pathology laboratory.			3		

TOTAL POINTS POSSIBLE 82

TOTAL POINTS POSSIBLE—2nd attempt 80

TOTAL POINTS EARNED _____

Points assigned reflect importance of step to meeting objective: Important = 1, Essential = 2, Critical = 3. Students will lose 2 points for repeated attempts. Failure results if any of the critical steps are omitted or performed incorrectly. If using a 100-point scale, determine score by dividing points earned by total points possible and multiplying the results by 100.

SCORE: _____

SKILL COMPETENCY ASSESSMENT

25-6 Dental Implant Surgery

Student's Name _____ Date _____

Instructor's Name _____

Skill: Routine steps should be followed for all treatment areas to maintain absolute clinical asepsis. This is a sterile procedure. The dental assistant transfers instruments and maintains the operating site.

Performance Objective: The student will follow a routine procedure that meets the regulations and protocol set forth by the dentist and regulatory agencies. The procedure is for placing an endosteal implant for a single tooth replacement. This is a two-stage procedure in which the appointments are scheduled 3 to 4 months apart. During the presurgery appointment, the treatment is explained in detail and the patient signs a written consent for the implant surgery. Radiographs are taken, impressions for the diagnostic cast are made, surgical templates (guides) are fabricated, and financial arrangements are completed. The patient is given intravenous sedation for this procedure. The dental assistant must be prepared and be thinking ahead of the dentist. (Assistant duties vary from state to state. Therefore, assistant performance below may be evaluated by action, verbal/ written responses, and/or combined responses and action.)

	Self-Evaluation	Student Evaluation	Possible Points	Instructor Evaluation	Comments
Equipment and Supplies First Surgical Procedure					
1. Intravenous sedation and local anesthetic setup			3		
2. Mouth mirror			2		
3. Surgical HVE tip			3		
4. Sterile gauze and cotton pellets			3		
5. Irrigating syringe and sterile saline solution			3		
6. Low-speed handpiece			3		
7. Sterile template			3		
8. Sterile surgical drilling unit			3		
9. Scalpel and blades			3		
10. Periosteal elevator			3		
11. Rongeurs			3		
12. Surgical curette			3		

	Self-Evaluation	Student Evaluation	Possible Points	Instructor Evaluation	Comments
13, Tissue forceps and scissors			3		
14. Cheek and tongue retractors			3		
15. Hemostat			3		
16. Bite-block			3		
17. Oral rinse			3		
18. Betadine			3		
19. Implant instrument kit			3		
20. Implant kit			3		
21. Suture setup			3		
Second Surgical Procedure 1. Items 1–7 from the first procedure			3		
2. Electrosurgical (cautery) unit and tips			3		
3. Hydrogen peroxide			2		
Competency Steps (*follow aseptic procedures*) **First Surgery for Endosteal Implants** **Anesthetic** 1. Prepare patient for IV sedation.			3		
2. Administer intravenous sedation.			3		
3. Prepare the materials necessary for local anesthetic.			3		
4. Assist in the administration of sedation and the anesthetic.			3		
Procedure 1. Pass the surgical template to the surgeon. State its purpose. Seat the template in the patient's mouth, with the target marked in soft tissue.			3		
2. Remove the template. Prepare the scalpel and blade.			3		

	Self-Evaluation	Student Evaluation	Possible Points	Instructor Evaluation	Comments
3. Transfer the scalpel and blade while maintaining the field of operation. State purpose of scalpel and blade.			3		
4. Transfer the periosteal elevator. State its purpose.			3		
5. Change burs as size increases. State their purpose.			3		
6. Irrigate with sterile saline as directed.			3		
7. Open the sterile implant and transfer it to the operator.			3		
8. Transfer a special inserting mallet or ratchet wrench.			3		
9. Ready the healing cap and the contra-angle screwdriver.			3		
10. Transfer the healing cap and the contra-angle screwdriver. Once the implant and healing cap are positioned, the flap is repositioned and sutured.			3		
Suturing 1. Prepare the suture materials.			3		
2. Place the suture in the needle holder.			3		
3. Transfer the suturing material.			3		
4. Retract the patient's cheeks while the surgeon sutures.			3		
5. Prepare the gauze pack (moist, folded, and ready) following suturing.			2		
6. Pass the gauze pack to the dentist.			2		
Postsurgery 1. Stay with the patient during recovery.			3		
2. Escort the patient when the patient is ready to leave.			3		

	Self-Evaluation	Student Evaluation	Possible Points	Instructor Evaluation	Comments
3. Give postoperative instructions orally and in writing.			3		
Second Surgical Procedure **Anesthetic** 1. Prepare the materials necessary for local anesthetic.			3		
2. Assist in the administration of the anesthetic.			3		
Procedure 1. Transfer the sterile template and sharp pointed instruments. State purpose.			3		
2. Receive the template.			3		
3. Evacuate as the electrosurgical loop is used.			3		
4. Once the tissue is excised, receive the healing screw in a gauze sponge.			3		
5. Prepare a cotton pellet and transfer it to the surgeon. Hydrogen peroxide is used on pellet.			3		
6. Transfer an abutment to the surgeon.			3		
Suturing 1. Prepare the suture material.			3		
2. Assist the surgeon during suturing.			3		
3. Give postoperative instructions and dismiss the patient.			2		

TOTAL POINTS POSSIBLE   169

TOTAL POINTS POSSIBLE—2nd attempt   167

TOTAL POINTS EARNED   ____

Points assigned reflect importance of step to meeting objective: Important = 1, Essential = 2, Critical = 3. Students will lose 2 points for repeated attempts. Failure results if any of the critical steps are omitted or performed incorrectly. If using a 100-point scale, determine score by dividing points earned by total points possible and multiplying the results by 100.

SCORE: _____

SKILL COMPETENCY ASSESSMENT

25-7 Treatment for Alveolitis

Student's Name _____ Date _____

Instructor's Name _____

Skill: Routine steps should be followed for all treatment areas to maintain absolute clinical asepsis. This is a sterile procedure. The dental assistant readies all materials as well as the tray setup.

Performance Objective: The student will follow a routine procedure that meets the regulations and protocol set forth by the dentist and regulatory agencies, keeping in mind that assistant duties vary from state to state. The assistant may be evaluated by action, verbal/written responses, and/or combined responses and action.

	Self-Evaluation	Student Evaluation	Possible Points	Instructor Evaluation	Comments
Equipment and Supplies 1. Mouth mirror			3		
2. Surgical HVE tip			3		
3. Local anesthetic setup (may be required)			3		
4. Surgical scissors			3		
5. Surgical curettes			3		
6. Irrigating syringe and warm sterile saline solution			3		
7. Iodoform gauze or sponge			3		
Competency Steps (*follow aseptic procedures*) **Anesthetic** 1. Prepare the materials, if necessary, for local anesthetic.			3		
2. Assist in the administration of the anesthetic.			3		
Procedure 1. Pass the suture scissors.			3		
2. Pass the surgical curette. State purpose.			3		
3. Prepare the irrigating syringe.			3		

	Self-Evaluation	Student Evaluation	Possible Points	Instructor Evaluation	Comments
4. Maintain the site area by retraction and suction.			3		
5. Prepare the medicated dressing. State preparation.			3		
6. Pass the dressing for surgeon to place.			3		
7. Give postoperative instructions (this includes doctor's prescription for pain control).			3		
8. Arrange for the patient to return in 1 to 2 days to repeat the above process.			3		

TOTAL POINTS POSSIBLE   51

TOTAL POINTS POSSIBLE—2nd attempt   49

TOTAL POINTS EARNED   ————

Points assigned reflect importance of step to meeting objective: Important = 1, Essential = 2, Critical = 3-Students will lose 2 points for repeated attempts. Failure results if any of the critical steps are omitted or performed incorrectly. If using a 100-point scale, determine score by dividing points earned by total points possible and multiplying the results by 100.

SCORE: ——————

SKILL COMPETENCY ASSESSMENT

25-8 Removal of Simple and Continuous Simple Sutures

Student's Name _____ Date _____

Instructor's Name _____

Skill: Routine steps should be followed for all treatment areas to maintain absolute clinical asepsis. This procedure is performed by the dentist and/or the expanded-function dental assistant. The patient returns to the office for suture removal. The dental assistant prepares the materials needed and the patient before beginning the procedure.

Performance Objective: The student will follow a routine procedure that meets the regulations and the protocol set forth by the dentist and regulatory agencies.

	Self-Evaluation	Student Evaluation	Possible Points	Instructor Evaluation	Comments
Equipment and Supplies					
1. Basic setup: mouth mirror, explorer, cotton pliers			3		
2. Suture scissors			3		
3. Hemostat			2		
4. Gauze sponges			2		
5. Air-water syringe tip, HVE tip			2		
Competency Steps (*follow aseptic procedures*) **Removal of Simple Sutures** 1. Prepare the materials, if necessary, for local anesthetic.			2		
2. Take the suture scissors and cut the thread below the knot, close to the tissue.			3		
3. Secure the knot with the cotton pliers and gently pull, lifting the suture out of the tissues.			3		
4. Place the suture on a gauze sponge.			2		

	Self-Evaluation	Student Evaluation	Possible Points	Instructor Evaluation	Comments
Removal of Continuous Simple Sutures 5. Cut each suture and remove individually.			3		
6. Loosen the suture with the cotton pliers, and while still holding the suture thread with the cotton pliers, cut the thread close to the tissue.			3		
7. As each suture is removed, place on a gauze sponge so that it can be counted when finished.			3		
TOTAL POINTS POSSIBLE			31		
TOTAL POINTS POSSIBLE—2nd attempt			29		
TOTAL POINTS EARNED			____		

Points assigned reflect the importance of the step in meeting the objective: Important = 1, Essential = 2, Critical = 3. Students will lose 2 points for repeated attempts. Failure results if any of the critical steps are omitted or performed incorrectly. If using a 100-point scale, determine score by dividing points earned by total points possible and multiplying the results by 100.

SCORE: _____

SKILL COMPETENCY ASSESSMENT

25-9 Removal of Sling and Continuous Sling Sutures

Student's Name _____ Date _____

Instructor's Name _____

Skill: Routine steps should be followed for all treatment areas to maintain absolute clinical asepsis. This procedure is performed by the dentist and/or the expanded-function dental assistant. The patient returns to the office for suture removal. The dental assistant prepares the materials needed and the patient before beginning the procedure.

Performance Objective: The student will follow a routine procedure that meets the regulations and the protocol set forth by the dentist and regulatory agencies.

	Self-Evaluation	Student Evaluation	Possible Points	Instructor Evaluation	Comments
Equipment and Supplies					
1. Suture scissors			3		
2. Cotton pliers			2		
3. Gauze sponges			2		
Competency Steps (*follow aseptic procedures*)					
1. Cut sling suture in two places.			2		
2. With cotton pliers, gently lift the suture on each side of the tooth to loosen the suture from the tissue.			2		
3. Lift suture thread on the other side of tooth near the tissue, and cut it as close to tissue as possible without cutting the tissue.			3		
4. Using cotton pliers, remove each thread carefully, pulling toward the opposite side, away from the flap.			2		
5. Place each thread of the suture on a gauze sponge to be counted.			3		

	Self-Evaluation	Student Evaluation	Possible Points	Instructor Evaluation	Comments
6. Examine the suture site.			2		

TOTAL POINTS POSSIBLE   21

TOTAL POINTS POSSIBLE—2nd attempt   19

TOTAL POINTS EARNED   ____

Points assigned reflect the importance of the step in meeting the objective: Important = 1, Essential = 2, Critical = 3. Students will lose 2 points for repeated attempts. Failure results if any of the critical steps are omitted or performed incorrectly. If using a 100-point scale, determine score by dividing points earned by total points possible and multiplying the results by 100.

SCORE: _____

SKILL COMPETENCY ASSESSMENT

25-10 Removal of Horizontal and Vertical Mattress Sutures

Student's Name _____ Date _____

Instructor's Name _____

Skill: Routine steps should be followed for all treatment areas to maintain absolute clinical asepsis. This procedure is performed by the dentist and/or the expanded-function dental assistant. The patient returns to the office for suture removal. The dental assistant prepares the materials needed and the patient before beginning the procedure.

Performance Objective: The student will follow a routine procedure that meets the regulations and the protocol set forth by the dentist and regulatory agencies.

	Self-Evaluation	Student Evaluation	Possible Points	Instructor Evaluation	Comments
Equipment and Supplies 1. Suture scissors			3		
2. Cotton pliers			2		
3. Gauze sponges			2		
Competency Steps (follow aseptic procedures) 1. Gently lift the knot with cotton pliers.			2		
2. Cut the suture below the knot, close to the tissue.			2		
3. Make the second cut on the opposite surface close to the tissue.			3		
4. Remove one piece of the suture by holding the knot with the cotton pliers, lifting gently. Remove remaining suture thread.			2		
5. Place each thread of the suture on a gauze sponge to be counted.			3		

	Self-Evaluation	Student Evaluation	Possible Points	Instructor Evaluation	Comments
6. Examine the suture site.			2		

TOTAL POINTS POSSIBLE 21

TOTAL POINTS POSSIBLE—2nd attempt 19

TOTAL POINTS EARNED _____

Points assigned reflect the importance of the step in meeting the objective: Important = 1, Essential = 2, Critical = 3. Students will lose 2 points for repeated attempts. Failure results if any of the critical steps are omitted or performed incorrectly. If using a 100-point scale, determine score by dividing points earned by total points possible and multiplying the results by 100.

SCORE: _____

CHAPTER 26

100%

Oral Pathology

SPECIFIC INSTRUCTIONAL OBJECTIVES

The student should strive to meet the following objectives and demonstrate an understanding of the facts and principles presented in this chapter:

1. Define oral pathology and identify the dental assistant's role in this specialty.

2. Characterize the process of inflammation.

3. Identify oral lesions according to placement.

4. Identify oral diseases and lesions related to biological agents.

5. Describe oral diseases and lesions related to physical agents.

6. Identify oral diseases and lesions related to chemical agents.

7. Identify oral conditions related to hormonal disturbances.

8. Identify oral conditions related to developmental disturbances.

9. Distinguish among oral conditions related to nutritional deficiencies.

10. Identify the conditions and the lesions of oral neoplasms.

11. Identify oral lesions related to HIV and AIDS.

12. Describe the conditions related to miscellaneous disorders affecting the oral cavity.

SUMMARY

The dental assistant, who sits opposite the dentist, has a different view of the patient's oral cavity. Anything that appears atypical should be brought to the dentist's attention, without alarming the patient.

The dental assistant does not diagnose oral pathological diseases but identifies abnormal conditions in the mouth. Further, the dental assistant must know how to prevent disease transmission, how the identified pathological condition may interfere with planned treatment, and what effect it will have on the overall health of the patient.

EXERCISES AND ACTIVITIES

Multiple Choice

1. Which disturbances will also show disease signs in the mouth?

   a. Hormonal

   b. Developmental

   c. Nutritional

   d. All of the above

2. An all-encompassing term for an abnormal structure in the oral cavity is

   a. plaque.

   b. histamine.

   c. antigen.

   d. lesion.

3. _____ is the surgical removal of a small amount of the suspicious lesion tissue.

   a. Etiology

   b. Biopsy

   c. Orifice

   d. Ankylosis

4. Which lesion is caused by bleeding from a ruptured blood vessel during an injection of oral anesthetic?

   a. Cyst

   b. Blister

   c. Hematoma

   d. Nodule

5. _____ is said to bring about inflammation.

   a. Etiology

   b. Histamine

   c. Antigenic

   d. Papule

6. Which of the following are diagnostic tools used to evaluate oral pathology?

   a. Radiographs

   b. Clinical diagnosis

   c. Genetic history

   d. All of the above

7. The dentist reads the radiographs to note which of the following?

   a. Absorption

   b. Cysts

   c. Abscesses

   d. All of the above

8. All of the following are included in the clinical diagnosis performed by the dentist *except*

   a. whether absorption is present.

   b. the location of the pathology.

   c. the size of the pathology.

   d. the shape of the pathology.

9. When a disease or disorder has no known cause, it is called

   a. therapeutic.

   b. idiopathic.

   c. differential.

   d. bulla.

10. At what stage can adults unknowingly pass the herpetic gingivostomatitis virus to children?

    a. During the onset

    b. During the vesicular stage

    c. During the crusted stage

    d. All of the above

11. Dental assistants must take care with patients who have herpes. Which of the following should the dental assistant avoid?

    a. Stretching the lesion

    b. Pulling the lesion

    c. Cross-contamination

    d. All of the above

12. In the second stage of syphilis, _____ occur(s).

    a. flu-like symptoms

    b. the emergence of lesions and mucous patches

    c. split papule

    d. All of the above

13. Which of the following is (are) included in the final stage of syphilis?

    a. Tertiary stage
    b. Third stage
    c. Gumma lesion
    d. All of the above

14. Which of the following lesions is associated with chronic inflammation and appears as a neoplasm filled with granulation tissue?

    a. Ecchymosis
    b. Granuloma
    c. Nodule
    d. Purpura

15. _____ is a bacterial infection that first causes painful swelling and later causes pus and yellow granule discharges.

    a. Herpes simplex
    b. Actinomycosis
    c. Herpes labialis
    d. Aphthous ulcer

16. The virus responsible for herpes simplex, which is transmitted through physical contact and is typically seen in children around the age of six, is called

    a. actinomycosis.
    b. herpes labialis.
    c. herpes zoster.
    d. herpetic gingivostomatitis.

17. Which herpetic virus can cause a crusting ulceration on the fingers, hands, or eyes that is extremely painful?

    a. Herpes labialis
    b. Herpes zoster
    c. Aphthous ulcer
    d. Herpetic whitlow

18. _____ appear(s) as painful lesions that can last up to 5 weeks; patients with HIV are predisposed to it.

    a. Canker sores
    b. Herpes simplex
    c. Herpes labialis
    d. Herpes zoster

19. Which bacterial disease has three primary stages, with bone and cartilage being destroyed in the final stage?

    a. Hutchinson's
    b. Mulberry
    c. Syphilis
    d. Thrush

20. An ill-fitting denture can cause small ulcers that, after continued irritation, become folds of excess tissue called

    a. hypoplasia.
    b. hyperplasia.
    c. thrush.
    d. granuloma.

21. The heat and the irritating effect of chemicals in tobacco can cause areas of tissue to first turn red. If the irritation continues, the epithelium tissue builds a layer of keratin as a protective coating. This tissue area is described as

    a. nicotine stomatitis.
    b. hyperkeratinized.
    c. hypokeratinized.
    d. aspirin burn.

22. The openings of the salivary glands are called

    a. infections.
    b. orifices.
    c. apexes.
    d. granulomas.

23. Numerous light yellow lesions are sometimes found in the oral cavity, most often on the buccal mucosa. These round lesions, which are sebaceous oil glands near the surface of the epithelium, are called

    a. exostoses.
    b. angular cheilitis.
    c. Fordyce's spots.
    d. dysplasic cells.

24. Which developmental disturbance appears as a wrinkled, deeply grooved surface on the tongue? It may be symmetrical or irregular in pattern.

    a. Fissured tongue

    b. Ankyloglossia

    c. Black hairy tongue

    d. Bifid tongue

25. Which of the following conditions is a result of a vitamin B complex deficiency and will form a lesion in the corner of the mouth?

    a. Herpes labialis

    b. Herpetic zoster

    c. Angular cheilitis

    d. Candida albicans

26. When a patient loses vertical dimensions of the face, saliva can pool in the corners of the mouth, and a fungal infection called _____ can occur.

    a. herpes labialis.

    b. herpes zoster.

    c. Candida albicans.

    d. angular cheilitis.

27. When an individual's immune system is depressed, it can be overcome by _____ infections such as herpes, hepatitis, tuberculosis, candidiasis, and pneumonia.

    a. innocuous

    b. opportunistic

    c. hormonal

    d. chemical

28. Which of the following lesions, according to its placement in the surface of the oral mucosa, is classified as above the surface?

    a. Cyst

    b. Ecchymosis

    c. Nodule

    d. Blister

29. A hematoma lesion is classified as

    a. above the surface of the oral mucosa.

    b. below the surface of the oral mucosa.

    c. even with the surface of the oral mucosa.

    d. flat with the surface of the oral mucosa.

30. Which of the following lesions is classified as below the surface of the oral mucosa?

    a. Bulla

    b. Pustule

    c. Abscess

    d. Granuloma

31. A macule lesion is

    a. a medical term for bruising of the tissue.

    b. a spot of different texture or color on the skin.

    c. small spots colored red or purple.

    d. caused by bleeding in underlying tissues.

32. Which four conditions are essential parts of the body's response to injury or disease?

    1. Biological agents
    2. Redness (erythema)
    3. Chemical agents
    4. Heat
    5. Swelling (edema)
    6. Hormonal agents
    7. Pain
    8. Physical agents

    a. 1, 4, 5, 8

    b. 1, 2, 3, 6

    c. 2, 4, 5, 7

    d. 2, 3, 4, 6

33. Which of the following lesions can be classified as flat or above the surface of the oral mucosa?

  1. Granuloma
  2. Petechiae
  3. Purpura
  4. Bulla
  5. Blister
  6. Neoplasm
  7. Plaque
  8. Nodule

  a. 2, 3, 5   c. 2, 3, 4
  b. 1, 6, 8   d. 6, 7, 8

34. Canker sores are associated with which of the following?

  1. Abscesses
  2. Heredity
  3. Trauma
  4. Plaque
  5. Stress
  6. Food allergens
  7. Hormonal changes
  8. Hematomas

  a. 1, 2, 4, 5, 8   c. 2, 3, 4, 7, 8
  b. 2, 3, 5, 6, 7   d. 1, 2, 3, 6, 7

35. A bulla is a large (greater than one-half inch in diameter), fluid-filled blister

  a. above the surface of the oral mucosa.   c. below the surface of the oral mucosa.
  b. flat with the surface of the oral mucosa. d. that is not found on the oral mucosa.

36. A papule (a type of lesion), whose surface may be pigmented in color and either smooth or warty in texture, is

  a. flat with the surface of the oral mucosa. c. below the surface of the oral mucosa.
  b. above the surface of the oral mucosa.   d. not found on the oral mucosa.

37. Ecchymosis, a medical term for bruising of the tissue, is

  a. even or flat with the surface of the oral mucosa. c. below the surface of the oral mucosa.
  b. above the surface of the oral mucosa.   d. not found on the oral mucosa.

38. Which virus is responsible for cold sores (painful blisters around the mouth that are commonly called fever blisters)?

  a. Aphthous ulcer   c. Stomatitis
  b. Herpes simplex   d. Cheilitis

39. An obturator is constructed to treat which of the following developmental disturbances?

  a. Cleft lip   c. Ankylosis
  b. Cleft palate   d. Anodontia

40. Teeth that are present at the time of birth or within the first month after birth are called

  a. microdontia.   c. supernumerary teeth.
  b. neonatal teeth.   d. anodontia.

Matching

Match the following term with its definition.

Term		Definition
1. ___ Papule		a. Capable of causing production of an antibody
2. ___ Plaque		b. Small, pus-containing blister
3. ___ Pustule		c. Small in diameter, solid, raised area of the skin
4. ___ Antigenic		d. Solid raised or flat patch in the oral mucosa

Critical Thinking

1. A dental assistant does not diagnose, but may alert the dentist to, abnormal conditions in the mouth. After an injection, what should the dental assistant monitor the injection site for? What is the cause?

2. Dental assistants must exert extreme care while working with patients who have herpes. Enumerate some protective measures.

3. The number of people who are seeking oral piercing is on the rise. In the dental office, various dental treatments may require the removal of oral cavity jewelry. List areas of the oral cavity where an oral piercing may be placed, and describe one of the most serious side effects of piercing.

 CASE STUDY 1

The dental assistant has a different viewpoint on the patient oral's cavity. Therefore, anything that appears atypical should be brought to the attention of the dentist.

1. List three different agents or disturbances that cause oral pathology.

2. Enumerate recognizable disease symptoms in the mouth.

3. List three disorders or reactions that can affect the oral cavity.

4. Describe oral pathology conditions of the mouth.

CASE STUDY 2

Oral structures must be closely observed. When a dental assistant believes that something is atypical in the patient's oral cavity, the dentist evaluates that area as well.

1. Explain the purpose of observing lesions.

2. Describe how the dentist examines a lesion.

3. Explain the biopsy procedure. What evidence will the biopsy provide?

4. Define etiology.

CASE STUDY 3

The dentist may use several diagnostic tools to identify oral pathology, including radiographs. The dental assistant takes radiographs, and the quality of these x-rays is an integral part of the evaluation process.

1. Explain other diagnostic tools that may be used to check for oral pathology.

2. Describe the use of radiographs in identifying oral pathology and what may be visualized on the radiograph.

3. Identify the clinical steps the dentist will use to assess the patient.

4. Explain additional diagnostic methods for assessing a patient's oral pathology.

CHAPTER 27

Orthodontics

SPECIFIC INSTRUCTIONAL OBJECTIVES

The student should strive to meet the following objectives and demonstrate an understanding of the facts and principles presented in this chapter:

1. Define orthodontics and describe the orthodontic setting.

2. Define the role of the dental assistant in an orthodontic setting.

3. Define and describe occlusion and malocclusion.

4. Identify the causes of malocclusion.

5. Describe preventive, interceptive, and corrective orthodontics.

6. Explain the process of tooth movement.

7. Describe the preorthodontic appointment for diagnostic records.

8. Describe the consultation appointment and the roles of the assistant, patient, and orthodontist.

9. Differentiate between fixed and removable appliances.

10. Identify and describe the function of basic orthodontic instruments.

11. Describe the stages of orthodontic treatment.

12. Explain the procedure for removing orthodontic appliances and how the teeth are kept in position after appliance removal.

SUMMARY

Orthodontics is an exciting specialty that provides many opportunities for the dental assistant. Depending on the size of the practice and the number of auxiliaries, the assistant assists the dentist, performs many chairside skills independently, motivates patients, provides oral hygiene instruction, does laboratory tasks, and may work with the orthodontist during case presentations/consultations.

The chapter covers the various appointments needed for orthodontic treatment, the materials and instruments used, and types of orthodontic appliances most commonly used. Each state regulates the education and the skills the dental assistant may perform directly and indirectly on the orthodontic patient. To become a certified orthodontic assistant, the assistant must pass a specialty examination administered by the Dental Assistant National Board and/or the individual state board of dentistry.

EXERCISES AND ACTIVITIES

Multiple Choice

1. Which dental specialty deals with the recognition, prevention, and treatment of malalignment and irregularities of the teeth, jaws, and face?

   a. Endodontics

   b. Radiology

   c. Oral pathology

   d. Orthodontics

2. The orthodontic team consists of the

   a. dentist.

   b. receptionist and business staff.

   c. assistant.

   d. laboratory technician.

   e. All of the above

3. Which orthodontic team member may pour and trim diagnostic models and construct orthodontic appliances?

   a. Laboratory technician

   b. Orthodontic assistant

   c. Office coordinator

   d. Business office staff

4. Which of the following is an ideal occlusion relationship?

   a. Transversion of one tooth

   b. Labioversion or buccoversion toward the lip

   c. Maxillary and mandibular teeth are in maximum contact and normally spaced

   d. Infraversion in the arch

5. The established system for classifying malocclusion is called (the) _____ classification.

   a. transversion

   b. Angle's

   c. Pasteur's

   d. interceptive

6. _____ is considered a common preventive or interceptive treatment.

   a. Treatment of adults

   b. Treatment of children in the last stage of mixed dentition

   c. Treatment of children entering full permanent dentition

   d. Extraction of teeth to prevent overcrowding

7. Which of the following common treatments fall under corrective orthodontics?

   a. Braces

   b. Bands

   c. Retainers

   d. All of the above

8. The process that allows teeth to be moved by eliminating tissue no longer needed by the body is called

   a. deposition.

   b. resorption.

   c. buccoversion.

   d. linguoversion.

9. _____ is (are) an example of a fixed orthodontic appliance.

   a. A retainer

   b. An activator

   c. Braces

   d. Headgear

10. Which fixed appliance is either welded to the bands or bonded directly to the teeth?

    a. Band

    b. Bracket

    c. Buccal tube

    d. Ligature wire

11. The function of (the) _____ is to apply force to move the teeth into or to hold the teeth in the desired positions.

    a. buccal tubes

    b. bracket

    c. arch wire

    d. springs

12. The _____ wraps around the bracket and is tightened by twisting.

    a. arch wire

    b. ligature wire

    c. spring

    d. separator

13. _____ are attached to hooks/buttons that are secured on the band/brackets.

    a. Springs

    b. Tooth positioners

    c. Elastic separators

    d. Elastics

14. After the premature loss of a primary tooth, which special fixed appliance is worn to maintain a space for the permanent tooth?

    a. Bracket

    b. Space maintainer

    c. Headgear

    d. Activator

15. Which removable appliance, usually worn for a specific number of hours each day, is used to apply force to move teeth, restrain or alter cranial-facial bone growth, and reinforce the stability of intraoral appliances?

    a. Space maintainer

    b. Headgear

    c. Activator

    d. Tooth positioner

16. Normal occlusion is a general term that includes the following:

    1. Mandibular teeth are in maximum contact with maxillary teeth.

    2. Teeth are slightly rotated and turned.

    3. Teeth are mesial to normal position.

    4. Anterior teeth overlap by 2 mm maxillary to mandibular.

    a. 1, 2, 3, 4

    b. 2, 3

    c. 1, 4

    d. 4, 2

17. The etiology of malocclusion can fall into one of three categories: genetic, systemic, or local. For which of the following might genetic factors be responsible?

    1. Systemic diseases

    2. Trauma

    3. Palatal clefts

    4. Supernumerary teeth

    5. Thumb sucking

    6. Nutritional disturbances

    a. 1, 2

    b. 3, 4

    c. 5, 6

    d. 3, 6

18. _____ means that the tooth is distal to normal position.

    a. Linguoversion

    b. Distoversion

    c. Mesioversion

    d. Infraversion

19. _____ means that the tooth is tipped toward the lip or cheek.

    a. Torsoversion

    b. Labioversion

    c. Transversion

    d. Linguoversion

20. _____ causes of malocclusion include systemic diseases and nutritional disturbances that upset the normal schedule of dentition development during infancy and early childhood.

   a. Local factor

   b. Systemic factor

   c. Developmental factor

   d. Environmental factor

21. The teeth are retained in position through the process of _____, which creates and deposits new cells.

   a. resorption

   b. deposition

   c. transposition

   d. disposition

22. _____ are placed in the contact areas between the teeth, forcing the teeth to spread to accommodate the orthodontic bands.

   a. Separators

   b. Plastic rings

   c. Brackets

   d. Springs

23. A(n) _____ is an abnormal relationship of a tooth or a group of teeth in one arch to the opposing teeth in the other arch.

   a. underjet

   b. cross-bite

   c. overjet

   d. open bite

24. When the vertical overlap of the maxillary teeth is greater than the incisal one-third of the mandibular anterior teeth, this is termed a(n)

   a. overjet.

   b. overbite.

   c. underjet

   d. cross-bite

25. An abnormal horizontal distance between the labial surface of the mandibular anterior teeth and the lingual surface of the maxillary anterior teeth is called a(an)

   a. overjet.

   b. overbite.

   c. open bite.

   d. cross-bite.

26. Which of the following is not considered a removable appliance?

   a. Headgear

   b. Palatal expansion appliance

   c. Retainer

   d. Activator

27. Name the appliance that is used to position the lower jaw forward and is used to encourage lower jaw growth.

   a. Herbst

   b. Frankel

   c. Bionator

   d. Angle

28. Which type of imaging has allowed orthodontists to provide treatment without the need to create study models?

   a. Magnetic resonance imaging

   b. Three-dimensional imaging

   c. Panoramic imaging

   d. Cephalometric imaging

29. Who invented the self-ligating bracket?

   a. Damon

   b. Angle

   c. Frankel

   d. Herbst

30. Which type of wire is most often used toward the end of treatment, when more control of tooth movement is needed?

   a. Beta-titanium

   b. Nickel-titanium

   c. Gold

   d. Stainless steel

Matching

Match the commonly used orthodontic instrument with its function.

1. _____ *c* Howe pliers
2. _____ *b* "Bird-beak" pliers
3. _____ *a* Three-prong pliers
4. _____ *d* Tweed loop pliers

a. Adjusts and bends wire *3*
b. Adjusts and bends clasps *2*
c. Utility plier *1*
d. Forms loops and springs *4*

Match the instrument in the photo with the proper name of the instrument.

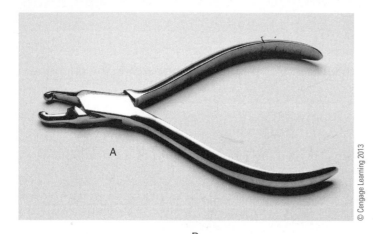

A

B

1. Pin and ligature cutter _____ *Band-contour pliers*

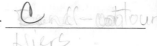

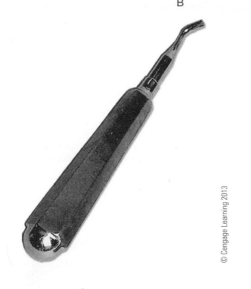

C

2. Posterior-band removing pliers _____ *band arm*

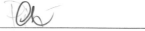

3. Band-contour pliers _____

4. Band driver (pusher) _____ b. _____

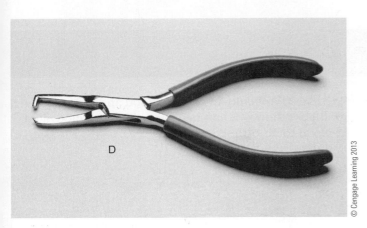

D

© Cengage Learning 2013

Critical Thinking

1. When reviewing job opportunities in the classifieds, Lila discovered that an orthodontic office was look-ing for a dental assistant. Name five intraoral tasks and five supportive tasks that an orthodontic assistant would likely perform.

2. Being efficient means that the assistant is ready to perform specific tasks in the orthodontic treatment se-quence. Name the steps in the orthodontic treatment sequence.

3. The orthodontic assistant must have knowledge and skills to prepare and manipulate various cements used in the band cementation procedure. Name some of these cements.

CASE STUDY 1

As a child Lynwood struggled with an overbite; he experienced difficulty in chewing food and kids teasing him. Now an adult, he is concerned about his facial profile for the work that he does, which has motivated him to seek help. The general dentist has referred Lynwood to an orthodontist.

1. Describe an overbite versus an overjet.

2. Enumerate what the clinical examination will consist of.

3. List the types of radiographs, what they will show, and how they might be used in the evaluation.

4. Explain what occurs during a consultation appointment.

CASE STUDY 2

The family of Cameron, age 5, has consulted with their general dentist for evaluation. The dentist's evaluation indicates that Cameron is losing his deciduous teeth to decay which leaves a space before the permanent dentition erupts. He is in a mixed dentition stage with the anterior teeth and when the permanent teeth erupt they are coming in lingually and are causing crowding. The dentist has referred Cameron to see an orthodontist for consultation.

1. Describe the process of preventive/interceptive orthodontics.

2. Provide the principles of maintaining space.

3. What is the main function of space maintainers?

Labeling

Label the instruments on the tray used for the placement and removal of elastic separators procedure.

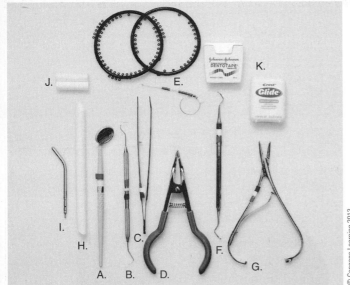

A. _____

B. _____

C. _____

D. _____

E. _____

F. _____

G. _____

H. _____

I. _____

J. _____

K. _____

SKILL COMPETENCY ASSESSMENT

27-1 Placement and Removal of Elastic Separators

Student's Name _____ Date _____

Instructor's Name _____

Skill: Routine steps should be followed for all treatment areas to maintain absolute clinical asepsis. The dental assistant must be prepared and thinking ahead to anticipate the dentist's needs. Elastic separators are small circular elastics that are stretched for placement. They fit around the contact area and, when released, apply constant pressure until the teeth move apart. The dental assistant may be permitted, in some states, to place and remove these separators.

Performance Objective: The student will follow a routine procedure that meets the regulations and protocol set forth by the dentist and regulatory agencies, keeping in mind that assistant duties vary from state to state. The assistant may be evaluated by actions, verbal/written responses, and/or combined responses and actions. After the diagnosis, the first treatment appointment is to place separators to prepare the teeth for the orthodontic bands. At the dentist's directions, the expanded-function assistant places the separators. The patient is scheduled to have the separators removed and the bands placed several days later.

	Self-Evaluation	Student Evaluation	Possible Points	Instructor Evaluation	Comments
Equipment and Supplies					
1. Basic setup: mouth mirror, explorer, and cotton pliers			3		
2. Separation pliers			3		
3. Separators (wire or elastic)			3		
4. Dental floss or tape (optional technique)			2		
5. Scaler			3		
Competency Steps (*follow aseptic procedures*) **Placement of Elastic Separators with Separating Pliers** 1. Examine the patient's mouth using the mouth mirror.			3		
2. Place the elastic separator over the beaks of the separating pliers.			3		
3. Squeeze the pliers to secure the elastic on the pliers.			3		

	Self-Evaluation	Student Evaluation	Possible Points	Instructor Evaluation	Comments
4. Further squeeze the pliers to stretch the elastic separator.			3		
5. Place the elastic between two teeth in a back-and-forth motion (similar to flossing).			3		
6. Insert one side of the elastic band below the contact in the interproximal space.			3		
7. Release the tension on the separating pliers.			3		
8. Remove the pliers.			3		
9. Repeat the process on all interproximal spaces around the teeth to receive the metal bands.			3		
Placement of Separators with Dental Floss 1. Place two lengths of dental floss through an elastic separator.			3		
2. Fold over each floss length until the ends meet.			3		
3. Pull each piece of floss by the ends to stretch the elastic.			3		
4. Using a back-and-forth motion, insert the separator.			3		
5. Once the separator is in place, release the floss and pull free.			3		
Removal of Elastic Separators 1. Using a scaler or explorer, insert one end into the ring of the elastic separator.			3		

	Self-Evaluation	Student Evaluation	Possible Points	Instructor Evaluation	Comments
2. Place a finger over the top of the separator to prevent the separator from snapping and injuring the patient.			3		
3. Pull gently on the instrument toward the occlusal until the elastic is free of the contact.			3		

TOTAL POINTS POSSIBLE 65

TOTAL POINTS POSSIBLE—2nd attempt 63

TOTAL POINTS EARNED ____

Points assigned reflect importance of step to meeting objective: Important = 1, Essential = 2, Critical = 3. Students will lose 2 points for repeated attempts. Failure results if any of the critical steps are omitted or performed incorrectly. If using a 100-point scale, determine score by dividing points earned by total points possible and multiplying the results by 100.

SCORE: _____

SKILL COMPETENCY ASSESSMENT

27-2 Placement and Removal of Steel Spring Separators

Student's Name _____ Date _____

Instructor's Name _____

Skill: Routine steps should be followed for all treatment areas to maintain absolute clinical asepsis. The dental assistant must be prepared and thinking ahead to anticipate the dentist's needs. The steel spring separators are metal coils that are stretched for placement. They fit under the contact area, and, when released, the coil will apply a constant pressure on the spring until the teeth move apart. The dental assistant may be permitted in some states to place and remove these separators.

Performance Objective: The student will follow a routine procedure that meets the regulations and the protocol set forth by the dentist and regulatory agencies. The dental assistant assists the dentist throughout this procedure. (Assistant duties vary from state to state. Therefore, performance of the following tasks may be evaluated by action, verbal/written responses, and/or combined responses and action.) After the diagnosis, the first treatment appointment is to place separators to prepare the teeth for the orthodontic bands. At the dentist's directions, the expanded-functions assistant places the designated separators. The patient is scheduled to have the separators removed and the bands placed several days later. This technique involves the placement and removal of the steel spring separators.

   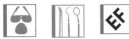

	Self-Evaluation	Student Evaluation	Possible Points	Instructor Evaluation	Comments
Equipment and Supplies 1. Basic setup: mouth 6mirror, explorer, and cotton pliers			3		
2. Dental floss			2		
3. Bird-beak or 139 pliers			3		
4. Steel spring separators			3		
Competency Steps (*follow aseptic procedures*) **Placement of Steel Spring Separators** 1. Use selected pliers.			3		
2. Grasp shortest side or leg of spring separator.			3		
3. Place curve-hook of spring separator under contact from the lingual side.			3		

	Self-Evaluation	Student Evaluation	Possible Points	Instructor Evaluation	Comments
4. Release short side of spring separator and slide it under contact.			3		
5. The coil is on facial side.			3		
6. Test placement by gently pressing on spring.			3		
Removal of Steel Spring Separator 1. Place finger of one hand over spring to prevent injury to patient.			3		
2. Place one end of scaler in coil.			3		
3. Lift scaler upward.			3		
4. Once spring is free from lingual embrasure, pull the coil toward the facial aspect.			3		
5. Pull coil toward facial aspect for removal.			3		

TOTAL POINTS POSSIBLE   44

TOTAL POINTS POSSIBLE—2nd attempt   42

TOTAL POINTS EARNED   ____

Points assigned reflect importance of step to meeting objective: Important = 1, Essential = 2, Critical = 3. Students will lose 2 points for repeated attempts. Failure results if any of the critical steps are omitted or performed incorrectly. If using a 100-point scale, determine score by dividing points earned by total points possible and multiplying the results by 100.

SCORE: _____

SKILL COMPETENCY ASSESSMENT

27-3 Placement and Removal of Brass Wire Separators

Student's Name _____ Date _____

Instructor's Name _____

Skill: Routine steps should be followed in all treatment areas to maintain absolute clinical asepsis. The dental assistant must be prepared and thinking ahead to anticipate the dentist's needs. The brass wire separators are brass wires that are bent into a "C" shape and placed. One end fits under the contact area and the other is placed over the contact area; the wire is then twisted. The wire will be twisted to apply a constant pressure on the contact until the teeth move apart. The dental assistant may be permitted in some states to place and remove these separators.

Performance Objective: The student will follow a routine procedure that meets the regulations and the protocol set forth by the dentist and regulatory agencies. The dental assistant assists the dentist throughout this procedure. (Assistant duties vary from state to state. Therefore, performance of the following tasks may be evaluated by action, verbal/written responses, and/or combined responses and action.) After the diagnosis, separators are placed during the first treatment appointment to prepare the teeth for the orthodontic bands. At the dentist's directions, the expanded-functions assistant places the designated separators. The separators are removed and the bands placed several days later. This technique involves the placement and removal of the brass wire separators.

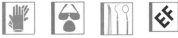

	Self-Evaluation	Student Evaluation	Possible Points	Instructor Evaluation	Comments
Equipment and Supplies 1. Basic setup: mouth mirror, explorer, and cotton pliers			3		
2. Spool of brass wire			3		
3. Hemostat			3		
4. Ligature-wire cutter			3		
5. Condenser			3		
Competency Steps (*follow aseptic procedures*) **Placement of Brass Wire Separators** 1. Bend brass wire into "C" shape leaving a "tail" portion.			3		

	Self-Evaluation	Student Evaluation	Possible Points	Instructor Evaluation	Comments
2. Starting from the lingual surface place one part of wire under contact using hemostat.			3		
3. Fold the other part of wire over the contact.			3		
4. Pull toward the facial.			3		
5. Bring ends of wire together.			3		
6. Twist ends.			3		
7. Cut twisted ends with ligature-cutting pliers.			3		
8. Tuck ends into the gingival embrasure.			3		
Removal of Brass Wire Separators 1. Lift brass wire carefully near occlusal surface on lingual side.			3		
2. Cut wire using ligature-cutting pliers.			3		
3. Use hemostat to remove both sections of wire from under contact on facial side.			3		

TOTAL POINTS POSSIBLE   48

TOTAL POINTS POSSIBLE—2nd attempt   46

TOTAL POINTS EARNED   _____

Points assigned reflect importance of step to meeting objective: Important = 1, Essential = 2, Critical = 3. Students will lose 2 points for repeated attempts. Failure results if any of the critical steps are omitted or performed incorrectly. If using a 100-point scale, determine score by dividing points earned by total points possible and multiplying the results by 100.

SCORE: _____

SKILL COMPETENCY ASSESSMENT

27-4 Cementation of Orthodontic Bands

Student's Name _____ Date _____

Instructor's Name _____

Skill: Routine steps should be followed for all treatment areas to maintain absolute clinical asepsis. The dental assistant must be prepared and thinking ahead to anticipate the dentist's needs. The assistant mixes cement according to the manufacturer's directions and loads the first band. The dental assistant must position the bands so that the orthodontist can pick up the bands in the order of placement. The orthodontist seats the band on the tooth.

Performance Objective: The student will follow a routine procedure that meets the regulations and protocol set forth by the dentist and regulatory agencies, keeping in mind that assistant duties vary from state to state. The assistant may be evaluated by action, verbal/written responses, and/or combined responses and action. The orthodontic bands are prepared specifically for the patient. The orthodontist places the bands on the teeth to accomplish the task needed to correct the patient's malocclusion. The dental assistant mixes the cement and prepares the band for seating.

	Self-Evaluation	Student Evaluation	Possible Points	Instructor Evaluation	Comments
Equipment and Supplies					
1. Basic setup: mouth mirror, explorer, and cotton pliers			3		
2. Cotton rolls and gauze			3		
3. Saliva ejector and HVE			3		
4. Low-speed handpiece with rubber cup and prophy paste			3		
5. Selected and prepared bands			3		
6. Band pusher			3		
7. Bite stick			3		
8. Scaler			3		
9. Cement of choice			3		
10. Paper pad or glass slab			3		
11. Cement spatula			3		
12. Plastic filling instrument (PFI)			3		

	Self-Evaluation	Student Evaluation	Possible Points	Instructor Evaluation	Comments
Competency Steps (*follow aseptic procedures*)					
1. Remove separators.			3		
2. Give teeth a rubber cup polish.			3		
3. Rinse patient's mouth thoroughly.			3		
4. Dry the teeth and place cotton rolls for isolation in areas where bands will be placed.			3		
5. Mix cement.			3		
6. Load the cement in the first band.			3		
7. Make transfer of the bands as easy as possible.			3		
8. Position the bands so that the orthodontist can pick them up in the order of placement.			3		
9. Pass the band driver and any other instruments that the orthodontist might request.			3		
10. Repeat the band procedure until all bands have been cemented or until the cement becomes too thick and a new mix is required.			3		
11. When a new mix is required, clean instruments with wet gauze or alcohol, and wipe and mix additional cement.			3		
12. Allow the cement to dry. (Clean up as in Step 11.)			3		
13. After the cement sets, remove excess cement with a scaler.			3		

	Self-Evaluation	Student Evaluation	Possible Points	Instructor Evaluation	Comments
14. When all cement has been removed, remove protective pins or wax from the brackets.			3		
15. Rinse the patient's mouth.			2		

TOTAL POINTS POSSIBLE — 80

TOTAL POINTS POSSIBLE—2nd attempt — 78

TOTAL POINTS EARNED — ____

Points assigned reflect importance of step to meeting objective: Important = 1, Essential = 2, Critical = 3. Students will lose 2 points for repeated attempts. Failure results if any of the critical steps are omitted or performed incorrectly. If using a 100-point scale, determine score by dividing points earned by total points possible and multiplying the results by 100.

SCORE: _____

SKILL COMPETENCY ASSESSMENT

27-5 Direct Bonding of Brackets

Student's Name _____ Date _____

Instructor's Name _____

Skill: Routine steps should be followed for all treatment areas to maintain absolute clinical asepsis. The dental assistant must be prepared and thinking ahead to anticipate the dentist's needs. The placement of brackets directly to the anterior teeth is a popular choice of treatment because it is more aesthetic and maintaining good oral hygiene is easier. The brackets are bonded to the tooth surface with a material and technique similar to that used to restore anterior teeth. The bonding material is prepared according to the manufacturer's directions. The dental assistant must position the brackets so that the orthodontist can pick up the brackets in the order of placement. The orthodontist seats the bracket on the tooth.

Performance Objective: The student will follow a routine procedure that meets the regulations and protocol set forth by the dentist and regulatory agencies, keeping in mind that assistant duties vary from state to state. The assistant may be evaluated by action, verbal/written responses, and/or combined responses and action. The orthodontic brackets are prepared specifically for the patient. The orthodontist places the brackets on the teeth to accomplish correction of the patient's malocclusion. This procedure involves bonding the brackets to the teeth; the dental assistant prepares the brackets for seating.

	Self-Evaluation	Student Evaluation	Possible Points	Instructor Evaluation	Comments
Equipment and Supplies					
1. Basic setup: mouth mirror, explorer, and cotton pliers			3		
2. Cotton rolls and gauze			3		
3. Saliva ejector and HVE			3		
4. Low-speed handpiece with rubber cup and pumice			3		
5. Bracket kit			3		
6. Retractors for the cheeks and lips			3		
7. Bracket forceps			3		
8. Acid etchant			3		
9. Bonding agent			3		
10. Scaler			3		

	Self-Evaluation	Student Evaluation	Possible Points	Instructor Evaluation	Comments
Competency Steps (*follow aseptic procedures*)					
1. Polish the teeth that are to receive brackets with a rubber cup and pumice (polishing paste without fluoride).			3		
2. Rinse and dry the patient's mouth.			3		
3. Place cotton rolls where brackets are to be bonded.			3		
4. Position retractors.			3		
5. Prepare the etchant.			3		
6. Pass the etchant to the operator.			3		
7. Place acid etchant on the enamel surface (follow manufacturer's directions to determine placement time).			3		
8. Maintain a dry operating field.			3		
9. Rinse the patient's mouth to ensure that all etchant is removed from the tooth surface (approximately 30 seconds).			3		
10. Dry the tooth or teeth (will have chalky appearance).			3		
11. Prepare bonding agent according to the manufacturer's directions.			3		
12. Apply bonding to the back of the bracket.			3		
13. Transfer the agent to the dentist for placement on the tooth.			3		
14. Transfer the bracket; the orthodontist positions it on the tooth.			3		

	Self-Evaluation	Student Evaluation	Possible Points	Instructor Evaluation	Comments
15. Remove excess bonding agent with a scaler or a similar instrument from around the bracket.			3		
16. Hold brackets in position on the tooth until the bonding material sets chemically or with a curing light.			3		
17. Remove the cotton rolls.			2		
18. Remove the retractors from the patient's mouth.			2		
TOTAL POINTS POSSIBLE			82		
TOTAL POINTS POSSIBLE—2nd attempt			80		
TOTAL POINTS EARNED			____		

Points assigned reflect importance of step to meeting objective: Important = 1, Essential = 2, Critical = 3. Students will lose 2 points for repeated attempts. Failure results if any of the critical steps are omitted or performed incorrectly. If using a 100-point scale, determine score by dividing points earned by total points possible and multiplying the results by 100.

SCORE: _____

SKILL COMPETENCY ASSESSMENT

27-6 Placement of the Arch Wire and Ligature Ties

Student's Name _____ Date _____

Instructor's Name _____

Skill: Routine steps should be followed for all treatment areas to maintain absolute clinical asepsis. The dental assistant must be prepared and thinking ahead to anticipate the dentist's needs. The orthodontist selects and shapes the arch wire so that once the bands and brackets are placed, the arch wire can be positioned and secured in place. The arch wire is commonly secured into the brackets with elastic or stainless steel ligatures (ties) and/or slot Damon SL.

Performance Objective: The student will follow a routine procedure that meets the regulations and protocol set forth by the dentist and regulatory agencies, keeping in mind that assistant duties vary from state to state. The assistant may be evaluated by action, verbal/written responses, and/or combined responses and action.

	Self-Evaluation	Student Evaluation	Possible Points	Instructor Evaluation	Comments
Equipment and Supplies 1. Basic setup: mouth mirror, explorer, and cotton pliers			3		
2. Cotton rolls and gauze			3		
3. Saliva ejector and HVE			3		
4. Selected arch wire			3		
5. Weingart pliers			3		
6. Bird-beak pliers			3		
7. Elastics or ligature wire			3		
8. Ligature-cutting pliers			3		
9. Ligature-tying pliers			3		
10. Distal-end cutting pliers			3		
11. Condenser			3		
Competency Steps (*follow aseptic procedures*) 1. Insert the arch wire into buccal tubes on molar bands using Weingart pliers.			3		

	Self-Evaluation	Student Evaluation	Possible Points	Instructor Evaluation	Comments
2. If the wire is too long, cut the ends off with distal-end cutting pliers.			3		
3. Place the arch wire in brackets' horizontal slots along the arch. This may be accomplished with elastic ties, ligature wire, or Damon SL bracket.			3		
Elastic Ties Placement					
1. Secure the arch wire in the brackets with elastic ties.			3		
2. Spread the ties and place them on the gingival extensions of the brackets.			3		
3. Pull the tie over the arch wire.			3		
4. Wrap the tie around the occlusal extensions of the brackets.			3		
Ligature Wire Ties Placement					
1. Hold the ligature wire between the thumb and index finger.			3		
2. Wrap the wire around the occlusal and gingival wings of the bracket in the distal-mesial direction.			3		
3. Cross the ends of the wire together.			3		
4. Using a hemostat or ligature tying pliers, twist the ends of the wire together for several rotations.			3		
5. Repeat the process to secure the arch wire.			3		
6. Cut the twisted ends of ligature wire, called the "pigtail," with ligature-wire cutting pliers at 3 to 4 mm.			3		
7. Bend the pigtail into the embrasure space with the condenser.			3		

	Self-Evaluation	Student Evaluation	Possible Points	Instructor Evaluation	Comments
8. When all pigtail ends have been tucked into place, run a finger over the area to check for sharp ends.			3		
9. Check the distal ends of the arch wire. Cut any excess with distal-end cutting pliers.			3		
Rubber Elastic Bands 1. Show the patient how to place and remove the elastic bands.			3		
2. Instruct the patient how often to change the rubber bands.			3		
3. Give the patient a sufficient number of bands with instructions to call the office for more if needed.			3		

TOTAL POINTS POSSIBLE   90

TOTAL POINTS POSSIBLE—2nd attempt   88

TOTAL POINTS EARNED   ____

Points assigned reflect importance of step to meeting objective: Important = 1, Essential = 2, Critical = 3. Students will lose 2 points for repeated attempts. Failure results if any of the critical steps are omitted or performed incorrectly. If using a 100-point scale, determine score by dividing points earned by total points possible and multiplying the results by 100.

SCORE: _____

SKILL COMPETENCY ASSESSMENT

27-7 Completion Appointment

Student's Name _____ Date _____

Instructor's Name _____

Skill: Routine steps should be followed for all treatment areas to maintain absolute clinical asepsis. The dental assistant must be prepared and thinking ahead to anticipate the dentist's needs. Once the teeth have moved into position and the orthodontist is satisfied with the treatment, the braces are removed. The patient receives a coronal polish, and an impression is taken for use in the construction of a retainer or a positioner to hold the teeth in position so that the alveolar bone can stabilize the new positions of the teeth.

Performance Objective: The student will follow a routine procedure that meets the regulations and protocol set forth by the dentist and regulatory agencies, keeping in mind that assistant duties vary from state to state. The assistant may be evaluated by action, verbal/written responses, and/or combined responses and action. When the orthodontist determines that the patient's teeth have moved to the desired positions, the appliances are removed.

	Self-Evaluation	Student Evaluation	Possible Points	Instructor Evaluation	Comments
Equipment and Supplies					
1. Basic setup: mouth mirror, explorer, and cotton pliers			3		
2. Cotton rolls and gauze			3		
3. Scaler			3		
4. Ligature-wire cutting pliers			3		
5. Hemostat			3		
6. Bracket and adhesive-removing pliers			3		
7. Posterior band remover			3		
8. Ultrasonic scaler (optional)			3		
9. Prophy angle, cups, and prophy paste			3		
10. Alginate impression material and selected tray			3		

	Self-Evaluation	Student Evaluation	Possible Points	Instructor Evaluation	Comments
Competency Steps (*follow aseptic procedures*) 1. Loosen the ligature ties with a scaler or an explorer.			3		
2. Cut the ligature with wire-cutting pliers.			3		
Elastic Bands 1. Remove the elastic ties with a scaler.			3		
2. Place the tip of the scaler explorer under the elastic.			3		
3. Roll the elastic over the bracket wings until the elastic is released.			3		
Ligature Wire Ties 1. Place the beaks of the ligature-wire cutting pliers where the wire is exposed.			3		
2. Cut the wire.			3		
3. Carefully remove the wire from the wings of the bracket.			3		
4. Repeat on each tooth until all ligature wires are removed.			3		
5. Using a hemostat, remove the arch wire from the brackets.			3		
6. Pull the arch wire from the buccal tube on one side.			3		
7. Hold the arch wire securely to prevent injury to the patient while removing the opposite end.			3		

	Self-Evaluation	Student Evaluation	Possible Points	Instructor Evaluation	Comments
Anterior Bracket Removal					
1. Use a bracket and adhesive-removal pliers.			3		
a. Place the lower beak of the pliers on the gingival edge of the bracket.			3		
b. Place the nylon tip of the pliers on the occlusal edge of the bracket.			3		
2. Squeeze the pliers to break the bond and remove some cement.			3		
Posterior Band Removal					
1. Place band-removing pliers with the cushioned end on the buccal cusp.			3		
2. Place the blade end of the pliers against the gingival edge of the band.			3		
3. Gently lift the band toward the occlusal surface.			3		
4. Repeat this process on the lingual surface until the band is free.			3		
Completion Phase					
1. Remove cement and direct bonding materials from tooth surfaces with a hand scaler, an ultrasonic scaler, and/or a finishing bur.			3		
2. Complete a rubber cup polish.			3		
3. Take photographs if needed.			2		
4. Take an alginate impression of both arches.			3		
5. Send impressions to the lab for construction of the retainer.			2		
6. Schedule the patient's next appointment for later that day or the next.			3		

	Self-Evaluation	Student Evaluation	Possible Points	Instructor Evaluation	Comments
7. Place a retainer or positioner.			3		
8. Instruct the patient on the placement and removal of the removable appliance and the wearing schedule.			3		

TOTAL POINTS POSSIBLE   112

TOTAL POINTS POSSIBLE—2nd attempt   110

TOTAL POINTS EARNED   ____

Points assigned reflect importance of step to meeting objective: Important = 1, Essential = 2, Critical = 3. Students will lose 2 points for repeated attempts. Failure results if any of the critical steps are omitted or performed incorrectly. If using a 100-point scale, determine score by dividing points earned by total points possible and multiplying the results by 100.

SCORE: _____

CHAPTER 28

Pediatric Dentistry and Enamel Sealants

SPECIFIC INSTRUCTIONAL OBJECTIVES

The student should strive to meet the following objectives and demonstrate an understanding of the facts and principles presented in this chapter:

1. Define pediatric dentistry as a specialty.
2. Describe the pediatric office and team members.
3. Explain the common behavior characteristics of children of various ages.
4. Describe child behavior management techniques.
5. Explain the role of the parent or guardian in pediatric dentistry.
6. Identify common procedures in pediatric dentistry.
7. Identify the equipment unique to pediatric dentistry.
8. Explain common emergencies in pediatric dentistry and the treatment for these emergencies.
9. Identify the signs of child abuse and the procedure for reporting suspected child abuse cases.

Advanced Chairside Functions

10. Explain the purpose of using dental sealants and where they are placed.
11. List the indications and contraindications of placing sealants.
12. Discuss the role of the dental assistant in the placement of dental sealants.
13. Describe the types of sealant materials.
14. List and describe the steps of the application procedure.

SUMMARY

The scope of pediatric treatment includes restoring and maintaining the primary, mixed, and permanent dentition, and applying preventive measures for dental caries, periodontal disease, and malocclusion. The primary focus of the pediatric dental practice is preventive treatment and dealing with the compromised child patient. The whole staff needs to enjoy working with children and be sincere and honest in their actions and feelings. To be effective in the management of children, the dental team must be upbeat, motivated, and aware.

The role of the dental assistant in the pediatric practice will vary according to areas of responsibility. One part that the assistant is involved in is managing the child. Another part is the tasks that the assistant performs at chairside. Depending on the state, when assistants work independently, they assume the authority role and must maintain control of the child. The dental assistant is also an educator of the child and parents.

Dental sealants are an excellent means of preventing and reducing tooth decay. Depending on individual state dental practice acts, the dental assistant may or may not place sealants. If dental assistants are allowed to place sealants, they must obtain additional education and skills needed. Sealants are placed mainly on permanent teeth, preferably just after they erupt in the mouth. The technique for placing sealants requires practice to become proficient.

EXERCISES AND ACTIVITIES

Multiple Choice

1. Which specialty practice provides dental care for children and the compromised child patient?

   a. Orthodontics
   b. Pedodontics
   c. Endodontics
   d. General dentistry

2. Which treatment area is designed with several chairs arranged in a single open area?

   a. Quiet room
   b. Prevention room
   c. Open bay
   d. Reading room

3. Fear is a major factor in children's behavior problems. Objective fears are based on

   a. suggestions from others.
   b. attitudes from others.
   c. concerns developed from others.
   d. the child's experiences.

4. A behavior management technique called _____ consists of telling the child the name of the instrument, showing it to the child, and then demonstrating how it is used.

   a. voice control
   b. tell, show, and do
   c. subjective
   d. nonverbal

5. The _____ behavior management technique pairs a timid child in the dental chair with a cooperative child of similar age.

   a. positive reinforcement
   b. distraction
   c. modeling
   d. nonverbal communication

6. Children who are involved in contact sports should be fitted for

   a. fixed space maintainers.
   b. removable space maintainers.
   c. dental matrices.
   d. mouth guards.

7. Behavior modification is sometimes necessary. Fixed appliances, such as cribs and rakes, are used to prevent

   a. thumb sucking.
   b. tongue thrust.
   c. modeling.
   d. pulpotomy.

8. Which custom matrix is designed for and used on primary teeth?

    a. T-band

    b. Tofflemire

    c. Space maintainer

    d. Stainless steel crown

9. Which custom-made matrix bands are used on primary teeth for Class II restorations?

    a. T-band

    b. Tofflemire

    c. Spot-welded

    d. Stainless steel crown

10. If the pulp has been exposed through mechanical or traumatic means, but there is a chance for a favorable response, which procedure is indicated?

    a. Direct pulp capping

    b. Pulpotomy

    c. Apexogenesis

    d. Pulpectomy

11. For the young permanent teeth, a pulpotomy maintains pulp vitality and allows enough time for the root end to develop and close. In these cases, the treatment is called

    a. direct pulp capping.

    b. pulpectomy.

    c. apexogenesis.

    d. avulsed.

12. Which procedure involves the complete removal of the dental pulp?

    a. Pulpectomy

    b. Apexogenesis

    c. Pulpotomy

    d. Pulp capping

13. Which condition occurs when the teeth are forcibly driven into the alveolus so that only a portion of the crown is visible?

    a. Displaced tooth

    b. Avulsed tooth

    c. Traumatic intrusion

    d. Apexogenesis

14. When a tooth has been completely removed from the mouth, it is called

    a. displaced.

    b. traumatic intrusion.

    c. apexogenesis.

    d. avulsed.

15. Dentists should report suspicious signs of child abuse to a

    a. social service agency.

    b. local police department.

    c. child protective service.

    d. All of the above.

16. The following general behavior characteristics fit children of which age?

    1. Can respond to the dentist's instructions

    2. Can understand simple explanations

    3. Likes to be with parents and siblings

    4. Likes to play, for example, "see the 'squirt gun'"

    a. 4 to 6

    b. 2 to 6

    c. 2 to 4

    d. 6 to 12

17. For which of the following reasons is the primary dentition restored?

    a. Primary teeth are needed to hold space for the permanent teeth.

    b. Primary teeth maintain the functions of the teeth in chewing, speech, and aesthetics.

    c. Primary teeth act as guides for the permanent dentition during eruption.

    d. All of the above.

18. Which of the following apply to sealants?

    a. Prevent tooth decay

    b. Reduce tooth decay

    c. Both a. and b.

    d. None of the above

19. Sealants are placed and the patient is instructed to have them checked once every

    a. 2 years.

    b. 6 months to a year.

    c. 5 years.

    d. None of the above.

20. The enamel surface is "etched" in preparation for sealant. Application time varies from

    a. 30 to 60 seconds.

    b. 30 to 90 seconds.

    c. 5 to 30 seconds.

    d. 15 to 30 seconds.

21. _____ sealant material is known as self-cure or auto polymerization.

    a. Light-cured

    b. Chemically cured

    c. Surgical

    d. Mechanical

22. The height for holding the curing light is _____ mm directly above the occlusal surface.

    a. 2

    b. 6

    c. 4

    d. 8

23. The sealant procedure area is kept dry by

    a. asking the patient to keep the tongue still.

    b. placing cotton rolls on both the buccal and lingual of the mandibular.

    c. placing cotton rolls on the buccal of the maxillary.

    d. All of the above.

24. The purpose of using Dri-Angles is to

    a. reduce saliva flow.

    b. assist in retracting the tongue.

    c. both a. and b.

    d. None of the above.

25. On the Frankl behavior scale, a child who is reluctant to listen and uncooperative would be rated as:

    a. 1; definitely negative

    c. 3; positive

    b. 2; negative

    d. 4; definitely positive

 Critical Thinking

1. Accepting a role as a pediatric assistant means different duties and responsibilities than in a general practice. Describe the dental assistant's role and responsibilities in a pediatric dental office.

2. In some states, dental assistants may perform the duty of placing sealants. The most likely cause of sealant failure is lack of moisture control. Describe ways that moisture control can be achieved during sealant placement.

3. A dental assistant is responding to a phone call regarding a patient who has had a gymnastic accident. An anterior tooth has been knocked out of the mouth. Provide instructions on what should be done for the patient.

CASE STUDY 1

Sometimes a child's parent asks, "Why fill a deciduous tooth? Won't an adult tooth eventually take its place?" In other words, why not simply extract the tooth, as this is less costly in terms of time and money. As discussed in Chapter 27, Orthodontics, maintaining the space needed for adult teeth to emerge is important. Assume that a young patient needs pulp therapy on a primary tooth.

1. Enumerate the conditions that lead to pulp therapy.

2. Define vital pulp therapy.

3. Describe IPT and DPC.

4. Describe "nonvital."

CASE STUDY 2

Joel, age 4, has kept his parents up at night with toothaches. His parents took him to their general dentist and it was not a pleasant experience! Joel would not open his mouth and he would scream when the dentist approached his mouth. The general dentist referred him to a pediatric dentist.

1. Name and describe some behavior management techniques.

2. Describe subjective fears versus objective fears.

3. Describe the dental assistant's role with the pediatric patient.

4. List some general behavior characteristics of children at ages 2 to 4.

CASE STUDY 3

Eric, age 7, has a toothache and is being seen by a dentist for the first time. One of the dental assistant's responsibilities is to observe the patient from his or her perspective opposite that of the dentist. The dental assistant observed that although the temperature outside was below freezing, the child lacked warm clothes, and his sandals were dirty and torn. The assistant also observed a fresh red handprint on the child's upper arm. Sharing this information with the dental team is a step in determining whether to report that Eric may be a victim of neglect or abuse.

1. Describe dental office team responsibilities in reporting child abuse.

2. List types of child abuse.

3. List agencies with which a child abuse report is filed.

4. Describe child abuse legislation in your state.

5. List the contents of a child abuse report.

SKILL COMPETENCY ASSESSMENT

28-1 T-Band Placement

Student's Name _____ Date _____

Instructor's Name _____

Skill: Routine steps should be followed for all treatment areas to maintain absolute clinical asepsis. The dental assistant must be prepared and thinking ahead to anticipate the dentist's needs. T-bands are designed to be used on primary teeth, and are available in various designs and sizes. They are often made of brass strips that are "crossed" at one end. The T-bands are adjustable, do not require a retainer, and can be secured on the tooth.

Performance Objective: The student will follow a routine procedure that meets the regulations and protocol set forth by the dentist and regulatory agencies, keeping in mind that assistant duties vary from state to state. The assistant may be evaluated by performance (actions), verbal/written responses, and/or combined responses and actions. For this procedure, the tooth has been prepared and the matrix is assembled and placed on the tooth.

	Self-Evaluation	Student Evaluation	Possible Points	Instructor Evaluation	Comments
Equipment and Supplies					
1. T-band assortment			3		
2. Burnisher			3		
3. Cotton pliers or hemostat			3		
4. Crown and collar scissors			3		
Competency Steps (*follow aseptic procedures*)					
1. Select an appropriately sized T-band (can be selected ahead of time).			3		
2. Loop the band to shape the approximate diameter of the tooth.			3		
3. Fold the "T" ends over the band loop, leaving a circle with a long tail or end.			3		
4. Place the band on the tooth in the interproximal space, while covering the margins of the preparation.			3		

	Self-Evaluation	Student Evaluation	Possible Points	Instructor Evaluation	Comments
5. Where the "T" is folded, place it on the buccal surface, away from the margins of the preparation.			3		
6. Tighten the band by pulling on the free end (tail) until the band is tight around the tooth.			3		
7. Bend the free end back toward the "T" to secure the band.			3		
8. Remove the excess band with scissors.			3		
9. Wedge and burnish the band.			3		
10. To remove the T-band, fold back the overlapping section of the band to loosen it.			3		
11. Use cotton pliers to remove the band from the tooth.			3		
TOTAL POINTS POSSIBLE			45		
TOTAL POINTS POSSIBLE—2nd attempt			43		
TOTAL POINTS EARNED			_____		

Points assigned reflect importance of step to meeting objective: Important = 1, Essential = 2, Critical = 3. Students will lose 2 points for repeated attempts. Failure results if any of the critical steps are omitted or performed incorrectly. If using a 100-point scale, determine score by dividing points earned by total points possible and multiplying the results by 100.

SCORE: _____

SKILL COMPETENCY ASSESSMENT

28-2 Spot-Welded Matrix Band Placement

Student's Name _____ Date _____

Instructor's Name _____

Skill: Routine steps should be followed for all treatment areas to maintain absolute clinical asepsis. The dental assistant must be prepared and thinking ahead to anticipate the dentist's needs. Custom-made bands are used for Class II restorations and on primary teeth. The matrix material comes in rolls of 1/4- to 3/16-inch width and 0.002-gauge thickness. This custom matrix does not require a retainer to be secured on the tooth, but a spot-welding machine is required. This band is made quickly at chairside.

Performance Objective: The student will follow a routine procedure that meets the regulations and the protocol set forth by the dentist and regulatory agencies. The dental assistant assists the dentist throughout this procedure. (Assistant duties vary from state to state. Therefore, the assistant may be evaluated by performance [actions], verbal/written responses, and/or combined responses and actions.) For this procedure, the tooth has been prepared for a restoration and the spot-welded matrix band is prepared by the dental assistant at chairside.

	Self-Evaluation	Student Evaluation	Possible Points	Instructor Evaluation	Comments
Equipment and Supplies					
1. Spot-welded matrix band material			3		
2. Crown and collar scissors			3		
3. Cotton pliers, hemostat, or Howe pliers			3		
4. Burnisher			3		
5. Spot-welding unit			3		
Competency Steps (*follow aseptic procedures*)					
1. Cut approximate length of matrix band material.			3		
2. Turn on spot-welding unit to warm up.			3		
3. Loop matrix material around tooth.			3		
4. Bring loop ends of material together on buccal surface.			3		

	Self-Evaluation	Student Evaluation	Possible Points	Instructor Evaluation	Comments
5. Pinch band tightly together with a hemostat, cotton pliers, or Howe pliers.			3		
6. Bend excess material to one side.			3		
7. Take band to spot-welding unit and spot weld the band together to form a circle measuring the diameter of the tooth.			3		
8. Trim off the excess and sharp edges of the band.			3		
9. Replace the band on the tooth with welded area on buccal surface.			3		
10. Place wedges in the interpro-ximal and contour.			3		
11. After amalgam has been placed, in preparation to remove the band, cut the lingual aspect of the band.			3		
12. Pull the band in an occlusal/buc-cal direction with cotton pliers.			3		

TOTAL POINTS POSSIBLE   51

TOTAL POINTS POSSIBLE—2nd attempt   49

TOTAL POINTS EARNED   _____

Points assigned reflect importance of step to meeting objective: Important = 1, Essential = 2, Critical = 3. Students will lose 2 points for repeated attempts. Failure results if any of the critical steps are omitted or performed incorrectly. If using a 100-point scale, determine score by dividing points earned by total points possible and multiplying the results by 100.

SCORE: _____

SKILL COMPETENCY ASSESSMENT

28-3 Pulpotomy

Student's Name _____ Date _____

Instructor's Name _____

Skill: Routine steps should be followed for all treatment areas to maintain absolute clinical asepsis. The dental assistant must be prepared and thinking ahead to anticipate the dentist's needs.

Performance Objective: The student will follow a routine procedure that meets the regulations and protocol set forth by the dentist and regulatory agencies, keeping in mind that assistant duties vary from state to state. The dental assistant prepares the treatment room, patient, equipment, and supplies. The tooth is opened and treated before a temporary restoration is placed. The assistant may be evaluated by performance (actions), verbal/written responses, and/or combined responses and actions.

	Self-Evaluation	Student Evaluation	Possible Points	Instructor Evaluation	Comments
Equipment and Supplies					
1. Amalgam setup			3		
2. Formocresol			3		
3. Sterile round burs			3		
4. Zinc oxide-eugenol cement (ZOE or IRM)			3		
Competency Steps (*follow aseptic procedures*)					
1. Administer anesthetic.			2		
2. Place the dental dam.			3		
3. Secure a high-speed handpiece with the bur in place.			3		
4. The operator removes the coronal portion of the pulp with a spoon excavator or round bur.			3		
5. Prepare a sterile cotton pellet, wetting it with Formocresol.			3		
6. Pass the pellet to the dentist for placement in the chamber for 5 minutes.			3		

	Self-Evaluation	Student Evaluation	Possible Points	Instructor Evaluation	Comments
7. After the hemorrhage is controlled, remove the cotton pellet and rinse and dry the pulp chamber.			3		
8. Mix zinc oxide–eugenol to base consistency.			3		
9. Pass the base to the dentist.			3		
10. Place the restoration of choice, such as amalgam.			3		
11. Remove the rubber dam.			3		
12. Check the occlusion.			3		
13. Alternatives to amalgam are a stainless steel crown and/or temporary restoration.			3		
TOTAL POINTS POSSIBLE			50		
TOTAL POINTS POSSIBLE—2nd attempt			48		
TOTAL POINTS EARNED			____		

Points assigned reflect importance of step to meeting objective: Important = 1, Essential = 2, Critical = 3. Students will lose 2 points for repeated attempts. Failure results if any of the critical steps are omitted or performed incorrectly. If using a 100-point scale, determine score by dividing points earned by total points possible and multiplying the results by 100.

SCORE: _____

SKILL COMPETENCY ASSESSMENT

28-4 Stainless Steel Crown Placement

Student's Name _____ Date _____

Instructor's Name _____

Skill: Routine steps should be followed for all treatment areas to maintain absolute clinical asepsis. The dental assistant must be prepared and thinking ahead to anticipate the dentist's needs. Stainless steel crowns come in a variety of sizes. The crown must fit the circumference of the prepared tooth and contact the adjacent teeth, mesially and distally. In expanded-function states, the dental assistant will assist the dentist in the selection.

Performance Objective: The student will follow a routine procedure that meets the regulations and protocol set forth by the dentist and regulatory agencies. The procedure is performed by the dentist and the dental assistant. The assistant maintains the operating field, mixes materials, and assists in the preparation of the stainless steel crown. (Assistant duties vary from state to state. Therefore, the assistant may be evaluated by performance/actions, verbal/written responses, and/or combined responses and actions.)

	Self-Evaluation	Student Evaluation	Possible Points	Instructor Evaluation	Comments
Equipment and Supplies					
1. Basic setup: mouth mirror, explorer, and cotton pliers			3		
2. Cotton rolls and gauze			2		
3. HVE and saliva ejector			3		
4. High-speed handpiece with selected burs			3		
5. Low-speed handpiece with green stone and rubber abrasive wheel			3		
6. Spoon excavator			3		
7. Selection of stainless steel crowns			3		
8. Crown and collar scissors			3		
9. Contouring and crimping pliers			3		
10. Mixing spatulas, paper pad, and permanent cement			3		
11. Articulating forceps and paper			3		
12. Dental floss			2		

	Self-Evaluation	Student Evaluation	Possible Points	Instructor Evaluation	Comments
Competency Steps (*follow aseptic procedures*) 1. Administer anesthetic.			2		
2. Secure a high-speed handpiece with tapered diamond burs.			3		
3. Prepare the tooth similar to a gold crown (reduce the circumference and height of the tooth).			3		
4. Transfer instruments as needed.			3		
5. Evacuate during tooth preparation.			3		
6. Remove decay via conventional methods, passing instruments and evacuating as needed.			3		
7. Select a stainless steel crown from the kit and try on the tooth. In states where the assistant is not allowed to perform this function, the dentist will do so.			3		
8. Once the crown is selected, use the crown and collar scissors to adjust the occlusal-gingival height. The gingival margin of the crown should extend 1 mm beyond the margin of the tooth preparation.			3		
9. Use green stone to smooth the crown's rough edges.			3		
10. Polish the edges of the crown with a rubber abrasive wheel.			3		
11. Place the crown on the tooth to check the patient's bite.			3		
12. Check the patient's occlusion with articulating paper.			3		

	Self-Evaluation	Student Evaluation	Possible Points	Instructor Evaluation	Comments
13. Make adjustments as necessary. Prepare articulating paper, dry the tooth, and pass paper. Receive the articulating forceps and paper and prepare the handpiece, if necessary.			3		
14. Use dental floss to check contacts.			2		
15. Use contouring and crimping pliers to contour the crown and crimp the cervical margins of the crown in toward the tooth.			3		
16. Remove the crown and dry the tooth thoroughly.			2		
17. Mix cement and place it in the crown.			3		
18. Pass the crown to the dentist for placement.			3		
19. Remove excess cement from around the crown and interproximal.			3		
20. Rinse the patient's mouth and dismiss the patient.			3		

TOTAL POINTS POSSIBLE — 91

TOTAL POINTS POSSIBLE—2nd attempt — 89

TOTAL POINTS EARNED — ____

Points assigned reflect importance of step to meeting objective: Important = 1, Essential = 2, Critical = 3. Students will lose 2 points for repeated attempts. Failure results if any of the critical steps are omitted or performed incorrectly. If using a 100-point scale, determine score by dividing points earned by total points possible and multiplying the results by 100.

SCORE: _____

SKILL COMPETENCY ASSESSMENT

28-5 Procedure for Placing Dental Sealants

Student's Name _____ Date _____

Instructor's Name _____

Skill: Routine steps should be followed for all treatment areas to maintain absolute clinical asepsis. The dental assistant is responsible for preparation of equipment and supplies needed for the appointment. The dentist will diagnose which teeth need dental sealants after a thorough examination that includes radiographs. Sealant kits usually contain everything needed to apply the sealant.

Performance Objective: The student will follow a routine procedure that meets the regulations and the protocol set forth by the dentist and regulatory agencies. (The assistant may be evaluated by performance/actions, verbal/written responses, and/or combined responses and actions.) This procedure is performed by the dental assistant, hygienist, or dentist depending on each state's Dental Practice Act. Before the sealant is placed, the tooth/teeth are polished with a rubber cup. Equipment and supplies for preparing the tooth/teeth and the sealant procedure are listed.

	Self-Evaluation	Student Evaluation	Possible Points	Instructor Evaluation	Comments
Equipment and Supplies					
1. Basic setup: mouth mirror, explorer, cotton pliers			3		
2. Air-water syringe tip, HVE tips, and saliva ejector			3		
3. Rubber cup or brush			3		
4. Low-speed handpiece with right-angle (prophy-angle) attachment			3		
5. Flour of pumice or prophy paste without fluoride, air polisher, dry toothbrush, or fissurotomy burs			3		
6. Dental dam setup, Dri-Angles or Garmer cotton roll holders, and short and long cotton rolls			3		
7. Etchant/conditioner			3		
8. Sealant material: a. Base material and catalyst (self-cure) b. Syringe or capsule (light cure)			3 3		

	Self-Evaluation	Student Evaluation	Possible Points	Instructor Evaluation	Comments
9. Applicators (micro-brush, small cotton tip applicators, or syringe) for etchant/conditioner and sealant			3		
10. Bonding agent			3		
11. Light-curing unit			3		
12. Articulating paper and forceps			3		
13. Assorted burs and/or stones for reducing high spots			3		
14. Floss			3		
Competency Steps (*follow aseptic procedures*) 1. Check tooth or teeth with explorer.			2		
2. Polish occlusal surface of teeth to receive sealant. a. Use flour of pumice or non-fluoride prophy paste with rubber cup or bristle brush. b. Clean occlusal surfaces. c. Rinse teeth and dry thoroughly. d. Check pits and fissures with explorer. e. Rinse and dry again.			3 3 3 3 3		
3. Perform isolation steps: a. Place dental dam. b. Place cotton rolls and/or Garmer clamps (long or short cotton rolls). c. Place cotton rolls on both buccal and lingual on the mandibular teeth and on only the buccal for the maxillary teeth. Place a dry angle on buccal mucosa.			3 3 3		

	Self-Evaluation	Student Evaluation	Possible Points	Instructor Evaluation	Comments
4. Dry and etch: a. After tooth/teeth are isolated, dry them. b. Apply etchant. Follow manufacturer's directions (use applicator, apply to occlusal surface, in pits and fissures, and two-thirds up the cuspid incline, using a dabbing motion while applying sealant). c. Time etchant, usually 15 to 30 seconds.			3 3 3		
5. Rinse 20 to 30 seconds; use evacuator tip to remove remaining acid and water (re-isolate with dry cotton rolls if this method was used).			3		
6. Dry all etched surfaces and examine appearance. Should appear dull and chalky white (if they do not, etch again for 15 to 30 seconds).			3		
7. Apply sealant material, place the sealant on the mesial occlusal to flow toward the distal. Applicator tip or a micro-brush can be used to carefully move sealant, while preventing air bubbles and reaching desired thickness (follow manufacturer's directions for preparation and application).			3		
8. Curing the sealant: a. Self-curing: allow to set (polymerize) according to manufacturer's directions. b. Light-curing: hold curing light 2 mm directly above occlusal surface, expose for appropriate time (materials differ, ranging from 20 to 60 seconds). Use tinted protective eyewear during curing process.			3		

	Self-Evaluation	Student Evaluation	Possible Points	Instructor Evaluation	Comments
9. Evaluate the sealant: a. With explorer, check to see if sealant has hardened and is smooth.			3		
b. In the event of irregularities or voids, repeat process to properly seal areas.			3		
c. If surface is free from saliva, additional sealant can be added without etching the tooth first.			3		
d. If saliva has contacted tooth, process must be completely repeated.			3		
10. Rinse the sealant after it has set; rinse or wipe surface with moist cotton roll/pellet to remove air-inhibited layer.			3		
11. Finishing the sealant: a. Remove cotton rolls or dental dam.			3		
b. Check contact with dental floss.			3		
c. Dry teeth and place articulating paper to evaluate any high spots.			3		
d. Perform occlusion reduction as needed.			3		
12. Apply fluoride: a. Apply fluoride to sealed tooth/teeth etched but not sealed.			3		
b. Record sealants on patient's chart.			3		
c. Instruct patient about having the sealants checked every 6 months.			3		

TOTAL POINTS POSSIBLE   131

TOTAL POINTS POSSIBLE—2nd attempt   129

TOTAL POINTS EARNED   ____

Points assigned reflect importance of step to meeting objective. Important = 1, Essential = 2, Critical = 3. Students will lose 2 points for repeated attempts. Failure results if any of the critical steps are omitted or performed incorrectly. If using a 100-point scale, determine score by dividing points earned by total points possible and multiplying the results by 100.

SCORE: _____

CHAPTER 29

Periodontics and Coronal Polish

The student should strive to meet the following objectives and demonstrate an understanding of the facts and principles presented in this chapter:

1. Describe the scope of periodontics.
2. Identify members of the periodontal team and their roles.
3. Describe the stages of periodontal disease.
4. Explain the diagnostic procedures involved in the patient's first visit to the periodontal office.
5. Identify and describe periodontal instruments and their uses.
6. Describe nonsurgical procedures and the dental assistant's role in each procedure.
7. Explain surgical procedures and dental assisting responsibilities.
8. Explain the purpose of periodontal dressing.
9. Identify the types of periodontal dressings and how they are prepared, placed, and removed.
10. Describe periodontal maintenance procedures and the patient's role relating to each.

Advanced Chairside Functions

11. Define coronal polish.
12. Describe and explain the rationale for each step in the coronal polish procedure.
13. Explain indications and contraindication for coronal polish.
14. Describe and identify dental deposits and stains.
15. List types of abrasives and explain characteristics of each type.

16. List and explain types of equipment and materials used to perform a coronal polish.

17. Explain how to maintain the oral cavity during a coronal polish.

18. List auxiliary polishing aids and explain their functions.

19. Describe steps in the coronal polish procedure.

SUMMARY

Periodontal disease is as old as the human race. According to the American Academy of Periodontology, three out of four adults will experience, to some degree, periodontal problems at some time in their lives. In children and adolescents, marginal gingivitis and gingival recession are the most prevalent conditions.

The dental assistant performs chairside assisting duties and the expanded functions allowed by the state dental practice act, including placing and removing periodontal dressing, removing sutures, and performing coronal polishes. The dental assistant takes radiographs, takes impressions for study models, and administers fluoride treatments. The assistant also gives pre- and postoperative instructions and prepares the treatment room for surgery. These functions are in addition to treatment room preparation and maintenance and sterilization procedures. The dental assistant is involved in educating and motivating the patient throughout the treatment. In some offices, the dental assistant may also perform laboratory tasks, such as pouring study models or making periodontal splints.

Performing a coronal polish, an expanded function, requires increased skill and responsibility. This task is delegated by the dentist according to the state dental practice act. Some states require additional education, certification, or registration to perform this function.

EXERCISES AND ACTIVITIES

Multiple Choice

1. Bacterial plaque forms around the margin of the gingiva; when left undisturbed, it mineralizes and appears as a yellow or brown deposit on the teeth called

   a. food.

   b. plaque.

   c. calculus.

   d. a stain.

2. A curved instrument is used to measure the destruction of the interradicular bone of multirooted teeth. The area where the roots divide is called the

   a. sulcus.

   b. furcation.

   c. mesiofacial.

   d. distofacial.

3. Gingival tissue is measured during the periodontal exam with a periodontal probe to evaluate

   a. plaque.

   b. calculus.

   c. mobility.

   d. recession.

4. Which calibrated instrument is used to measure the depth of periodontal pockets?

   a. Curette

   b. Periodontal knives

   c. Periodontal hoe

   d. Periodontal probe

5. Which hand instrument is used to remove hard deposits of supragingival and subgingival calculus from teeth? Note: the working end has two sharp edges that come to a point.

   a. Scaler

   b. Periodontal hoe

   c. Orban knives

   d. Curette

6. Which hand instrument has a working end that has a cutting edge on one or both sides of the blade and a rounded end? It is used primarily for removing subgingival calculus.

   a. Scaler
   b. Periodontal hoe
   c. Orban knife
   d. Curette

7. _____ interdental knives are used to remove soft tissue interproximally using long and narrow blades.

   a. Orban
   b. Scalpel
   c. Kirkland
   d. Pocket marking plier

8. Which fast and effective instrument can be used as an adjunct to manual scaling procedures? Note: its water spray cools and flushes the area.

   a. Electrosurgery unit
   b. Ultrasonic unit
   c. Surgical scalpel
   d. Universal curette

9. Which instrument is used to coagulate blood during the incising of gingival tissue?

   a. Ultrasonic unit
   b. Electrosurgery unit
   c. Universal curette
   d. Gracey curette

10. When the beaks of the _____ are pinched together, the gingival tissue is perforated, leaving small pinpoint markings.

   a. periodontal probe
   b. pocket-marking pliers
   c. cotton forceps
   d. periosteal elevator

11. Which instrument reflects soft tissue away from the bone?

   a. Periodontal probe
   b. Pocket-marking pliers
   c. Curette
   d. Periosteal elevator

12. In a routine _____, deposits above and below the gingival margins are removed, and the coronal surfaces of the teeth are polished with rubber cups and brushes.

   a. root planing
   b. curettage
   c. prophylaxis
   d. scaling

13. _____ is the process of planing or shaving the root surface to leave a smooth root surface.

   a. Root planing
   b. Curettage
   c. Osteoplasty
   d. Ostectomy

14. The process that involves reshaping the gingival tissue to remove deformities is (a)

   a. gingivectomy.
   b. gingivoplasty.
   c. frenectomy.
   d. mucogingival surgery.

15. Periodontal flap surgery involves surgically separating the _____ from the underlying tissue.

   a. bone
   b. tooth
   c. gingiva
   d. sulcus

16. _____ is reconstructive surgery on the gingiva and/or mucosa tissues.

   a. A frenectomy
   b. Mucogingival surgery
   c. Gingival grafting
   d. An ostectomy

17. Which procedure involves taking tissue from one site and placing it on another?

   a. Frenectomy
   b. Mucogingival surgery
   c. Gingival grafting
   d. Ostectomy

18. Which procedure is a complete removal of the frenum, including the attachment to the underlying bone?

    a. Frenectomy

    b. Mucogingival surgery

    c. Gingival grafting

    d. Ostectomy

19. The periodontium includes which of the following?

    1. Calculus
    2. Food
    3. Debris
    4. Sulcus
    5. Gingiva
    6. Epithelial attachment
    7. Bone
    8. Plaque

    a. 1, 2, 3, 8

    b. 4, 5, 6, 7

    c. 2, 3, 4, 8

    d. 2, 3, 5, 6

20. Causes and indications of gingivitis include which of the following?

    1. Plaque buildup
    2. Calculus buildup
    3. Periodontal pocket
    4. Loose teeth (mobility)
    5. Tissues reddish in color
    6. Halitosis

    a. 1, 2, 5

    b. 3, 4, 6

    c. 1, 2, 3

    d. 2, 3, 6

21. _____ is described as follows: the margins of the gingiva and periodontal fibers recede and the supporting bone becomes inflamed and destroyed.

    a. Gingivitis

    b. Periodontitis

    c. Alveolitis

    d. Pulpitis

22. When tissues become reddish, interdental papilla may be swollen and bulbous, and tissues may bleed after brushing and flossing. This condition is called

    a. gingivitis.

    b. periodontitis.

    c. alveolitis.

    d. pulpitis.

23. Periodontal probing is measuring the depth of the periodontal pocket with a periodontal probe. Each tooth will have _____ sites probed and recorded.

    a. three

    b. six

    c. two

    d. four

24. Which surgical procedure reduces the height of the gingival tissue by removing diseased gingival tissue that forms the periodontal pocket?

    a. Gingivoplasty

    b. Gingivectomy

    c. Osteoplasty

    d. Ostectomy

25. Which procedure reshapes the gingival tissue to remove such deformities as clefts, craters, and enlargements?

    a. Gingivoplasty

    b. Gingivectomy

    c. Osteoplasty

    d. Ostectomy

26. Which type of osseous surgery reshapes the bone?

    a. Osteoplasty

    b. Ostectomy

    c. Gingivoplasty

    d. Gingivectomy

27. Which type of osseous surgery removes bone?

    a. Osteoplasty

    b. Ostectomy

    c. Gingivoplasty

    d. Gingivectomy

28. Sharp hand instruments that are used to remove hard deposits above the gingiva treat the _____ area.

    a. supragingival

    b. subgingival

    c. intragingival

    d. infragingival

29. When a laser is being used, primary safety measures require that the _____ wear protective eyewear.

    a. dentist

    b. staff

    c. patient

    d. All of the above

30. Tissue is moved from one area to another in the _____ procedure.

    a. gingival grafting

    b. frenectomy

    c. flap surgery

    d. gingivectomy

31. Once a manual sharpening stone has been used, proper care of it includes

    a. cleaning by scrubbing with a stiff brush.

    b. cleaning with soap and rinsing.

    c. ultrasonic cleaning.

    d. All of the above

32. Auxiliary polishing aids include

    a. bridge threaders.

    b. abrasive polishing strips.

    c. soft wood points.

    d. All of the above

33. The rubber cup used in polishing should have all of the following qualities except being

    a. soft.

    b. rough.

    c. flexible.

    d. adaptable to contours.

34. Select from the following statements the one that best describes the particle hardness characteristic of abrasives.

    a. Sharp-edged particles are more abrasive than dull ones.

    b. Harder particles abrade faster; particles must be harder than the surfaces they are used on.

    c. Particle should resist breakage during polishing.

    d. The larger the particle, the more abrasive it is.

35. According to the classification system that describes the severity of chronic periodontitis by the amount of clinical attachment loss, which of the following measurements describes moderate loss?

    a. 1 or 2 mm

    b. 3 or 4 mm

    c. 5 mm

    d. All of the above

36. _____, which are relatively new instruments in dentistry, are used to sever the periodontal ligament prior to atraumatic extractions and to prepare the tissue for dental implants.

    a. Lasers

    b. Periotomes

    c. Orbans

    d. Air abrasion tools

37. What anatomical feature is characterized by a fissure or elongated opening that extends toward the root of the tooth?

    a. Epithelial attachment

    b. Gingival cleft

    c. Sulcus

    d. Periodontal ligament

38. Which evaluation method was developed by the ADA and the AAP to standardize a system of screening for periodontal disease?

    a. Periodontal probing system
    c. Periodontal screening and reporting system
    b. Occlusal equilibration system
    d. Suppuration assessment system

39. _____ is a method of polishing the crown and root surface by use of a fine powder abrasive, air under pressure, and water.

    a. Jet polishing
    c. Ultrasonic polishing
    b. Electrosurgery
    d. Sickle scaling

40. How long should patients refrain from smoking after a periodontal surgical procedure?

    a. 1 to 2 hours
    c. 12 to 72 hours
    b. 6 to 24 hours
    d. 24 to 48 hours

Matching

Identify the following attachments and accessories in the figure.

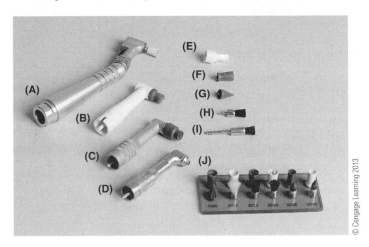

© Cengage Learning 2013

1. Assortment of cups, brushes, and points _____

2. Contra-angle with latch _____

3. Disposable prophy angle cup _____

4. Latch brush _____

5. Right angle with snap-on prophy cup _____

6. Right angle (prophy angle) for screw cup _____

7. Rubber point _____

8. Screw-on prophy burs _____

9. Snap-on prophy brush _____

10. Screw-on prophy cup _____

Identify the periodontal instruments in the figure.

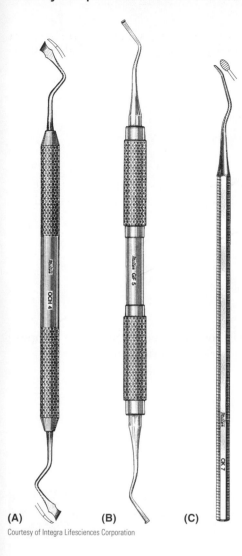

(A)   (B)   (C)

a. _____

b. _____

c. _____

Critical Thinking

1. The dental assistant may be able to perform coronal polishing. List methods for using the dental handpiece that help to avoid operator fatigue.

2. Stains are discoloration of the teeth and are caused by many things. The dental assistant will evaluate stains and determine whether the stains can be removed. Explain intrinsic versus extrinsic stains and exogenous versus endogenous stains.

3. Various materials are used for periodontal dressings. The dental assistant will need to be able to competently mix and apply these dressings. List the four common types of periodontal dressings.

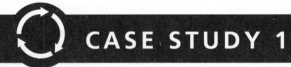

CASE STUDY 1

Dental assistant Jill is preparing to perform a coronal polish. Her skill and knowledge of the oral characteristics of various types of stains will be useful in determining whether a stain is removable and in selecting the correct abrasive agent.

1. List three types of intrinsic stains and three types of extrinsic stains.

2. List three characteristics of abrasives.

3. Describe the rate of abrasion.

CASE STUDY 2

Joan has agreed to treatment to correct gum defects that includes bone reshaping during surgery. Some of the damage was caused by periodontal disease.

1. Describe osseous surgery.

2. Describe osteoplasty.

3. Explain the difference between additive and subtractive surgery.

4. List the differences between a bone graft, a mucogingival surgery, and a gingival graft.

CASE STUDY 3

The purpose of the first periodontal appointment, which includes a clinical exam, is to gather information. The dental assistant's role is to interpret the dentist's findings and to chart them precisely.

1. List the periodontal probing measurements, sites, and depth.

2. List three other conditions that are recorded during the clinical exam.

3. Explain the radiographic interpretation of vertical bone resorption and horizontal bone resorption.

CASE STUDY 4

Training regarding dental lasers is available for dental assistants and hygienists. Staff members must be able to explain the benefits of using such lasers to the patient.

1. List four benefits of lasers in dentistry.

2. List required safety measures during laser use.

3. List four uses of the dental laser.

SKILL COMPETENCY ASSESSMENT

29-1 Occlusal Adjustment

Student's Name _____ Date _____

Instructor's Name _____

Skill: Occlusal adjustment or equilibration is a procedure that involves adjusting the occlusal surface to eliminate detrimental forces and to provide functional forces to stimulate a healthy periodontium. The dental assistant must be prepared and able to think ahead to anticipate the dentist's needs. Routine steps should be followed for all treatment areas to maintain absolute clinical asepsis.

Performance Objective: The student will follow a routine procedure that meets the regulations and protocol set forth by the dentist and regulatory agencies. The dental assistant assists the dentist throughout this procedure. Assistant duties vary from state to state. Therefore, assistant performance may be evaluated by performance criteria, verbal/written responses, and/or combined responses and performance criteria. This procedure, which is performed by the periodontist, involves marking the patient's bite and adjusting the occlusal surfaces of the teeth. The dental assistant prepares the articulating paper or wax; maintains the operating field; and changes burs, discs, and stones in the handpiece.

	Self-Evaluation	Student Evaluation	Possible Points	Instructor Evaluation	Comments
Equipment and Supplies 1. Basic setup: mouth mirror, explorer, cotton pliers			3		
2. Cotton rolls and 2 × 2 gauze sponges			2		
3. Saliva ejector, HVE tip, air-water syringe tip			3		
4. Articulation forceps and articulating paper and/or occlusal wax			3		
5. Low-speed handpiece			3		
6. Diamond burs, various discs, and stones			3		
7. Polishing wheels and discs			3		
Competency Steps (*follow aseptic procedures*) 1. Seat and prepare the patient for the occlusal adjustment procedure.			2		

	Self-Evaluation	Student Evaluation	Possible Points	Instructor Evaluation	Comments
2. Prepare the articulating forceps with paper or wax and transfer them to the dentist.			3		
3. Dry the quadrant with an air syringe or a gauze sponge.			2		
4. Place articulating paper over the occlusal surfaces and instruct the patient to bite down and grind the teeth side to side.			3		
5. Remove the articulating paper and evaluate the colored marks left by the paper.			3		
6. Change burs, discs, and stones as requested by the dentist.			3		
7. Transfer the handpiece to the dentist.			3		
8. Use the air-water syringe and the evacuator to keep the area clean and clear during the procedure.			3		
9. Repeat this process until the teeth occlude evenly over the quadrant.			2		
10. Evaluate and adjust each quadrant.			2		

TOTAL POINTS POSSIBLE   46

TOTAL POINTS POSSIBLE—2nd attempt   44

TOTAL POINTS EARNED   ____

Points assigned reflect importance of step to meeting objective: Important = 1, Essential = 2, Critical = 3. Students will lose 2 points for repeated attempts. Failure results if any of the critical steps are omitted or performed incorrectly. If using a 100-point scale, determine score by dividing points earned by total points possible and multiplying the results by 100.

SCORE: _____

SKILL COMPETENCY ASSESSMENT

29-2 Scaling, Curettage, and Polishing

Student's Name _____ Date _____

Instructor's Name _____

Skill: The purpose of scaling is to remove plaque, calculus, and stains from the surfaces of the teeth. Gingival curettage, also known as soft tissue curettage, involves scraping the inner gingival walls of the periodontal pockets to remove inflamed tissue and debris. Supragingival as well as subgingival deposits are removed with scalers and curettes. After this process, the coronal surfaces of the teeth are polished with rubber cups, brushes, an abrasive, porte polishers, and dental tape. Depending on the state Dental Practice Act, dental assistants can remove supragingival deposits and/or perform the coronal polish. The dental assistant must be prepared and thinking ahead to anticipate the dentist's and/or dental hygienist's needs. Routine steps should be followed for all treatment areas to maintain absolute clinical asepsis.

Performance Objective: The student will follow a routine procedure that meets the regulations and protocol set forth by the dentist and regulatory agencies, keeping in mind that assistant duties vary from state to state. The assistant may be evaluated by performance, verbal/written responses, and/or combined responses and actions. The procedure is performed by the dentist or the dental hygienist. A dental hygiene assistant assists during this procedure. Responsibilities include instrument transfer, rinsing the oral cavity, evacuating with the HVE, removing debris from instruments, retracting, and patient comfort.

	Self-Evaluation	Student Evaluation	Possible Points	Instructor Evaluation	Comments
Equipment and Supplies					
1. Basic setup: mouth mirror, explorer, cotton pliers			3		
2. Saliva ejector, HVE tip, air-water syringe tip			3		
3. Cotton rolls and 2 × 2 gauze sponges			2		
4. Periodontal probe			3		
5. Scalers: Jacque and Shepherd's hook			3		
6. Curettes: universal and Gracey			3		
7. Dental floss and dental tape			3		
8. Prophy angle—rubber cups and brushes			3		

	Self-Evaluation	Student Evaluation	Possible Points	Instructor Evaluation	Comments
9. Prophy paste			2		
10. Optional—disclosing solution or tablets					
Competency Steps (*follow aseptic procedures*) 1. Examine the oral cavity.			3		
2. Use scalers and curettes to remove calculus and debris from around teeth (clean all surfaces of the teeth in one quadrant before moving to next quadrant). The operator polishes teeth after all calculus is removed.			3		
3. Keep the area clean and clear with HVE and air-water syringe as directed.			3		
4. Transfer instruments as directed.			3		
5. Polish teeth with prophy paste, a rubber cup, and a brush. Some practices use a prophy jet spray (spray salt water) as an alternative to rubber cup polish.			3		
6. Use dental tape and prophy paste to clean interproximal areas.			3		
7. Floss and rinse the entire mouth.			3		

TOTAL POINTS POSSIBLE   46

TOTAL POINTS POSSIBLE—2nd attempt   44

TOTAL POINTS EARNED   _____

Points assigned reflect importance of step to meeting objective: Important = 1, Essential = 2, Critical = 3. Students will lose 2 points for repeated attempts. Failure results if any of the critical steps are omitted or performed incorrectly. If using a 100-point scale, determine score by dividing points earned by total points possible and multiplying the results by 100.

SCORE: _____

SKILL COMPETENCY ASSESSMENT

29-3 Gingivectomy

Student's Name _____ Date _____

Instructor's Name _____

Skill: This surgical procedure reduces the height of the gingival tissue, which provides visibility and access to remove irritants and smooth the root surface. Depending on the state Dental Practice Act, dental assistants may place and remove the periodontal dressing. The dental assistant must be prepared and thinking ahead to anticipate the dentist's needs. Routine steps should be followed for all treatment areas to maintain absolute clinical asepsis.

Performance Objective: The student will follow a routine procedure that meets the regulations and protocol set forth by the dentist and regulatory agencies, keeping in mind that assistant duties vary from state to state. The assistant may be evaluated by performance, verbal/written responses, and/or combined responses and actions. The procedure is performed by the periodontist to remove diseased gingiva and to clean periodontal pockets. The dental assistant prepares the instruments and materials, prepares the patient, and performs assisting responsibilities during the procedure.

	Self-Evaluation	Student Evaluation	Possible Points	Instructor Evaluation	Comments
Equipment and Supplies					
1. Basic setup: mouth mirror, explorer, cotton pliers			3		
2. Periodontal probe			3		
3. Cotton rolls and 2 × 2 gauze sponges			2		
4. Saliva ejector, HVE tip, air-water syringe tip, surgical aspirator tip			3		
5. Anesthetic setup			3		
6. Pocket marker			3		
7. Periodontal knives—broad bladed and interproximal			3		
8. Scalpel, blades, and diamond burs			3		
9. Scalers and curettes			3		
10. Soft tissue rongeurs and surgical scissors			3		

	Self-Evaluation	Student Evaluation	Possible Points	Instructor Evaluation	Comments
11. Hemostat			3		
12. Suture needle and thread			3		
13. Periodontal dressing materials			3		
Competency Steps (*follow aseptic procedures*) 1. Administer anesthetic to anesthetize tissues and reduce blood flow to the area.			3		
2. Examine area with the periodontal probe.			3		
3. Mark the depths of pockets with the pocket marker.			3		
4. Transfer instruments as directed.			3		
5. Use broad-bladed knife or scalpel to incise the marked gingival area.			3		
6. Evacuate the area and transfer instruments.			3		
7. Use interdental knives to remove interproximal tissue.			3		
8. Use scissors, rongeurs, and burs to remove tissue tags.			3		
9. Have gauze ready to receive any tissue from instruments and to clean the area of debris.			3		
10. After tissue is removed, the periodontist scales and planes the root surface.			3		
11. Continue to pass instruments and evacuate the area.			3		
12. Use sterile saline solution to irrigate, as needed.			2		
13. If sutures are needed, prepare the suture needle and thread and position in a hemostat or needle holder.			3		

	Self-Evaluation	Student Evaluation	Possible Points	Instructor Evaluation	Comments
14. Pass the hemostat and transfer scissors as needed.			3		
15. Retract tissue as needed.			3		
16. After sutures are placed, irrigate the area with sterile saline solution.			3		
17. Evacuate the area.			3		
18. Prepare the periodontal dressing.			3		
19. Assist the dentist with periodontal dressing placement.			3		
20. Give the patient postoperative instructions.			3		
21. Make sure that the patient has no debris on his or her face.			2		
22. Dismiss the patient.			2		

TOTAL POINTS POSSIBLE   101

TOTAL POINTS POSSIBLE—2nd attempt   99

TOTAL POINTS EARNED   ____

Points assigned reflect importance of step to meeting objective: Important = 1, Essential = 2, Critical = 3. Students will lose 2 points for repeated attempts. Failure results if any of the critical steps are omitted or performed incorrectly. If using a 100-point scale, determine score by dividing points earned by total points possible and multiplying the results by 100.

SCORE: _____

SKILL COMPETENCY ASSESSMENT

29-4 Osseous Surgery

Student's Name _____ Date _____

Instructor's Name _____

Skill: This surgical procedure removes defects/deformities in the bone caused by periodontal disease and related conditions. In additive osseous surgery, bone or bone substitute is added to fill in areas. In subtractive osseous surgery, the bone is removed with chisels, rongeurs, files, diamond burs, and stones. The dental assistant must be prepared and thinking ahead to anticipate the dentist's needs. Routine steps should be followed for all treatment areas to maintain absolute clinical asepsis.

Performance Objective: The student will follow a routine procedure that meets the regulations and protocol set forth by the dentist and regulatory agencies. The dental assistant assists the dentist throughout this procedure. Assistant duties vary from state to state. Therefore, assistant performance may be evaluated by performance criteria, oral/written responses, and/or responses and performance criteria. The procedure is performed by the periodontist, and involves removing and recontouring diseased and defective bone tissue. The extent of the periodontal disease process determines the amount and type of surgery performed. The dental assistant prepares the instruments and materials, prepares the patient, and performs assisting responsibilities during the procedure.

	Self-Evaluation	Student Evaluation	Possible Points	Instructor Evaluation	Comments
Equipment and Supplies					
1. Basic setup: mouth mirror, explorer, cotton pliers			3		
2. Periodontal probe			3		
3. Cotton rolls and 2 × 2 gauze sponges			2		
4. Saliva ejector, HVE tip, air-water syringe tip, surgical aspirator tip			3		
5. Anesthetic setup			3		
6. Scalpel and blades			3		
7. Periodontal knives—broad bladed and interproximal			3		
8. Tissue retractor			3		
9. Periosteal elevator			3		
10. Diamond burs and stones			3		

	Self-Evaluation	Student Evaluation	Possible Points	Instructor Evaluation	Comments
11. Bone rongeurs, bone chisels, and files			3		
12. Scalers and curettes			3		
13. Hemostat and surgical scissors			3		
14. Suture setup			3		
15. Periodontal dressing materials			3		
Note: During flap surgery, soft tissue is incised and reflected to expose bone for reshaping and/or removal. **Competency Steps (follow aseptic procedures)** 1. Administer anesthetic.			3		
2. Operator incises soft tissue and loosens from underlying bone.			3		
3. Transfer instruments.			3		
4. Maintain good visibility for the operator.			3		
5. Reflect and stabilize the tissue flap with tissue retractors.			3		
6. Retract and hold tissue.			3		
7. Operator exposes the bone and excises diseased bone tissue.			3		
8. Use scalers and curettes to remove calculus and diseased tissue and plane roots.			3		
9. Transfer instruments.			3		
10. Rinse the area with sterile saline solution as needed.			3		
11. Evacuate the area.			3		
12. Keep the instruments clean by removing debris from instruments with a gauze sponge.			2		

	Self-Evaluation	Student Evaluation	Possible Points	Instructor Evaluation	Comments
13. Operator shapes and contours bone using diamond burs and stones, rongeurs, chisels, and files.			3		
14. Pass burs, stones, and instruments as needed.			3		
15. Operator replaces the tissue flap and positions it over the alveolar bone.			3		
16. Prepare and transfer the suture.			3		
17. Stabilize the tissue with tissue forceps during suturing procedure.			3		
18. Prepare the periodontal dressing.			3		
19. Assist the dentist with periodontal dressing placement.			3		
20. Give the patient postoperative instructions.			3		
21. Make sure that the patient has no debris on his or her face.			2		
22. Dismiss the patient.			2		

TOTAL POINTS POSSIBLE   107

TOTAL POINTS POSSIBLE—2nd attempt   105

TOTAL POINTS EARNED   ____

Points assigned reflect importance of step to meeting objective: Important = 1, Essential = 2, Critical = 3. Students will lose 2 points for repeated attempts. Failure results if any of the critical steps are omitted or performed incorrectly. If using a 100-point scale, determine score by dividing points earned by total points possible and multiplying the results by 100.

SCORE: _____

SKILL COMPETENCY ASSESSMENT

29-5 Preparation and Placement of Noneugenol Periodontal Dressing

Student's Name _____ Date _____

Instructor's Name _____

Skill: Periodontal dressings or packs are placed after periodontal surgical procedures. The dressing has no medicinal qualities but acts like a bandage to protect the tissue during healing. Zinc oxide-eugenol and non-eugenol materials are the most common materials used for periodontal dressings. The dental assistant must be prepared and thinking ahead to anticipate the dentist's needs. Routine steps should be followed for all treatment areas to maintain absolute clinical asepsis.

Performance Objective: The student will follow a routine procedure that meets the regulations and protocol set forth by the dentist and regulatory agencies, keeping in mind that assistant duties vary from state to state. The assistant may be evaluated by performance, verbal/written responses, and/or combined responses and actions. The dentist routinely places the dressing, but in some states the dental assistant is allowed to place and remove the periodontal dressing. The dressing is placed after the surgery to protect the tissues and promote the healing process.

	Self-Evaluation	Student Evaluation	Possible Points	Instructor Evaluation	Comments
Equipment and Supplies 1. Basic setup: mouth mirror, explorer, and cotton pliers			3		
2. Gauze sponges			2		
3. Noneugenol periodontal dressing material (base and accelerator)			3		
4. Paper pad and tongue depressor			3		
5. Lubricant			3		
6. Instrument to contour dressing (spoon excavator, sickle scaler)			3		
Competency Steps (*follow aseptic procedures*) 1. Lightly coat the patient's lips with Vaseline (after the hemorrhaging is controlled).			3		

	Self-Evaluation	Student Evaluation	Possible Points	Instructor Evaluation	Comments
2. Dispense dressing materials into equal lengths.			3		
3. Mix dressing materials with a tongue blade until they are homogeneous.			3		
4. Allow the material to set for 2 to 3 minutes or until the tackiness is gone.			3		
5. Lubricate gloved fingers with Vaseline so the putty-like material can be easily handled.			3		
6. Dressing comes with a retardant to slow the setting time, if necessary. Mold it easily for 3 to 5 minutes and work it for 15 to 20.			3		
7. Mold the dressing into a thin strip slightly longer than the surgical site.			3		
8. Divide the strip into two equal lengths, one for the facial surface and one for the lingual.			3		
9. Begin placement; form the end of one strip into a hook shape.			3		
10. Wrap the hook around the distal of the most posterior tooth.			3		
11. Adapt the rest of the strip along the facial surface, gently pressing the pack into interproximal areas.			3		

	Self-Evaluation	Student Evaluation	Possible Points	Instructor Evaluation	Comments
12. Apply the second strip to the lingual surface in the same manner. Wrap pack around the last posterior tooth and adapt it to the lingual surface, moving it toward the midline.			3		
13. Use the pack to cover the gingiva evenly without interfering with occlusion, tongue movement, or frenum attachment.			3		
14. Check dressing for overextensions.			3		
15. Remove excess dressing with a spoon excavator or a scaler.			3		
16. Gently press the instrument into the dressing to detach extra material.			3		
17. Smooth the pack and evaluate for even thickness.			3		
18. Ask the patient how the pack feels.			2		
19. Have the patient move the tongue, cheeks, and lips to mold the pack.			2		
20. Make adjustments, ensuring the dressing is securely in place, trimmed, and contoured.			3		

	Self-Evaluation	Student Evaluation	Possible Points	Instructor Evaluation	Comments
21. Give patient instructions:					
a. Keep the pack on for one week after surgery.			2		
b. The pack will harden in a few hours and withstand normal chewing stresses.			2		
c. The pack may chip and break off during the week but should remain intact as long as possible.			2		
d. If the patient experiences pain when pieces of the pack come off or become rough, the patient should call the office.			2		
e. The patient should brush the occlusal surfaces of the teeth involved in the surgery.			2		
f. Continue to brush and floss the rest of the teeth as normal.			2		

TOTAL POINTS POSSIBLE   87

TOTAL POINTS POSSIBLE—2nd attempt   85

TOTAL POINTS EARNED   _____

Points assigned reflect importance of step to meeting objective: Important = 1, Essential = 2, Critical = 3. Students will lose 2 points for repeated attempts. Failure results if any of the critical steps are omitted or performed incorrectly. If using a 100-point scale, determine score by dividing points earned by total points possible and multiplying the results by 100.

SCORE: _____

SKILL COMPETENCY ASSESSMENT

29-6 Removal of the Periodontal Dressing

Student's Name _____ Date _____

Instructor's Name _____

Skill: Periodontal dressings or packs are placed after periodontal surgical procedures. The dressings do not have any medicinal qualities but act like a bandage to protect the tissue during the healing process. Routine steps should be followed for all treatment areas to maintain absolute clinical asepsis.

Performance Objective: The student will follow a routine procedure that meets the regulations and protocol set forth by the dentist and regulatory agencies. This procedure is performed by the periodontist or the dental assistant depending on the expanded functions. Assistant duties vary from state to state. Therefore, the assistant may be evaluated by performance criteria, verbal/written responses, and/or combined responses and performance criteria. The patient has worn the dressing for a week to 10 days. The patient's mouth is examined before removing the dressing to check for areas where the dressing may have come loose or come off completely.

	Self-Evaluation	Student Evaluation	Possible Points	Instructor Evaluation	Comments
Equipment and Supplies					
1. Basic setup: mouth mirror, explorer, cotton pliers			3		
2. Saliva ejector, HVE tip, air-water syringe tip			3		
3. Gauze sponges and tissue scissors			3		
4. Instruments to remove the dressing (spoon excavator, sickle explorer, surgical hoe)			3		
Competency Steps (*follow aseptic procedures*)					
1. Seat the patient.			2		
2. Evaluate the surgical site.			3		
3. Insert the surgical hoe or spoon excavator along the margin. Apply lateral pressure to pry the dressing away from the tissue. (The pack may come off in large pieces.)			3		

	Self-Evaluation	Student Evaluation	Possible Points	Instructor Evaluation	Comments
4. Use scalers and floss to remove any particles from interproximal areas and tooth surfaces.			3		
5. Use cotton pliers to remove particles of dressing that are embedded in the surgical site.			3		
6. Gently rinse the entire area with warm water to remove any debris. Use the air-water syringe, if used carefully.			3		

TOTAL POINTS POSSIBLE   29

TOTAL POINTS POSSIBLE—2nd attempt   27

TOTAL POINTS EARNED   _____

Points assigned reflect importance of step to meeting objective: Important = 1, Essential = 2, Critical = 3. Students will lose 2 points for repeated attempts. Failure results if any of the critical steps are omitted or performed incorrectly. If using a 100-point scale, determine score by dividing points earned by total points possible and multiplying the results by 100.

SCORE: _____

SKILL COMPETENCY ASSESSMENT

29-7 Polishing with Rubber Cup

Student's Name _____ Date _____

Instructor's Name _____

Skill: Routine steps should be followed for all treatment areas to maintain absolute clinical asepsis. The dental assistant is responsible for preparation of equipment and supplies needed for the appointment. The coronal polish procedure involves removing soft deposits and extrinsic stains from the surfaces of the teeth and restorations. This is accomplished with an abrasive, dental handpiece, rubber cup, brush, and dental tape and floss. Developing a sequence that is always followed is recommended when polishing the entire mouth.

Performance Objective: The student will follow a routine procedure that meets the regulations and the protocol set forth by the dentist and regulatory agencies. Therefore, the assistant may be evaluated by performance criteria, verbal/written responses, and/or combined responses and performance criteria. This procedure is performed by the dental assistant, hygienist, or dentist. The following procedure for polishing with the rubber cup explains the positioning techniques and the action of the rubber cup.

	Self-Evaluation	Student Evaluation	Possible Points	Instructor Evaluation	Comments
Equipment and Supplies					
1. Basic setup: mouth mirror, explorer/periodontal probe, cotton pliers			3		
2. Saliva ejector, HVE tip, air-water syringe tip			3		
3. 2 × 2 gauze sponges, cotton-tipped applicator			3		
4. Dappen dish			3		
5. Lip lubricant			3		
6. Disclosing solution (optional)			3		
7. Low-speed handpiece			3		
8. Prophy angle attachment			3		
9. Assortment of rubber cups and brushes			3		

	Self-Evaluation	Student Evaluation	Possible Points	Instructor Evaluation	Comments
10. Prophy paste of various grits and finger rings (finger rings to hold paste cups)			3		
11. Dental tape and dental floss			3		
Competency Steps (*follow aseptic procedures*) 1. Seat patient and prepare for coronal polishing procedure: a. Offer lip lubricant for patient comfort. b. Review patient's medical history. c. Inspect oral cavity for amount of extrinsic stain. d. Select grit of abrasive to be used.			3 3 3 3 3		
2. Assistant may dry teeth and place disclosing solution on teeth (easier to detect plaque).			3		
3. After drying teeth, use cotton tip applicator to place solution on all surfaces of teeth (one quadrant, one arch, or one side at a time).			3		
4. After placing abrasive polishing agent in cup, place handpiece in patient's mouth and start the handpiece. Place cup near gingival sulcus, establish a fulcrum. Use correct cup placement and fulcrum for each arch (cup as far into mesial/distal surface as possible; fulcrum as close to tooth being polished as possible).			3		
5. Apply light pressure to flex cup, flare into sulcus (1 to 2 mm).			3		
6. Sweep rubber cup toward incisal or occlusal edge (if crown of tooth is long, lift cup halfway up tooth and make second stroke toward occlusal).			3		

	Self-Evaluation	Student Evaluation	Possible Points	Instructor Evaluation	Comments
7. At incisal or occlusal edge, lift cup slightly off tooth and replace it near gingiva to repeat the stroke, moving toward the opposite side of tooth.			3		
8. Repeat stroke, overlapping each time, until entire tooth surface is polished			3		
9. When finished with one tooth, move to adjacent tooth using same steps until surfaces of all teeth have been polished.			3		
10. For the patient's comfort, rinse mouth frequently (at least after polishing each quadrant).			3		
11. When all teeth are polished, rinse and evacuate patient's mouth thoroughly, removing all debris.			3		

TOTAL POINTS POSSIBLE   78

TOTAL POINTS POSSIBLE—2nd attempt   76

TOTAL POINTS EARNED   ____

Points assigned reflect importance of step to meeting objective: Important = 1, Essential = 2, Critical = 3. Students will lose 2 points for repeated attempts. Failure results if any of the critical steps are omitted or performed incorrectly. If using a 100-point scale, determine score by dividing points earned by total points possible and multiplying the results by 100.

SCORE: _____

SKILL COMPETENCY ASSESSMENT

29-8 Using Prophy Brush

Student's Name _____ Date _____

Instructor's Name _____

Skill: Routine steps should be followed for all treatment areas to maintain absolute clinical asepsis. The dental assistant is responsible for preparation of equipment and supplies needed for the appointment. The coronal polish procedure involves removing soft deposits and extrinsic stains from the surfaces of the teeth and restorations. This is accomplished with an abrasive, dental handpiece, rubber cup, brush, and dental tape and floss. Developing a sequence that is always followed is recommended when polishing the entire mouth.

Performance Objective: The student will follow a routine procedure that meets the regulations and the protocol set forth by the dentist and regulatory agencies. Therefore, the assistant may be evaluated by performance criteria, verbal/written responses, and/or combined responses and performance criteria. This procedure is performed by the dental assistant, hygienist, or dentist. The prophy brush follows the rubber cup polish, and includes techniques for manipulating and positioning the brush.

	Self-Evaluation	Student Evaluation	Possible Points	Instructor Evaluation	Comments
Equipment and Supplies					
1. Basic setup: mouth mirror, explorer/periodontal probe, cotton pliers			3		
2. Saliva ejector, HVE tip, air-water syringe tip			3		
3. 2 × 2 gauze sponges, cotton-tipped applicator			3		
4. Dappen dish			3		
5. Lip lubricant			3		
6. Disclosing solution (optional)			3		
7. Low-speed handpiece			3		
8. Prophy angle attachment			3		

	Self-Evaluation	Student Evaluation	Possible Points	Instructor Evaluation	Comments
9. Assortment of rubber cups and brushes			3		
10. Prophy paste of various grits and finger rings (finger rings to hold paste cups)			3		
11. Dental tape and dental floss			3		
Competency Steps (*follow aseptic procedures*) 1. Place softened brush on prophy angle, and apply prophy paste to tooth.			3		
2. Establish fulcrum close to posterior tooth to be polished.			3		
3. Move brush bristles toward mesial buccal cusp tip and continue until brush comes off occlusal surface.			3		
4. Replace brush bristles in central fossa.			3		
5. Apply slight pressure again, move brush up toward distal buccal cusp and brush comes off occlusal surface.			3		
6. Repeat this procedure on occlusal surfaces of posterior tooth until all of the occlusal surface is cleaned.			3		
7. Repeat this process on occlusal surfaces of all teeth.			3		
8. For the lingual surface of the anterior teeth, place prophy brush in lingual pit above the cingulum.			3		

	Self-Evaluation	Student Evaluation	Possible Points	Instructor Evaluation	Comments
9. Apply light pressure to flex and spread bristles of brush.			3		
10. Move brush toward incisal edge to polish lingual surface.			3		
11. Repeat on all lingual surfaces that have deep pits and grooves.			3		
12. When finished with brush, rinse and evacuate the oral cavity thoroughly.			3		

TOTAL POINTS POSSIBLE   69

TOTAL POINTS POSSIBLE—2nd attempt   67

TOTAL POINTS EARNED   _____

Points assigned reflect importance of step to meeting objective: Important = 1, Essential = 2, Critical = 3. Students will lose 2 points for repeated attempts. Failure results if any of the critical steps are omitted or performed incorrectly. If using a 100-point scale, determine score by dividing points earned by total points possible and multiplying the results by 100.

SCORE: _____

SKILL COMPETENCY ASSESSMENT

29-9 Polishing with Dental Tape and Floss

Student's Name _____ Date _____

Instructor's Name _____

Skill: Routine steps should be followed for all treatment areas to maintain absolute clinical asepsis. The dental assistant is responsible for preparation of equipment and supplies. The coronal polish procedure involves removing soft deposits and extrinsic stains from the surfaces of the teeth and restorations. This is accomplished with an abrasive, dental handpiece, a rubber cup, a brush, and dental tape and floss. Developing a sequence that is always followed is recommended when polishing the entire mouth. When using dental tape or floss, care must be taken not to damage the interdental papilla and free gingiva margins.

Performance Objective: The student will follow a routine procedure that meets the regulations and the protocol set forth by the dentist and regulatory agencies. Therefore, the assistant may be evaluated by performance criteria, verbal/written responses, and/or combined responses and performance criteria. This procedure is performed routinely by the dental assistant and dental hygienist. The procedure describes the portion of a coronal polish and the protocol for performing polishing with dental tape and dental floss, including preparation of materials, the patient, positioning of the operator and the patient, sequence of procedure, and evaluating the procedure. The details of use of the rubber cup and brush have been described previously in this section. Dental tape is used with an abrasive agent on the interproximal surfaces of the teeth. The dental floss is placed interproximally, wrapped around the tooth, and moved in an up-and-down motion.

	Self-Evaluation	Student Evaluation	Possible Points	Instructor Evaluation	Comments
Equipment and Supplies					
1. Basic setup: mouth mirror, explorer, cotton pliers			3		
2. Saliva ejector, HVE tip, air-water syringe tip			3		
3. 2 × 2 gauze sponges, cotton-tipped applicators, tongue blade, and cotton rolls			3		
4. Dappen dish			3		
5. Lip lubricant			3		
6. Disclosing solution (optional)			3		
7. Low-speed handpiece			3		
8. Prophy angle attachment			3		

	Self-Evaluation	Student Evaluation	Possible Points	Instructor Evaluation	Comments
9. Prophy cups and brushes			3		
10. Prophy pastes, various grits, and finger ring holder			3		
11. Dental tape and dental floss			3		
Competency Steps (*follow aseptic procedures*) 1. Cut off a piece of dental tape 12 to 18 inches long.			3		
2. Wipe some abrasive agent into the interproximal contact areas of teeth in a quadrant, with a cotton tip or finger.			3		
3. Wrap the tape around the middle fingers of both hands, leaving a length of tape just long enough to wrap around the tooth while maintaining control.			3		
4. Take tape through contact at an oblique angle (\) in a back-and-forth motion, using gentle pressure and holding the tape against the tooth. Prevent snapping through contact and damaging gingiva.			3		
5. Wrap tape around the tooth to cover the line angles of the tooth on both buccal and lingual.			3		
6. When **proximal** surface of one tooth is completed, lift tape up and over the interdental papilla without removing the tape through the contact and readapt the tape on the proximal surface of adjacent tooth.			3		

	Self-Evaluation	Student Evaluation	Possible Points	Instructor Evaluation	Comments
7. Polish this surface with the tape and abrasive and then remove tape through contact. (If tape is pulled through the embrasure area, be careful not to injure gingival tissues.)			3		
8. Continue around each tooth in both arches until all surfaces have been polished (includes most distal surface of each quadrant; use different areas of tape as needed, rinse area thoroughly, and evacuate all debris).			3		
9. Follow the taping using dental floss to remove any debris left. Floss all areas and rinse thoroughly.			3		

TOTAL POINTS POSSIBLE 60

TOTAL POINTS POSSIBLE—2nd attempt 58

TOTAL POINTS EARNED _____

Points assigned reflect importance of step to meeting objective: Important = 1, Essential = 2, Critical = 3. Students will lose 2 points for repeated attempts. Failure results if any of the critical steps are omitted or performed incorrectly. If using a 100-point scale, determine score by dividing points earned by total points possible and multiplying the results by 100.

SCORE: _____

SKILL COMPETENCY ASSESSMENT

29-10 Coronal Polishing Procedure

Student's Name _____ Date _____

Instructor's Name _____

Skill: Routine steps should be followed for all treatment areas to maintain absolute clinical asepsis. The dental assistant is responsible for preparation of equipment and supplies needed for the appointment. The coronal polish procedure involves removing soft deposits and extrinsic stains from the surfaces of the teeth and restorations. This is accomplished with an abrasive, a dental handpiece, a rubber cup, a brush, and dental tape and floss. Developing a sequence that is always followed is recommended when polishing the entire mouth.

Performance Objective: The student will follow a routine procedure that meets the regulations and the protocol set forth by the dentist and regulatory agencies. Therefore, the assistant may be evaluated by performance criteria, verbal/written responses, and/or combined responses and performance criteria. This procedure is performed routinely by the dental assistant and dental hygienist. The procedure describes the protocol for performing a coronal polish including preparation of materials and the patient, positioning of the operator and the patient, sequence of procedure, and evaluating the procedure. The details of using the rubber cup, brush, dental tape, and floss have been described previously in this section.

	Self-Evaluation	Student Evaluation	Possible Points	Instructor Evaluation	Comments
Equipment and Supplies					
1. Basic setup: mouth mirror, explorer, cotton pliers			3		
2. Saliva ejector, HVE tip, air-water syringe tip			3		
3. 2 × 2 gauze sponges, cotton-tipped applicators, tongue blade, and cotton rolls			3		
4. Lip lubricant and disclosing solution in dappen dish			3		
5. Low-speed handpiece with prophy angle attachment			3		
6. Prophy cups and brushes (dappen dish with warm water to soak brushes in)			3		
7. Prophy pastes, various grits, and finger ring holder			3		

	Self-Evaluation	Student Evaluation	Possible Points	Instructor Evaluation	Comments
8. Dental tape and dental floss			3		
9. Auxiliary aids as needed			3		
The following are necessary off-tray items:					
1. Patient's chart			3		
2. Red/blue pencil, lead pencil, and pen			3		
3. Barriers for the dental unit			3		
4. Patient bib and bib chain			3		
5. Patient safety glasses			3		
6. Patient hand mirror			3		
Competency Steps (*follow aseptic procedures*)					
1. Gather equipment and materials, prepare operatory for patient, and review patient's records.			3		
2. Prepare the patient: a. Follow established procedure, seat patient, and review/update patient's records. b. Explain procedure to patient. c. Follow aseptic procedures, and prepare patient for coronal polish. d. Evaluate patient's condition, perform oral inspection. e. After examining teeth, select abrasive agents to be used. f. Lubricate patient's lips, dry teeth, and apply disclosing agent with cotton tip applicator. g. Adjust dental unit light for good vision.			3 3 3 3 3 3 3		

	Self-Evaluation	Student Evaluation	Possible Points	Instructor Evaluation	Comments
3. Position operator and patient. a. Demonstrate position of operator and patient.			3		
b. Demonstrate position of patient's head. • Patient's head is turned away from operator when operator is polishing maxillary/mandibular right facial and maxillary/mandibular left lingual.			3		
• Patient's head is turned toward operator when operator is polishing maxillary/mandibular right lingual and maxillary/mandibular left facial.			3		
4. Sequence of procedure: a. Begin polish on quadrant that you decided would be beginning point.			3		
b. Follow appropriate criteria on use of abrasives, rubber cup, prophy brush, tape, and floss.			3		
c. Rinse patient's mouth after each quadrant (or as needed).			3		
5. Evaluating the coronal polish: a. Once all steps of coronal polish are complete, rinse patient's mouth thoroughly with spray from air-water syringe and evacuate.			3		
b. Apply disclosing solution to detect any missed areas of plaque or stain.			3		
c. Using mouth mirror and air syringe, inspect each surface for any remaining soft deposits and/or stains.			3		
d. Note these areas on the chart for future reference.			3		

	Self-Evaluation	Student Evaluation	Possible Points	Instructor Evaluation	Comments
e. Polish areas missed with prophy cup and/or brush.			3		
f. Rinse patient's mouth to remove all abrasive agent.			3		
g. Inspect teeth for lustrous shine with no debris or extrinsic stains; soft tissues should be free of abrasion or trauma.			3		
h. The patient is ready for fluoride treatment.			3		
i. The dentist may want to see patient before patient is dismissed.			3		
6. Charting the coronal polish: a. Assistant must record coronal polish completely and accurately on patient's dental chart.			3		
b. Chart entries are recorded in ink, dated, and signed or entered into computer system.			3		
c. Include any comments about condition of patient's mouth and type(s) of material(s)used.			3		

TOTAL POINTS POSSIBLE   123

TOTAL POINTS POSSIBLE—2nd attempt   121

TOTAL POINTS EARNED   _____

Points assigned reflect importance of step to meeting objective: Important = 1, Essential = 2, Critical = 3. Students will lose 2 points for repeated attempts. Failure results if any of the critical steps are omitted or performed incorrectly. If using a 100-point scale, determine score by dividing points earned by total points possible and multiplying the results by 100.

SCORE: _____

CHAPTER 30

Fixed Prosthodontics and Gingival Retraction

SPECIFIC INSTRUCTIONAL OBJECTIVES

The student should strive to meet the following objectives and demonstrate an understanding of the facts and principles presented in this chapter:

1. Define the scope of fixed prosthodontics.

2. Explain the dentist's considerations when recommending various prostheses to a patient.

3. Describe various types of fixed prostheses and their functions.

4. Describe dental materials used in fixed prostheses.

5. Identify and explain the CAD/CAM restorative system.

6. Explain the involvement of the laboratory technician in the fabrication of fixed prostheses.

7. Describe the role of the dental assistant in all phases of fixed prosthodontic treatment.

8. Explain techniques for retaining the prosthesis when there is little or no crown on the tooth.

9. Describe implant retainer prostheses.

10. Explain techniques for maintaining fixed prostheses.

Advanced Chairside Functions

11. Explain the function of gingival retraction.

12. Describe the different types of gingival retraction.

13. Explain the steps of placing and removing gingival retraction cord.

SUMMARY

Fixed prosthodontics encompasses replacement of missing teeth or parts of teeth with extensive restorations. There are many types of fixed prostheses and a variety of materials used for preparation, fabrication, and cementation. The dental assistant is involved in all stages of fixed prosthodontic treatment. It is important to understand the sequence of the procedure and the various types of restorations when assisting the dentist.

The goal of this chapter is to assess the more common procedures to give the dental assistant the background and sequence to assist the dentist.

Restorations routinely take at least two appointments to complete. The assistant explains the steps of the procedure to the patient, answers questions, and provides postoperative and home care instructions.

Gingival retraction is an important step when preparing the tooth for the final impression. Margins of the preparations must be exposed so that the impression will reflect an accurate image of the tooth and preparation, and thus insure that the fixed prosthesis will fit perfectly. Learning about the various materials and techniques helps the dental assistant become more skilled when working with the dentist.

EXERCISES AND ACTIVITIES

Multiple Choice

1. Replacing missing teeth will benefit the patient by

   a. restoring masticatory function.

   b. improving aesthetics.

   c. improving speech.

   d. All of the above

2. The artificial part that replaces a missing tooth is called a

   a. retention pin.

   b. retention core.

   c. retention post.

   d. prosthesis.

3. A(n) _____ covers the entire coronal surface of the tooth.

   a. full-cast crown

   b. partial crown

   c. three-quarter crown

   d. onlay

4. Which cast restoration covers the area between the cusps in the middle of the tooth, the proximal surfaces that are involved, and the cusp ridges?

   a. Full-cast crown

   b. Partial crown

   c. Three-quarter crown

   d. Onlay

5. Which cast restoration covers three or more, but not all, surfaces of the tooth?

   a. Full-cast crown

   b. Partial crown

   c. Three-quarter crown

   d. Onlay

6. Which restoration replaces the missing tooth structure of a mesio-occlusal surface?

   a. Onlay

   b. Inlay

   c. Three-quarter crown

   d. Partial crown

7. The Maryland bridge is used to replace _____ tooth (teeth).

   a. one

   b. two

   c. three

   d. four

8. _____ are thin layers of tooth-colored material that cover much of the facial surface.

   a. Porcelain-fused-to-metal crowns

   b. Implant retainer prostheses

   c. Core buildups

   d. Veneers

9. Dental casting alloy uses a combination of metals, including

   a. silane.

   b. polysiloxane.

   c. platinum.

   d. polyether.

10. A _____, a treatment performed for vital teeth that have very little crown structure, is made of amalgam, composite, or a silver alloy/glass ionomer combination.

    a. veneer

    b. core buildup

    c. retention pin

    d. post-retained core

11. The dentist performs an examination to determine whether a patient is a candidate for a fixed prosthesis. Which of the following methods are included in this examination?

    1. Exam of intra- and extraoral tissues
    2. Number of inlays
    3. Radiographs
    4. Retention pins
    5. Diagnostic casts made
    6. Implant retainer prosthesis

       a. 1, 4, 6

       b. 1, 3, 5

       c. 2, 3, 6

       d. 2, 4, 5

12. A bridge is a restoration that spans the space of a missing tooth or teeth. The teeth adjacent to the missing tooth are called

    a. pontics.

    b. abutments.

    c. inlays.

    d. onlays.

13. Each unit of a bridge represents a tooth. The missing tooth is replaced by a(n)

    a. pontic.

    b. abutment.

    c. inlay.

    d. onlay.

14. Which of the following are included among new chemical retraction alternatives?

    a. Topical hemostatic solution

    b. Astringent with dento-infusion tubes

    c. Plastic Luer-Lok syringe

    d. All of the above

15. Which of the following is defined by the term "ischemia"?

    a. Cauterization of tissues

    b. Shrinking of tissues

    c. Surgical removal of tissue

    d. Mechanical treatment of tissue

16. An astringent used in the retraction cord could bring on tachycardia, and thus is a contraindication for individuals with which of the following conditions?

    a. Heart disease

    b. Diabetes

    c. Hyperthyroidism

    d. All of the above

17. The proper position of the tucked retraction cord is _____ mm into the crevice.

    a. 1/2

    b. 1 to 3

    c. 5

    d. Both a. and c.

18. Instruments used on dental implants are

    a. stainless steel.

    b. titanium.

    c. plastic coated.

    d. gold.

19. Retraction cord is available in a variety of configurations, such as

    a. twisted.

    b. braided.

    c. woven.

    d. All of the above

20. Which of the following are contraindications for the use of electrosurgery?

    a. Receiving radiation therapy

    b. Cardiac pacemakers

    c. Any disease that is slow healing

    d. All of the above

 Critical Thinking

1. After a tooth is prepared for a crown, gingival retraction is performed. During this process, all hemorrhaging must be arrested. List the types of retraction that can be used and any contraindications.

2. The dental assistant provides the patient with instructions and tips on maintaining the new crown or bridge. List some of the aids that the patient will need to know how to use.

3. Sometimes additional retention is needed during tooth preparation to improve the overall restoration. Explain when additional retention is needed, and describe the retention options.

CASE STUDY 1

During the tooth preparation stage, the preparation goes deep and below the gingival. The gingiva are bleeding. The dentist opts for use of an electrosurgery unit during the retraction cord phase and final impression for this patient.

1. What is the function of an electrosurgery unit?

2. Describe how electrosurgery works.

3. Describe the dental assistant's tasks during use of the electrosurgery unit.

4. When is the use of electrosurgery contraindicated?

CASE STUDY 2

Because the dental assistant is involved in all stages of fixed prosthodontic treatment, understanding the sequence, preparation, and procedure is important.

1. Describe the overall sequence of dental assistant tasks during fixed prosthodontic treatment.

2. List responsibilities of the dental assistant in the preparation of equipment and supplies.

3. List expanded functions that may be available for assistants in certain states.

4. Describe other tasks for which the dental assistant may be responsible.

CASE STUDY 3

Diane needs a crown procedure, but she does not have much time for treatment as her family is leaving on an extended trip in the near future. A dental staff member consults with the dentist and Diane about using CEREC 3, an alternative to fixed prosthodontics. The patient accepts and the procedure appointment is scheduled.

1. List dental staff commitments when using CAD/CAM restorative systems.

2. Name the two pieces of hardware that come with the system.

3. Describe various ceramic materials available to the dentist.

4. Describe the benefits of these restorative systems to the patient.

5. List the basic steps of CEREC restoration.

SKILL COMPETENCY ASSESSMENT

30-1 Porcelain Veneers

Student's Name _____ Date _____

Instructor's Name _____

Skill: The porcelain veneer technique is sensitive to shade selection and gingival margin adaptation if the veneer is to look natural and adapt well. Porcelain veneers are similar to indirect resin veneers in that they require two appointments and are fabricated in the dental laboratory. Routine steps should be followed for all treatment areas to maintain absolute clinical asepsis. The dental assistant must be prepared and thinking ahead to anticipate the dentist's needs.

Performance Objective: The student will follow a routine procedure that meets the regulations and protocol set forth by the dentist and regulatory agencies, keeping in mind that assistant duties vary from state to state. The procedure is completed in two appointments. During the first appointment, the tooth is prepared and impressions are taken; at the second appointment, the porcelain veneer is seated. Between the two appointments, the impressions are sent to a dental laboratory where the porcelain veneer is fabricated. The assistant may be evaluated by performance, verbal/written responses, and/or combined responses and actions.

	Self-Evaluation	Student Evaluation	Possible Points	Instructor Evaluation	Comments
Preparation Appointment (first appointment)					
Equipment and Supplies (*for the preparation appointment*)					
1. Basic setup: mouth mirror, explorer, and cotton pliers			3		
2. Cotton rolls, 2 × 2 gauze			2		
3. HVE tip, air-water syringe tip			3		
4. Anesthetic setup			3		
5. High-speed handpiece and assorted burs			3		
6. Shade guide			3		
7. Spoon excavator			3		
8. Low-speed handpiece with prophy angle, rubber cup, and pumice			3		

	Self-Evaluation	Student Evaluation	Possible Points	Instructor Evaluation	Comments
9. Retraction cord and placement instrument			3		
10. Bite registration materials			3		
11. Alginate impression materials for model of opposing arch			3		
12. Final impression materials (polysiloxane or polyether)			3		
13. Temporary veneer (optional)			2		
14. Laboratory prescription form			2		
Competency Steps (*follow aseptic procedures*) **Preparation (First Appointment)** 1. Take the bite registration.			2		
2. Take the opposing arch impression.			3		
3. Clean the teeth with a rubber cup and pumice (to remove extrinsic stains).			3		
4. The dentist selects the shade (determines how light the patient wants the veneers and how light the finished shade will be).			3		
5. Prepare the teeth according to the design of the veneer (prepare incisal edge and cervical margin carefully so that the finished veneer will be even with the gingival crest or just slightly subgingival).			3		
6. Place retraction cord (achieve hemostasis and visualize margins).			3		

	Self-Evaluation	Student Evaluation	Possible Points	Instructor Evaluation	Comments
7. Take the final impression with a dimensionally stable material (polysiloxane or polyether).			3		
8. Place temporary veneers, if necessary.			3		
9. Remove the retraction cord after the temporary veneers are placed.			3		
10. Inform the patient that the gums will be tender for several days from the retraction cord placement.			2		
11. Dismiss the patient.			2		
Laboratory Fabrication					
1. Send impressions to the dental laboratory with a laboratory prescription.			3		
2. The laboratory will follow the dentist's prescription on length of veneer, shade, thickness, and texture (color photos of the patient are helpful in the design and shade process).			3		
3. The laboratory fabricates the veneers and returns them to the office.			3		
Cementation Appointment (Second Appointment) **Equipment and Supplies** 1. Basic setup: mouth mirror, explorer, and cotton pliers			3		
2. Cotton rolls, 2 × 2 gauze, cheek and lip retractors			3		
3. Saliva ejector, HVE tip, air-water syringe tip			3		
4. Porcelain veneers from the laboratory			3		

	Self-Evaluation	Student Evaluation	Possible Points	Instructor Evaluation	Comments
5. Low-speed handpiece with prophy angle, rubber cup, and pumice			3		
6. Silane coupling agent and small applicator (brush)			3		
7. Retraction cord and placement instrument			3		
8. Chlorhexidine soap			2		
9. Plastic or ultra-thin metal strips			2		
10. Etchant and applicator			3		
11. Bonding agent and curing light			3		
Competency Steps (*follow aseptic procedures*) 1. Schedule the appointment (coordinated as close as possible to first appointment and laboratory work, and delivery scheduled so that turnaround time is minimal).			3		
2. Complete preliminary cleaning of the teeth with pumice (remove plaque and stains).			3		
3. Try veneers on the tooth and make adjustments with finishing diamonds (veneers are fragile; handle with care). Once all adjustments are completed, clean the veneers.			3		
4. Clean and dry inside of the veneer thoroughly (use acid etch to clean and decontaminate the inside of the veneer).			3		

	Self-Evaluation	Student Evaluation	Possible Points	Instructor Evaluation	Comments
5. Apply a thin layer of silane coupling agent (this material allows bonding to porcelain).			3		
6. Place light-cured bonding agent in the veneers (make sure that all air bubbles have been eliminated).			3		
7. Fill the veneer with material and spread it evenly.			3		
8. Place veneers in a light-protected area or box until the teeth are prepared.			3		
9. Prepare the teeth for bonding: a. Place retraction cord on the facial surface. b. Clean the facial surface with chlorhexidine soap. c. Use a prophy cup or brush with Step b.			3 3 3		
10. Isolate the teeth being bonded. a. Cotton rolls b. Cheek and lip retractors c. Saliva ejector d. Plastic or ultra-thin metal strips			2 2 2 2		
11. Etch the teeth being bonded (follow directions of adhesive system manufacturer).			3		
12. Apply adhesive to the teeth being bonded.			3		
13. Seat each veneer in the correct position.			3		
14. In some cases, spot cure veneer and remove excess cement.			3		
15. Light cure each veneer in place.			3		

	Self-Evaluation	Student Evaluation	Possible Points	Instructor Evaluation	Comments
16. Remove excess cement with a scalpel.			3		
17. Contour and refine margins with finishing diamonds or burs.			3		
18. Polish veneers with rubber wheels, cups, and polishing paste.			3		

TOTAL POINTS POSSIBLE   174

TOTAL POINTS POSSIBLE—2nd attempt   172

TOTAL POINTS EARNED   _____

Points assigned reflect importance of step to meeting objective: Important = 1, Essential = 2, Critical = 3. Students will lose 2 points for repeated attempts. Failure results if any of the critical steps are omitted or performed incorrectly. If using a 100-point scale, determine score by dividing points earned by total points possible and multiplying the results by 100.

SCORE: _____

SKILL COMPETENCY ASSESSMENT

30-2 Preparation for Porcelain-Fused-to-Metal Crown

Student's Name _____ Date _____

Instructor's Name _____

Skill: The dental assistant assists the dentist in all aspects of the procedure, from selecting the shade of the tooth to general chairside assisting. The dental assistant is responsible for preparing the equipment and supplies needed for both appointments. Each tray setup is arranged according to the sequence of the procedure, with auxiliary instruments and materials close at hand. The procedure includes many different types of dental materials that the dental assistant will prepare and/or use throughout the procedure. The assistant coordinates the patient's appointments and the laboratory schedule. In some offices, the assistant may perform some laboratory functions. In some states with advanced functions, the qualified assistant can perform procedures such as placing retraction cord, placement and removal of temporaries, taking preliminary impressions, and removing excess cement.

Performance Objective: The student will follow a routine procedure that meets the regulations and protocol set forth by the dentist and regulatory agencies, keeping in mind that assistant duties vary from state to state. The procedure is performed by the dentist and dental assistant. Like the veneer procedure, this process involves two appointments. The following sequence of procedures for a patient needing a porcelain-fused-to-metal crown encompasses the steps in the preparation appointment, including retention procedures, and the steps in the cementation appointment. Each step is explained and the dental assistant's responsibilities are described. The patient is seated and prepared for the procedure. The assistant may be evaluated by performance, verbal/written responses, and/or combined responses and actions.

	Self-Evaluation	Student Evaluation	Possible Points	Instructor Evaluation	Comments
Equipment and Supplies					
1. Basic setup: mouth mirror, explorer, and cotton pliers			3		
2. Cotton rolls, gauze, dental floss, articulating paper, and forceps			3		
3. HVE tip, saliva ejector, and three-way syringe tip			3		
4. Anesthetic setup			3		
5. Dental dam setup			3		
6. High-speed handpiece with selection of diamonds, discs, and burs			3		
7. Irreversible hydrocolloid (alginate) impression materials			3		

	Self-Evaluation	Student Evaluation	Possible Points	Instructor Evaluation	Comments
8. Spoon excavator, scaler, plastic-filling instrument, and cement spatula			3		
9. Tooth shade guide (optional)			2		
10. Retention materials, depending on amount of tooth structure retained; core buildup materials and postretention pins (optional)			3		
11. Gingival retraction cord and placement instrument			3		
12. Final impression material and tray (stock or custom tray)			3		
13. Bite registration materials			3		
14. Crown and collar scissors			3		
15. Provisional (temporary) coverage materials			3		
16. Low-speed handpiece with burs, discs, and stones			3		
17. Laboratory prescription and container for impressions (off-tray item)			3		

Competency Steps (*follow aseptic procedures*)
1. Administer local anesthetic:
  a. Prepare the syringe.
  b. Transfer the syringe to the dentist.
  c. Observe the patient.
			
			3
			3
			3		

2. Take alginate impressions for types of temporaries and a model of the opposing arch:
  a. Select trays.
  b. Mix the irreversible hydrocolloid.
  c. Take the impression.
  d. Properly store and/or pour impressions in plaster or stone.
			
			3
			3
			3
			
			3		

	Self-Evaluation	Student Evaluation	Possible Points	Instructor Evaluation	Comments
3. Make a tooth shade guide selection (shading can be variegated): a. Prepare the shade guide (moisten). b. Help select a shade (hold close to tooth under natural light). c. Record the shade selection in the patient's chart and laboratory prescription.			2 2 3		
4. Prepare the crown with a high speed handpiece and various diamonds and burs.			3		
5. Finish the margins of the preparation: a. Prepare the chamfer or shoulder. b. Prepare and pass the high-speed handpiece. c. Evacuate and maintain the operating field with an air-water syringe. d. Retract and exchange instruments, such as the spoon excavator. Abutment teeth are prepared.			3 3 3 3		
6. Place retraction cord (once the tooth is prepared): a. Pass a piece of retraction cord in cotton pliers to the dentist. b. Pass the appropriate cord-condensing instrument (plastic filling instrument).			3 3		
7. Keep the retraction cord in place for 5 minutes.			3		
8. The dentist selects the tray and impression material.			3		

	Self-Evaluation	Student Evaluation	Possible Points	Instructor Evaluation	Comments
9. Take the final impression: a. Transfer cotton pliers to remove the retraction cord. b. Transfer syringe material. c. Receive cotton pliers and cord. d. Mix and load the heavier material into the tray. e. The prosthodontist will seat the tray. f. Move the light from the patient's face and clean up impression materials. g. Final impression: rinse, disinfect, and place impression materials in a plastic laboratory container.			3 3 3 3 3 2 3		
10. Take the bite registration: a. Prepare bite registration materials. b. Pass the bite registration to the prosthodontist (in some states, the dental assistant can legally take the bite impression). c. After the bite registration is taken, rinse the patient's mouth. d. Rinse, disinfect, and place materials in a plastic laboratory container.			2 2 2 3		
11. The provisional (temporary) restoration meets the following needs: a. The purpose of temporary is to protect prepared teeth. b. Temporary restoration function is to protect occlusal margins. c. Aesthetic purposes are to help patient look natural between appointments. d. A temporary may be worn for 7 to 10 days.			3 3 3 3		
12. Temporary types: a. Crown forms (identification) b. Custom made (identification)			3 3		

	Self-Evaluation	Student Evaluation	Possible Points	Instructor Evaluation	Comments
13. The prosthodontist or assistant will make the temporary restoration depending on expanded functions laws:					
a. Prepare materials and trays as dictated by technique.			3		
b. Ready equipment and supplies:			3		
• Crown and bridge scissors			3		
• Crimping and contour pliers			3		
• Burs, discs, and stones to contour and finish			3		
c. Pass and receive instruments.			3		
d. Keep area rinsed and dried.			3		
e. Mix the temporary cement.			3		
f. Place the temporary cement in the crown.			2		
g. Pass the bite stick for the patient to bite on.			2		
h. Pass 2 × 2 gauze sponge to wipe off any excess.			2		
14. Once the cement is dry, remove the bite stick.			2		
15. Use scaler to remove excess dry cement.			3		
16. Pass dental floss to check the interproximal contacts.			3		
17. Hold articulating paper in articulating forceps for the patient to bite on to test bite.			2		
18. If adjustments are needed, pass the low-speed handpiece with finishing bur.			3		
19. Rinse and evacuate the patient's mouth before the patient is dismissed.			3		
20. After the patient is dismissed, patient's impressions, models, and laboratory prescription are readied for laboratory pick-up.			3		

	Self-Evaluation	Student Evaluation	Possible Points	Instructor Evaluation	Comments
21. Laboratory prescription includes the following:					
a. Patient's name			3		
b. Description of the prosthesis			3		
c. Types of materials chosen by dentist for prosthesis construction			3		
d. Shade or shading desired			3		
e. Prosthodontist name, license number, address, telephone number, fax number, and signature			3		
f. Completion date, when the case will be delivered to the dental office			3		

TOTAL POINTS POSSIBLE   217

TOTAL POINTS POSSIBLE—2nd attempt   215

TOTAL POINTS EARNED   _____

Points assigned reflect importance of step to meeting objective: Important = 1, Essential = 2, Critical = 3. Students will lose 2 points for repeated attempts. Failure results if any of the critical steps are omitted or performed incorrectly. If using a 100-point scale, determine score by dividing points earned by total points possible and multiplying the results by 100.

SCORE: _____

SKILL COMPETENCY ASSESSMENT

30-3 Cementation of Porcelain-Fused-to-Metal Crown

Student's Name _____ Date _____

Instructor's Name _____

Skill: The dental assistant is responsible for preparation of equipment and supplies needed for the appointment. The procedure includes removing the temporary restoration and cementation of the permanent prosthesis.

Performance Objective: The student will follow a routine procedure that meets the regulations and protocol set forth by the dentist and regulatory agencies, keeping in mind that assistant duties vary from state to state. The temporary is removed, the permanent prosthesis is evaluated, and the final cementation is completed. The assistant may be evaluated by performance, verbal/written responses, and/or combined responses and actions.

	Self-Evaluation	Student Evaluation	Possible Points	Instructor Evaluation	Comments
Equipment and Supplies					
1. Basic setup: mouth mirror, explorer, and cotton pliers			3		
2. Cotton rolls, gauze, dental floss, articulating paper, and forceps			3		
3. HVE tip, saliva ejector, and air-water syringe tip			3		
4. Low-speed handpiece with finishing burs, discs, and stones			3		
5. Anesthetic setup			3		
6. Spoon excavator and scaler			3		
7. Plastic filling instrument (PFI) and cement spatula			3		
8. Orangewood bite stick (crown remover, crown seater, and mallet are optional)			3		
9. Final cementation materials (glass ionomer cement, polycarboxylate cement, resin cements, or zinc phosphate cement)			2		

	Self-Evaluation	Student Evaluation	Possible Points	Instructor Evaluation	Comments
10. Porcelain-fused-to-metal crown from laboratory			3		
Competency Steps (*follow aseptic procedures***)** 1. The day before the appointment, make sure that the laboratory has completed the crown and that it has been delivered to the office.			3		
2. Prepare topical and local anesthetic.			3		
3. Transfer the syringe to the dentist.			3		
4. Observe the patient.			3		
5. Rinse and evacuate the mouth.			3		
6. Remove the provisional coverage with a crown remover, scaler, and other instruments of choice (ones that fit under the margin of the temporary).			3		
7. Assist during removal of the temporary and excess cement removal by transferring instruments and keeping the area clean and free of debris.			3		
Or, as part of expanded functions: 8. Remove the temporary.			3		
9. Remove excess cement.			3		
10. Rinse and dry the area and ready the crown.			3		

	Self-Evaluation	Student Evaluation	Possible Points	Instructor Evaluation	Comments
11. Casting the try-in: a. Transfer instruments. b. Transfer dental floss. c. Transfer articulating paper and forceps. d. Keep the area dry. e. Pass the low-speed handpiece with finishing burs, discs, and stones. f. If casting has to be returned to the laboratory, disinfect the crown and prepare it to return to the laboratory.			3 2 2 3 3 3		
12. Before cementation, isolate the area with cotton rolls and protective liners and/or place a cavity varnish.			3		
13. Prepare permanent cement materials (to be mixed according to manufacturer's directions).			3		
14. Mix permanent cement when the dentist is ready.			3		
15. Place some cement in the crown and pass it to the dentist.			3		
16. Pass the plastic filling instrument to the prosthodontist to place cement on the preparation.			3		
17. Receive PFI and pass the crown.			3		
18. Pass the bite stick for the patient to bite.			2		
19. After the cement has hardened, excess cement is removed with a scaler or an explorer.			3		
20. Rinse and evacuate the patient's mouth.			2		

	Self-Evaluation	Student Evaluation	Possible Points	Instructor Evaluation	Comments
21. Use dental floss to remove excess cement interproximally.			3		
22. Instruct the patient on brushing and flossing.			3		
23. Document the procedure, and dismiss the patient.			3		

TOTAL POINTS POSSIBLE   109

TOTAL POINTS POSSIBLE—2nd attempt   107

TOTAL POINTS EARNED   _____

Points assigned reflect importance of step to meeting objective: Important = 1, Essential = 2, Critical = 3. Students will lose 2 points for repeated attempts. Failure results if any of the critical steps are omitted or performed incorrectly. If using a 100-point scale, determine score by dividing points earned by total points possible and multiplying the results by 100.

SCORE: _____

SKILL COMPETENCY ASSESSMENT

30-4 Placing and Removing Retraction Cord

Student's Name _____ Date _____

Instructor's Name _____

Skill: Routine steps should be followed for all treatment areas to maintain absolute clinical asepsis. The dental assistant is responsible for preparation of equipment and supplies needed for the appointment. The tissue must be retracted horizontally to allow room for sufficient impression material, and displaced vertically to wholly expose the margin. Retraction may be done chemically, mechanically, surgically, or by a combination of these.

Performance Objective: The student will follow a routine procedure that meets the regulations and the protocol set forth by the dentist and regulatory agencies. Therefore, the assistant may be evaluated by performance criteria, verbal/written responses, and/or combined responses and performance criteria. This procedure is performed by the dentist or an expanded-function dental assistant. After the tooth has been prepared, the retraction cord is placed. The equipment and supplies are included as part of the crown/bridge tray setup. The specific items needed to place and remove the retraction cord are listed.

	Self-Evaluation	Student Evaluation	Possible Points	Instructor Evaluation	Comments
Equipment and Supplies 1. Mouth mirror, explorer, cotton pliers			3		
2. HVE tip and air-water syringe tip			3		
3. Scissors			3		
4. Hemostat			3		
5. Retraction cord(s)			3		
6. Retraction cord placement instrument or plastic instrument			3		
7. Cotton rolls, 2 × 2 gauze sponges			3		
Competency Steps (*follow aseptic procedures*) 1. Prosthodontist prepares tooth for crown.			3		
2. Dental assistant rinses and dries area in preparation for placement of retraction cord.			3		

	Self-Evaluation	Student Evaluation	Possible Points	Instructor Evaluation	Comments
3. Cotton rolls placed on facial (if mandibular-lingual) surface; area is carefully dried.			3		
4. Prosthodontist selects retraction cord(s) to be placed on tooth.			3		
5. Length of cord needed is determined by circumstances of prepared tooth.			3		
6. Cord is cut to appropriate length; for anterior tooth, wrap around little finger, and for posterior tooth, wrap around larger finger.			3		
7. Assistant twists cord ends to compress fibers.			3		
8. Cord is looped and placed in hemostat or cotton pliers.			3		
9. Cord is looped and placed around margin of prepared tooth, tightened slightly; end of cord is toward buccal surface for easy access.			3		
10. Hemostat or cotton pliers release, leaving cord in sulcus.			3		
11. Retraction cord is packed into position with a packing instrument or plastic instrument.			3		
12. Cord is gently packed around cervical area, apical to preparation.			3		
13. Cord is packed around tooth and overlaps usually on facial surface.			3		
14. A tip of cord is left showing out of sulcus in order for easy removal just prior to taking impression.			3		

	Self-Evaluation	Student Evaluation	Possible Points	Instructor Evaluation	Comments
15. Retraction cord is left in place for 5 minutes when chemical retraction cord is used (10 to 15 minutes for mechanical retraction).			3		
16. End of retraction cord is grasped and removed in a circular motion just prior to impression material being placed.			3		

TOTAL POINTS POSSIBLE   69

TOTAL POINTS POSSIBLE—2nd attempt   67

TOTAL POINTS EARNED   ____

Points assigned reflect importance of step to meeting objective: Important = 1, Essential = 2, Critical = 3. Students will lose 2 points for repeated attempts. Failure results if any of the critical steps are omitted or performed incorrectly. If using a 100-point scale, determine score by dividing points earned by total points possible and multiplying the results by 100.

SCORE: _____

CHAPTER 31

Cosmetic Dentistry and Teeth Whitening

SPECIFIC INSTRUCTIONAL OBJECTIVES

The student should strive to meet the following objectives and demonstrate an understanding of the facts and principles presented in this chapter:

1. Define cosmetic dentistry and describe what is involved in cosmetic dentistry.

2. Describe who performs cosmetic dentistry and education requirements.

3. Explain the role of the dental assistant in cosmetic dentistry.

4. Explain the scope of cosmetic dentistry.

5. Describe fundamental principles that the cosmetic dentist must learn when creating the perfect smile.

6. Discuss the basic elements of psychology and sociology that are considered for cosmetic treatment.

7. Explain what the patient should consider when selecting a dentist for cosmetic treatment.

8. Identify and describe specific procedures performed in cosmetic dentistry, including diagnosis and treatment planning, legal forms, and documentation.

9. Describe the role that oral photography has in cosmetic dentistry, the equipment needed, and how the patient is set up for the photographs to be taken.

10. Describe why soft tissue surgery may be needed in cosmetic dentistry, how it is performed, and how lasers and electrosurgery are involved.

11. Explain why the dental team needs to know about occlusion in cosmetic dentistry.

12. Describe the types of restorations that are placed and materials used for cosmetic restorations.

13. Describe the marketing techniques for cosmetic dentistry.

Advanced Chairside Functions

14. Explain how teeth are whitened, and causes of intrinsic and extrinsic tooth staining.

15. Explain the benefits of whitening techniques used in dentistry.

16. Describe the role of the dental assistant in the whitening process.

17. List and describe types of whitening techniques.

18. Describe the procedures for dental office whitening for vital and nonvital teeth, and for home whitening and over-the-counter whitening materials.

19. Explain information given to the patient concerning outcomes, procedure, responsibilities, and precautions related to teeth whitening.

SUMMARY

Cosmetic dentistry can be a life-changing experience for both the patient and the dental team. These procedures involve many and varied aspects of dentistry and provide esthetic services to patients. Cosmetic dentistry involves very detailed, comprehensive treatments that can involve orthodontics, oral maxillofacial surgery, occlusion adjustments, endodontic treatment, and periodontics. The fundamentals of cosmetic dentistry are discussed as well as the psychology of working with patients interested in improving their smile.

Tooth whitening may also be a part of esthetic treatments desired by patients to improve the appearance of their teeth. Various materials and techniques are discussed including nonvital and vital tooth whitening, in-office and home whitening techniques, and available OTC products.

The dental assistant plays an important role in all cosmetic and tooth-whitening procedures. The assistant must be educated and trained to assist the dentist and be actively involved in providing information to the patient.

EXERCISES AND ACTIVITIES

Multiple Choice

1. The _____ is the largest dental organization dedicated to the art and science of cosmetic dentistry.

   a. ADA

   b. AACD

   c. OTC

   d. CD

2. Veneers used in cosmetic dentistry are a part of which of the following specialties?

   a. Periodontics

   b. Orthodontics

   c. Fixed prosthetics

   d. Endodontics

3. Implants used in cosmetic dentistry are a part of which of the following specialties?

   a. Fixed prosthetics

   b. Oral and maxillofacial surgery

   c. Periodontics

   d. Orthodontics

4. Tooth color has three dimensions. _____ is (are) the term(s) for the color.

   a. Chroma

   b. Value

   c. Hue

   d. Both a. and b.

5. _____ is the intensity or quality of the tooth color.

   a. Hue

   b. Chroma

   c. Value

   d. Translucency

6. _____ is the brightness of a tooth shade.

   a. Value

   b. Chroma

   c. Hue

   d. Opacity

7. In manipulating _____, areas in the light appear to come forward while areas in the dark recede.

   a. horizontal

   b. vertical

   c. depth

   d. Both a. and b.

8. The need to understand a patient's feelings concerning his or her appearance includes knowledge of the patient's

   a. personality.

   b. motivations.

   c. expectations.

   d. All of the above.

9. Which of the following documentation activities would be included as part of routine procedure for all cosmetic dentistry treatments?

   a. Document that a conclusive treatment plan was given to the patient, and a consent form was signed before treatment began.

   b. Document any adverse occurrences or problems that arose during the course of treatment.

   c. Document instances when the patient did not follow home-care instructions.

   d. All of the above

10. The extraoral view includes which of the following?

    a. Full face

    b. Profile

    c. Both a. and b.

    d. None of the above

11. Oral photography is a new skill in cosmetic dentistry. Oral photographs are used in

    a. patient records.

    b. insurance claim documentation.

    c. laboratory communications.

    d. All of the above.

12. Intraoral photo techniques involve using retraction means and mirrors. However, retractors are not used for the _____ view, thereby making it more relaxed and casual.

    a. semi-upright position with mouth open

    b. occlusal

    c. natural smile line

    d. centric occlusion

13. The oral photo shows the patient's centric occlusion.

    a. anterior-view

    b. maxillary occlusal-view

    c. buccal-view

    d. mandibular occlusal-view

14. All of the following are indications for soft tissue contouring treatment except

    a. incomplete passive eruption of one or more teeth.

    b. value in color.

    c. hypertrophied papilla.

    d. hypertrophied gingival tissue from drug therapy.

15. Superoxol solution, which is _____ % hydrogen peroxide, is placed as a whitening agent in the un-filled pulp chamber of a nonvital tooth.

    a. 10 to 15
    b. 30 to 35

    c. 15 to 20
    d. 20 to 25

16. _____ whitening is used to lighten an endodontically treated tooth.

    a. Walking
    b. Assisted

    c. OTC
    d. Power

17. Power whitening is accomplished on _____ teeth.

    a. nonvital
    b. vital

    c. endodontic
    d. None of the above

18. All of the following are commonly used whitening agents except

    a. sodium perborate.
    b. sodium bicarbonate.

    c. hydrogen peroxide.
    d. carbamide peroxide.

19. Which of the following can be side effects of OTC whitening materials?

    a. Temporary tooth sensitivity
    b. Temporary gingival sensitivity

    c. Irreversible tooth damage
    d. All of the above

20. All of the following are OTC whitening products except

    a. strips.
    b. chewing gum.

    c. composite resin.
    d. toothpaste.

21. Whitening agents used in toothpaste include

    a. hydrogen peroxide.
    b. calcium peroxide.

    c. sodium percarbonate.
    d. All of the above.

22. Creating the "perfect smile" is the focus of _____ dentistry.

    a. pediatric
    b. cosmetic/aesthetic

    c. endodontics
    d. oral surgery

23. The preliminary evaluation to determine the elements of the "perfect smile" includes the

    a. shape of the teeth compared to the adjacent teeth.
    b. position of the teeth compared to the adjacent teeth.

    c. color of the teeth compared to the adjacent teeth.
    d. All of the above

24. Gingival tissue enlargement may make the teeth appear shorter than normal. What procedure could be performed to improve the appearance of a patient with this condition?

    a. Crown lengthening
    b. Placement of veneers

    c. Gingivectomy
    d. Gingival grafting

25. What type of restoration would be used in an area of heavy occlusal stress?

    a. Composite resin restoration
    b. Amalgam restoration

    c. Porcelain restoration
    d. Ceramometal restoration

Matching

When a patient inquires about teeth whitening, the dental assistant needs to be knowledgeable about various options. Match each term with its description.

1. _____ OTC

2. _____ assisted

3. _____ power

4. _____ "walking"

a. Liquids/gels, with applications of heat or curing light

b. Thick paste, placed in coronal portion of nonvital tooth

c. Whitening products that can be purchased over the counter

d. Whitening procedure begins in office

 ## Critical Thinking

1. Name the steps in the whitening procedure and anticipated outcomes.

2. The dental office plays an important part in the process of enhancing a person's smile. List dental assistant duties in a cosmetic procedure.

3. Describe the role of the general dentist and the role of the cosmetic dentist in cosmetic dentistry.

4. Learning how patients select a cosmetic dentist is useful. List areas that patients should consider when selecting a cosmetic dentist.

CASE STUDY 1

There are multiple causes of teeth staining or discoloration, as well as multiple lightening techniques. Elizabeth wants to know the differences between treatment of internal staining and treatment of external staining.

1. Explain the causes of tooth staining.

2. Describe nonvital teeth whitening.

3. Name two general whitening methods.

4. Describe the advantages and disadvantages with each method stated in question 3.

CASE STUDY 2

Although whitening procedures have been proven safe and effective through the ADA and the Federal Drug Administration, research is continually being done and the office must keep up-to-date. Patients will see new advertisements in various media, requiring the dental team to be prepared for their questions.

1. List the ways in which teeth are whitened.

2. List the three most commonly used materials in the whitening process.

3. Explain the role of the dental assistant in the whitening process.

4. Describe factors that determine the relative success of whitening procedures.

CASE STUDY 3

Cosmetic dentistry includes many procedures that improve a person's smile and overall appearance, as well as how he or she feels about the same.

1. List considerations useful in gaining a comprehensive picture of the patient's teeth and gingival tissues.

2. Explain the importance of the type of lighting used during shade selection of teeth.

3. Describe the principles of color and how color is interpreted.

4. Explain illusion and how it may affect the appearance of teeth.

5. Describe how certain qualities of a tooth determine perception of its shape and form.

SKILL COMPETENCY ASSESSMENT

31-1 Nonvital Whitening

Student's Name _____ Date _____

Instructor's Name _____

Skill: Routine steps should be followed for all treatment areas to maintain absolute clinical asepsis. The dental assistant is responsible for preparation of equipment and supplies needed for treatment. Endodontically treated teeth sometimes turn dark due to blood, pulpal debris, and restorative materials that are used to fill the canal. These teeth can be lightened by both internal and external whitening.

Performance Objective: The student will follow a routine procedure that meets the regulations and the protocol set forth by the dentist and regulatory agencies. Therefore, the assistant may be evaluated by performance criteria, verbal/written responses, and/or combined responses and performance criteria. This procedure is performed by the dentist. The patient has received information about the procedure and the possible outcome before the procedure begins. Multiple treatments may be necessary.

	Self-Evaluation	Student Evaluation	Possible Points	Instructor Evaluation	Comments
Equipment and Supplies					
1. Basic setup: mouth mirror, explorer, cotton pliers			3		
2. Cotton rolls, gauze sponges, cotton pellets			3		
3. HVE tip, air-water syringe tip, saliva ejector			3		
4. Dental dam setup			3		
5. Protective gel			3		
6. Waxed dental floss			3		
7. High-speed handpiece and assorted burs			3		
8. Low-speed handpiece			3		
9. Prophy brush			3		
10. Cement base materials			3		

	Self-Evaluation	Student Evaluation	Possible Points	Instructor Evaluation	Comments
11. Whitening materials			3		
12. Heat source			3		
13. Temporary coverage and cement			3		
14. Finishing burs			3		
Competency Steps (*follow aseptic procedures*) 1. Examination and evaluation: dentist examines root canal–treated tooth.			3		
2. Isolation a. Place dental dam and ligature of waxed dental floss on designated tooth/teeth. b. Add additional gel to seal dam.			3 3		
3. Open tooth: remove excess restoration and any debris in crown. (With crown of tooth open, some dentists will scrub chamber with soap solution and prophy brush or cotton pellet.)			3		
4. The root canal is sealed with 2 to 3 mm of thick base cement or light-cured resin ionomer or bonded composite (tooth must be sealed to prevent whitening from penetrating the root).			3		

	Self-Evaluation	Student Evaluation	Possible Points	Instructor Evaluation	Comments
5. Whitening the tooth					
a. Gel whitening in the office					
• Involves chamber being filled for 30 minutes.			3		
• Change whitening gel every 10 minutes.			3		
• Then place a cotton pellet and temporary crown.			3		
• Patient is scheduled for appointment in 3 to 7 days for evaluation.			3		
b. "Walking" whitening					
• Thick mixture of whitening agents is placed in crown.			3		
• Covered with temporary cement.			3		
• Patient scheduled for appointment in 2 to 5 days.			3		
c. Combination of techniques			3		
6. Restore tooth. Desired results should be achieved in three appointments. If tooth remains too dark, a veneer should be considered.					
a. Temporary filling removed.			3		
b. Chamber rinsed and evacuated.			3		
c. Etching applied to inside of crown.			3		
d. Rinse.			3		
e. Apply dental adhesive.			3		
f. Fill chamber with restorative material.			3		
g. Light cure.			3		

	Self-Evaluation	Student Evaluation	Possible Points	Instructor Evaluation	Comments
7. Polish tooth and finish restoration with finishing burs and polish.			3		
8. At the next appointment in a few days, have patient evaluate the color, and the possibility of a veneer.			3		

TOTAL POINTS POSSIBLE   108

TOTAL POINTS POSSIBLE—2nd attempt   106

TOTAL POINTS EARNED   ____

Points assigned reflect importance of step to meeting objective: Important = 1, Essential = 2, Critical = 3. Students will lose 2 points for repeated attempts. Failure results if any of the critical steps are omitted or performed incorrectly. If using a 100-point scale, determine score by dividing points earned by total points possible and multiplying the results by 100.

SCORE: _____

SKILL COMPETENCY ASSESSMENT

31-2 In-Office Whitening for Vital Teeth

Student's Name _____ Date _____

Instructor's Name _____

Skill: Routine steps should be followed for all treatment areas to maintain absolute clinical asepsis. The dental assistant is responsible for preparation of equipment and supplies needed for the appointment. Whitening vital teeth in the office involves the application of whitening liquids or gels, often with the application of heat and a curing light.

Performance Objective: The student will follow a routine procedure that meets the regulations and the protocol set forth by the dentist and regulatory agencies. Therefore, the assistant may be evaluated by performance criteria, verbal/written responses, and/or combined responses and performance criteria. This procedure is performed by the dentist in the dental office. The assistant explains the procedure and possible outcomes to the patient.

	Self-Evaluation	Student Evaluation	Possible Points	Instructor Evaluation	Comments
Equipment and Supplies					
1. Protective gel			3		
2. Rubber dam setup			3		
3. Waxed dental floss			3		
4. High-speed handpiece and assorted burs			3		
5. Low-speed handpiece			3		
6. Prophy brush			3		
7. Cement base materials			3		
8. Whitening materials			3		
9. Heat source			3		
10. Temporary coverage and cement			3		
11. Finishing burs			3		

	Self-Evaluation	Student Evaluation	Possible Points	Instructor Evaluation	Comments
Competency Steps *(follow aseptic procedures)* 1. Patient is prepared; procedure is explained; videos, photos, and pamphlets may be available for patient; and teeth and surrounding tissues are examined			3		
2. Isolation: a. Cover all surrounding tissues with protective gel. b. Place dental dam and ligature of waxed dental floss on designated tooth/teeth (pull floss toward the cervix and secure). c. Add additional gel to seal dam.			3 3 3		
3. Polish crowns of teeth to remove plaque debris that might interfere with whitening process (with prophy paste or flour of pumice).			3		
4. Whitening procedure: a. Mix material to thick consistency (follow manufacturer's instructions for specific steps). b. Place on facial and lingual surfaces of tooth or in a tray. c. Apply whitening heat and/or light source (approximately 30 minutes). d. No-heat materials are applied every 10 minutes, with fresh materials mixed each time for three to four applications. e. Rinse and evacuate between each application. f. Remove bulk of whitening gel.			3 3 3 3 3 3		
5. Remove isolation materials: a. Thoroughly rinse area. b. Cut ligatures and interseptal dam. c. Remove dental dam from patient's mouth. d. Rinse again. e. Remove any protective gel with floss and wet gauze.			3 3 3 3 3		
6. Polish teeth using composite resin polishing cup or fluoride prophy paste.			3		

	Self-Evaluation	Student Evaluation	Possible Points	Instructor Evaluation	Comments
7. Examine area and check patient's tissues. Patient is instructed to avoid substances that may stain teeth, and is warned that the teeth may be sensitive following whitening (usually three appointments 1 to 2 weeks apart are required to reach desired shade).			3		

TOTAL POINTS POSSIBLE   87

TOTAL POINTS POSSIBLE—2nd attempt   85

TOTAL POINTS EARNED   _____

Points assigned reflect the importance of the step in meeting the objective: Important = 1, Essential = 2, Critical = 3. Students will lose 2 points for repeated attempts. Failure results if any of the critical steps are omitted or performed incorrectly. If using a 100-point scale, determine score by dividing points earned by total points possible and multiplying the results by 100.

SCORE: _____

SKILL COMPETENCY ASSESSMENT

31-3 Home Whitening

Student's Name _____ Date _____

Instructor's Name _____

Skill: Routine steps should be followed for all treatment areas to maintain absolute clinical asepsis. The dental assistant is responsible for preparing the equipment and supplies needed for the appointment. Home whitening involves the patient applying a whitening agent, usually carbamide peroxide or diluted hydrogen peroxide, in a custom-fit tray for specific amounts of time. There are multiple materials and the techniques vary greatly; the dental office team must become familiar with materials being prescribed for their patients.

Performance Objective: The student will follow a routine procedure that meets the regulations and protocol set forth by the dentist and regulatory agencies. Therefore, the assistant may be evaluated by performance criteria, verbal/written responses, and/or combined responses and performance criteria. This procedure is performed by the patient at home after an examination by the dentist. The patient is given a whitening kit and step-by-step instructions from the dentist. The procedure is divided into appointments and steps that occur between appointments.

	Self-Evaluation	Student Evaluation	Possible Points	Instructor Evaluation	Comments
Equipment and Supplies 1. Basic setup: mouth mirror, explorer, cotton pliers			3		
2. Alginate			3		
3. Rubber mixing bowl and spatula			3		
4. Impression trays			3		
5. Camera for photographs			3		
6. Custom-fit, vacuum-formed tray			3		
7. Home whitening kit			3		
8. Shade guide for before-and-after color comparison			3		

	Self-Evaluation	Student Evaluation	Possible Points	Instructor Evaluation	Comments
Competency Steps (*follow aseptic procedures*)					
First Appointment					
1. Exam and consultation:					
a. The dentist examines teeth.			3		
b. The dentist considers teeth shade, sensitivity, restorations, areas of abrasion, and erosion.			3		
c. Complete general procedures before whitening.			3		
d. Explain whitening techniques to the patient.			3		
e. Select the best procedure for the patient's needs.			3		
2. Take impressions and photographs:					
a. Take alginate impressions of arches being bleached.			3		
b. Take "before" photographs of the patient.			3		
Between Appointments					
1. Pour alginate impressions in stone.			3		
2. Make a custom-fit, vacuum-formed tray (can be done in the office lab or commercial lab).			3		
Second Appointment					
1. With home technique, the patient tries tray to ensure fit.			3		
2. Instructions include when and for how long to wear trays.			3		
a. How to prepare materials			3		
b. Place custom-fit tray			3		
c. What to do in case gingiva becomes irritated			3		
d. How to handle other side effects			3		
3. In some cases, the patient receives one whitening in the office before whitening at home.			3		
4. Polish the teeth and prepare the whitening agent (place in tray).			3		

	Self-Evaluation	Student Evaluation	Possible Points	Instructor Evaluation	Comments
5. Insert trays in the patient's mouth for 30 to 60 minutes.			3		
6. Remove the trays, and suction teeth and rinse thoroughly.			3		
Follow-Up Appointment 1. Follow up on patient's progress and examine tissues. This appointment is usually within 2 weeks of second appointment.			3		

TOTAL POINTS POSSIBLE   84

TOTAL POINTS POSSIBLE—2nd attempt   82

TOTAL POINTS EARNED   ____

Points assigned reflect importance of step to meeting objective: Important = 1, Essential = 2, Critical = 3. Students will lose 2 points for repeated attempts. Failure results if any of the critical steps are omitted or performed incorrectly. If using a 100-point scale, determine score by dividing points earned by total points possible and multiplying the results by 100.

SCORE: _____

CHAPTER 32

Removable Prosthodontics

The student should strive to meet the following objectives and demonstrate an understanding of the facts and principles presented in this chapter:

1. Define removable prostheses and list the reasons for using them.
2. Describe considerations about the patient related to removable prosthetic treatment.
3. Explain the dental assistant's role in removable prosthetic treatment.
4. Outline steps of the diagnostic appointment and list materials needed.
5. Describe the consultation appointment and materials required for case presentation.
6. Describe advantages and disadvantages of the partial denture, the components, and the appointment schedule.
7. Describe the complete denture, considerations about the patient, and the appointment schedule.
8. Explain the types and steps of denture reline procedures.
9. Describe the procedure for a denture repair.
10. List steps to polish a removable prosthetic appliance.
11. Explain the overdenture and the advantages and disadvantages related to it.

SUMMARY

Removable prosthodontics, like fixed prosthodontics, refers to the replacement of missing teeth and tissues with artificial structures, or prostheses. With removable prosthodontics, however, the prosthesis can be removed from the mouth of the patient. Most patients prefer to have fixed prostheses, but in some cases it may not be the treatment of choice due to existing conditions.

The dental assistant's main functions are to prepare materials, record measurements and details for the fabrication of the denture, provide patient education and support, and perform some laboratory procedures. The procedures in removable prosthodontics do not require many instrument exchanges, and the assistant does not continually maintain the oral cavity throughout the appointment with the air-water syringe and the HVE. The steps in removable prosthodontics involve as many extraoral as intraoral procedures. The dental assistant has all the items prepared so that the dentist can explain to the patient the diagnosis, the proposed treatment plan, and the prognosis.

Both full dentures and partial dentures are discussed including advantages, disadvantages, the components of both prostheses, and the appointment schedules. Steps of a denture reline and repairs are described, as well as how to polish a removable appliance. The overdenture procedure is explained along with the advantages and disadvantages relating to it.

EXERCISES AND ACTIVITIES

True or False

1. A person is said to be edentulous when all the natural teeth are lost and no teeth remain.

    a. True
    b. False

2. A patient's posterior teeth have been extracted and dentures are constructed. Only the anterior teeth remain. Then, the anterior teeth are extracted, an alveolectomy is performed, and the denture is seated. This is called an immediate denture.

    a. True
    b. False

3. A complete denture is a type of fixed prosthesis.

    a. True
    b. False

4. One of the benefits of a removable partial denture is that it can be used in children and adolescents and can be easily replaced to accommodate the child's growth.

    a. True
    b. False

5. Once a denture is constructed and fitted, it will be good for the life of the patient and will not require any adjustments.

    a. True
    b. False

Multiple Choice

1. To be successful with a removable prosthetic appliance, a patient should

    a. have a positive attitude.
    b. be cooperative.
    c. be able to maintain good oral hygiene.
    d. All of the above

2. Which of the following is a benefit of a removable partial appliance?

    a. If teeth are lost, they can be added to the partial.
    b. No oral hygiene maintenance is required.
    c. There is no support for teeth standing alone.
    d. Frequent adjustment.

3. Before choosing a partial denture, the dentist must determine whether

    a. the remaining teeth have adequate root structure.
    b. the patient can maintain good oral health.
    c. the alveolar bone structure is adequate.
    d. All of the above

4. The _____ are the part of the removable partial denture that are positioned on the occlusal, incisal, or cingulum surfaces.

   a. connectors

   b. stress-breakers

   c. retainers

   d. rests

5. Which of the following is not a portion of the metal framework skeleton on a removable partial?

   a. Rests

   b. Acrylic base material

   c. Connectors

   d. Retainers

6. Which portion of the metal framework holds the working parts in proper position?

   a. Rests

   b. Stress-breaker

   c. Connectors

   d. Clasps

7. Which portion of the partial is most often made of acrylic resin and holds the denture teeth in the dental base?

   a. Stress-breaker

   b. Connector

   c. Retainer

   d. Saddle

8. The _____ is where the metal framework of the partial rests must be prepared before the final impressions are taken.

   a. saddle

   b. border molding

   c. abutment teeth

   d. centric occlusion

9. The dental laboratory _____ the appliance on models to simulate how it will occlude and mesh in various jaw positions.

   a. relines

   b. articulates

   c. trims

   d. cleans

10. Which of the following is a characteristic of anatomical posterior denture teeth?

    a. Resemble natural teeth with cusps

    b. No detailed anatomy on occlusal

    c. Concave

    d. Flat

11. The patient moves the mouth, lips, cheeks, and tongue to establish the accurate length for the periphery and adjacent tissues to be included in the final impression. This is called

    a. bite rim.

    b. centric occlusion.

    c. muscle trimming.

    d. vertical dimension.

12. What is the preformed, semirigid, acrylic resin material that temporarily represents the denture base?

    a. Baseplate

    b. Bite rim

    c. Vertical dimension

    d. Centric occlusion

13. In the natural dentition, the length of the crowns of the teeth determines the distance between the upper and lower jaws. This distance is called the

    a. centric occlusion.

    b. vertical dimension.

    c. border molding.

    d. denture base.

14. The _____ is determined when the jaws are closed in a position that produces maximum contact between the occluding surfaces of the maxillary and mandibular arch.

    a. centric occlusion

    b. vertical dimension

    c. border molding

    d. denture base

15. When pressure from a complete or partial denture causes the supporting tissues to shrink and change in size, the procedure to improve the fit of the denture and comfort of the patient is called

    a. overdenture.

    b. try-in.

    c. relining.

    d. muscle trimming.

16. Which of the following items are required for a consultation appointment?

    1. Baseplate
    2. Try-in
    3. Study models of patient's mouth
    4. Radiographs mounted on viewbox
    5. Contour pliers
    6. Proposed treatment plan

    a. 1, 2, 5
    b. 3, 4, 6

    c. 2, 3, 5
    d. 1, 3, 4

17. When a patient is considering a partial denture, the dentist should consider all of following factors except

    a. there must be a number of sufficiently positioned teeth in the arch.
    b. patient photographs.

    c. adequate root structure of the remaining teeth.
    d. whether the alveolar bone is able to support the partial denture.

18. This metal device relieves pressure on the abutment teeth of a removable partial.

    a. Retainer
    b. Stress-breaker

    c. Hinge
    d. Both b. and c.

19. The _____ clasp encircles and adapts to the contours of the abutment tooth.

    a. bar-type
    b. circumferential-type

    c. retainer
    d. hinge

20. This partial is an aesthetic choice and adapts well with the natural tissues of the mouth.

    a. Ethnic
    b. Natural

    c. Acrylic
    d. Flexible base resin

21. Which denture appointment is the last time the dentist can make adjustments before the denture is constructed?

    a. Final impressions appointment
    b. Jaw relationship appointment

    c. Oral surgery appointment
    d. Try-in appointment

22. At which appointment are radiographs and preliminary impressions taken?

    a. Examination and diagnosis appointment
    b. Jaw relationship appointment

    c. Oral surgery appointment
    d. Try-in appointment

23. What is the name of the device that is used to take measurements for determining the relationship of the maxillary dentition to the temporomandibular joint?

    a. Facebow
    b. Articulator

    c. Retainer
    d. Bite rims

24. What term is used to describe the movement of the mandibular from the centric position to a lateral or protrusive position?

    a. Retrusion
    b. Protrusion

    c. Lateral Excusion
    d. Vertical dimension

25. What is anterior movement called?

    a. Intercuspation
    b. Retrusion

    c. Protrusion
    d. Occlusion

Labeling

Identify the parts of a mandibular partial denture in the photo.

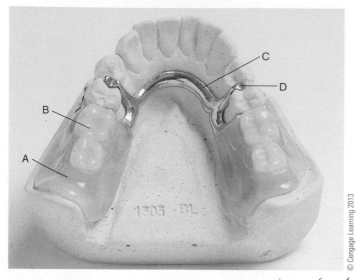

© Cengage Learning 2013

A. ~~Denture Sase~~ *Material*

B. Denture teeth.

C. Conectbate

D. occlusal rest

Critical Thinking

1. Explain the final denture construction in the laboratory before the try-in appointment.

2. Fred will receive a full maxillary denture. Because he still has anterior teeth and is concerned about going without any teeth while continuing to work, he selected an immediate insertion denture. Explain how the base plate, rim, and jaw relationship measurements are taken.

3. A sequence of appointments helps the patient and the dental assistant to be ready for each step of the process. List the suggested series of appointments for a complete denture.

CASE STUDY 1

Sally, age 58, has a loose denture; when delivering a speech, sometimes her denture floats and slurs her words. She should see her dentist and inquire about new methods that are used to correct a loose-fitting denture. For instance, if Sally has adequate bone density, an endosseous implant and an overdenture for the implant may work.

1. Describe an endosseous implant for retained teeth.

2. Describe the process for retained teeth.

3. Describe the implant process.

4. List selection choices for retained teeth or implant attachments.

5. Explain the advantages and disadvantages of implants.

CASE STUDY 2

After a recent luncheon with friends, during which she was anxious about her denture becoming loose, Rachel decided that she needed to consult with her dentist. Following an examination, the dentist recommended a denture reline.

1. Describe how the reline will benefit Rachel.

2. Explain tissue conditioning.

3. Describe the benefits of a soft reline.

4. Explain the differences between a laboratory reline and a soft reline.

CASE STUDY 3

The dental assistant's functions include recording measurements and details for the fabrication of the denture, as well as providing education and support to patients. Ester is coming in for a very detailed examination in preparation for a complete denture.

1. What features are examined during an intraoral cavity examination?

2. In addition to the results of the intraoral cavity examination, list other supportive documentation that will assist in the overall evaluation.

3. Describe the use of current photographs as a diagnostic tool.

4. List the types of data collected and used in devising the final treatment plan.

SKILL COMPETENCY ASSESSMENT

32-1 Final Impressions for Partial Denture

Student's Name _____ Date _____

Instructor's Name _____

Skill: The dental assistant is responsible for preparing the equipment and supplies needed for the appointment. The procedure includes preparing the abutment teeth, taking final impressions, taking the bite or occlusal registration, and selecting the shade and mold of the artificial teeth. Sometimes, restorative, periodontal, endodontic, or surgical procedures must be completed before the final impressions can be completed.

Performance Objective: The student will follow a routine procedure that meets the regulations and protocol set forth by the dentist and regulatory agencies. Therefore, the assistant may be evaluated by performance criteria, verbal/written responses, and/or combined responses and performance criteria. The procedure is performed by the dentist. After preparing the materials for the final impressions, the dental assistant greets and seats the patient. A protective drape is placed on the patient and the procedure is explained to the patient.

	Self-Evaluation	Student Evaluation	Possible Points	Instructor Evaluation	Comments
Equipment and Supplies					
1. Basic setup: mouth mirror, explorer, and cotton pliers			3		
2. Mouthwash			2		
3. Custom tray or stock tray			3		
4. Contouring wax for the impression trays			3		
5. Impression materials— spatula and mixing pad or dispensing gun and tips			3		
6. Wax or silicon bite registration materials			3		
7. Tooth shade and mold guides			3		
8. Laboratory prescription form			3		
9. Disinfectant the container for impressions and bite registration			3		

	Self-Evaluation	Student Evaluation	Possible Points	Instructor Evaluation	Comments
Competency Steps (*follow aseptic procedures*) 1. The dentist examines the oral cavity, and the assistant transfers a custom or stock tray for trying in the mouth (wax may be required for borders).			3		
2. Once the tray is contoured to fit, prepare tray by painting it with an adhesive.			3		
3. As directed by the dentist, prepare, mix, and load material into a tray and transfer the tray to the dentist (mix will be according to manufacturer's directions).			3		
4. Once the final impression is completed, receive final impressions and either disinfect them right away or set them aside to disinfect after the procedure is completed.			3		
5. Prepare the materials for the occlusal or bite registration.			3		
6. Soften bite wax in warm water, folding it several times before placing it in the patient's mouth.			3		
7. Mix other bite materials on a paper pad and place them on a quadrant tray placed in the patient's mouth or dispensed directly in the oral cavity with a dispensing gun and tip.			3		
8. After bite materials are set and are removed from the mouth, the dentist transfers them to the assistant to disinfect and place with the final impression.			3		

	Self-Evaluation	Student Evaluation	Possible Points	Instructor Evaluation	Comments
9. Assist the dentist in shade selection and recording. Shade is taken with a moistened shade guide under natural light.			3		
10. Make sure that the patient's face is clean of impression materials, and dismiss the patient.			3		
11. The dentist completes the laboratory prescription with details of the partial denture design. These data are also recorded in the patient's chart.			3		

TOTAL POINTS POSSIBLE   59

TOTAL POINTS POSSIBLE—2nd attempt   57

TOTAL POINTS EARNED   _____

Points assigned reflect importance of step to meeting objective: Important = 1, Essential = 2, Critical = 3. Students will lose 2 points for repeated attempts. Failure results if any of the critical steps are omitted or performed incorrectly. If using a 100-point scale, determine score by dividing points earned by total points possible and multiplying the results by 100.

SCORE: _____

SKILL COMPETENCY ASSESSMENT

32-2 Try-In Appointment for Partial Denture

Student's Name _____ Date _____

Instructor's Name _____

Skill: The dental assistant is responsible for preparing the equipment and supplies needed for the appointment. The dental laboratory has followed the dentist's instructions and has constructed an appliance that consists of the cast framework and the denture teeth set in wax. The partial denture is articulated on models to simulate how the appliance will occlude and mesh in various jaw positions. The laboratory has sent the partial to the dental office for the try-in and adjustments.

Performance Objective: The student will follow a routine procedure that meets the regulations and protocol set forth by the dentist and regulatory agencies. Therefore, the assistant may be evaluated by performance criteria, verbal/written responses, and/or combined responses and performance criteria. The procedure is performed by the dentist. The dental assistant prepares the materials and prepares the patient.

	Self-Evaluation	Student Evaluation	Possible Points	Instructor Evaluation	Comments
Equipment and Supplies					
1. Basic setup: mouth mirror, explorer, and cotton pliers			3		
2. Hand mirror for patient viewing			2		
3. Articulating paper and forceps			3		
4. Adjustment instruments, including wax spatula, pliers, and a heat source			3		
5. Low-speed handpiece with burs, discs, and stones			3		
6. Contour pliers			3		
7. Partial denture from the laboratory			3		
Competency Steps (*follow aseptic procedures*)					
1. Place appliance in the patient's mouth (or transfer appliance to the dentist); adjustments are made.			3		

	Self-Evaluation	Student Evaluation	Possible Points	Instructor Evaluation	Comments
2. Prepare the spatula by warming it in a heat source (an alcohol torch or a Bunsen burner).			3		
3. Transfer the spatula to the dentist.			3		
4. Transfer articulating paper as the occlusion is being evaluated.			2		
5. Transfer the handpiece and burs as needed to adjust the occlusion.			3		
6. Give the patient a hand mirror for viewing and commenting.			2		
7. Dismiss the patient.			2		
8. Assistant disinfects the partial to prepare it for the laboratory.			3		

TOTAL POINTS POSSIBLE   41

TOTAL POINTS POSSIBLE—2nd attempt   39

TOTAL POINTS EARNED   _____

Points assigned reflect importance of step to meeting objective: Important = 1, Essential = 2, Critical = 3. Students will lose 2 points for repeated attempts. Failure results if any of the critical steps are omitted or performed incorrectly. If using a 100-point scale, determine score by dividing points earned by total points possible and multiplying the results by 100.

SCORE: _____

SKILL COMPETENCY ASSESSMENT

32-3 Delivery Appointment for Partial Denture

Student's Name _____ Date _____

Instructor's Name _____

Skill: The dental assistant is responsible for preparing the equipment and supplies needed for the appointment. The dental laboratory has followed the dentist's instructions and has completed final construction of the partial denture. The laboratory has now sent the partial to the dental office for the final insertion.

Performance Objective: The student will follow a routine procedure that meets the regulations and protocol set forth by the dentist and regulatory agencies. Therefore, the assistant may be evaluated by performance criteria, verbal/written responses, and/or combined responses and performance criteria. The procedure is performed by the dentist with the assistance of the dental assistant. The partial denture is returned from the laboratory in a sealed container.

	Self-Evaluation	Student Evaluation	Possible Points	Instructor Evaluation	Comments
Equipment and Supplies 1. Basic setup: mouth mirror, explorer, and cotton pliers			3		
2. Partial denture			3		
3. Articulating paper and forceps			3		
4. Low-speed handpiece with acrylic burs and finishing burs			3		
Competency Steps (*follow aseptic procedure*) 1. Seat the patient (preparation for patient completed, materials and equipment similar to try-in appointment except wax adjustment instruments).			3		
2. If patient is wearing an appliance, place it in a cup of water.			3		
3. Rinse and transfer the new partial to the dentist for insertion.			3		

	Self-Evaluation	Student Evaluation	Possible Points	Instructor Evaluation	Comments
4. Transfer articulating paper as the occlusion is being evaluated.			2		
5. Transfer a low-speed handpiece with finishing or acrylic burs as needed to adjust the occlusion.			3		
6. Transfer contouring pliers for adjusting metal clasps.			3		
7. Dentist instructs/observes the patient on how to insert/remove partial. Explanation is also given on the care of the partial and supporting teeth.			3		
8. Dismiss the patient.			2		
9. Instruct the patient to call the office if sore spots develop, and that adjustments are expected.			3		

TOTAL POINTS POSSIBLE   37

TOTAL POINTS POSSIBLE—2nd attempt   35

TOTAL POINTS EARNED   _____

Points assigned reflect importance of step to meeting objective: Important = 1, Essential = 2, Critical = 3. Students will lose 2 points for repeated attempts. Failure results if any of the critical steps are omitted or performed incorrectly. If using a 100-point scale, determine score by dividing points earned by total points possible and multiplying the results by 100.

SCORE: _____

SKILL COMPETENCY ASSESSMENT

32-4 Final Impression Appointment

Student's Name _____ Date _____

Instructor's Name _____

Skill: The dental assistant is responsible for preparing the equipment and supplies needed for the appointment. Between the consultation and the final impression appointment, the alginate impressions are poured in plaster or stone. Custom acrylic trays are constructed based on these models.

Performance Objective: The student will follow a routine procedure that meets the regulations and protocol set forth by the dentist and regulatory agencies, keeping in mind that assistant duties vary from state to state. The assistant may be evaluated by performance criteria, verbal/written responses, and/or combined responses and performance criteria. The procedure is performed by the dentist. Materials are prepared and transferred to the dentist by the dental assistant.

	Self-Evaluation	Student Evaluation	Possible Points	Instructor Evaluation	Comments
Equipment and Supplies					
1. Basic setup: mouth mirror, explorer, and cotton pliers			3		
2. HVE tip, air-water syringe tip			3		
3. Cotton rolls and gauze			3		
4. Mouthwash for patient to rinse before impressions are taken			3		
5. Custom tray			3		
6. Compound wax and Bunsen burner for border molding the tray rims			3		
7. Laboratory knife to trim border molding			2		
8. Impression materials, such as spatulas and mixing pads or dispensing gun and tips			3		
9. Laboratory prescription form			2		

	Self-Evaluation	Student Evaluation	Possible Points	Instructor Evaluation	Comments
10. Disinfectant the container for impressions and bite registration			3		
Competency Steps 1. Insert the custom tray in the patient's mouth (the assistant may transfer the tray to the dentist) and evaluate it for fit. Preparation for final impression.			3		
2. Conduct the border molding or muscle trimming. (Heat the impression compound, place it along the borders of the custom tray, and then cool the tray and place it in the patient's mouth. While the tray is in the patient's mouth, move the lips, cheeks, and tongue to establish the accurate length of the periphery and the adjacent tissue to be included in the final impression.)			3		
3. Prepare the final impression material and place it in the tray.			3		
a. Evaluate maxillary impression. (Include tuberosities, frenum attachments, and other landmarks of the arch.)			3		
b. Evaluate the mandibular impression (include the retromolar pads, oblique ridge, mylohyoid ridge, and frenum attachments).			3		
4. Remove tray once the material has set.			3		
5. Rinse the patient's mouth thoroughly.			3		

	Self-Evaluation	Student Evaluation	Possible Points	Instructor Evaluation	Comments
6. Repeat the impression procedure for the opposing arch if the full denture is being fabricated for both arches.			3		
7. Disinfect and prepare impressions for the laboratory.			3		
8. Prepare the prescription form and send it to the laboratory.			2		
9. Dismiss the patient.			2		
TOTAL POINTS POSSIBLE			59		
TOTAL POINTS POSSIBLE—2nd attempt			57		
TOTAL POINTS EARNED			____		

Points assigned reflect importance of step to meeting objective: Important = 1, Essential = 2, Critical = 3. Students will lose 2 points for repeated attempts. Failure results if any of the critical steps are omitted or performed incorrectly. If using a 100-point scale, determine score by dividing points earned by total points possible and multiplying the results by 100.

SCORE: _____

SKILL COMPETENCY ASSESSMENT

32-5 Jaw Relationship Appointment

Student's Name _____ Date _____

Instructor's Name _____

Skill: The dental assistant is responsible for preparing equipment and supplies. Between the final impressions and measurement appointments, the dental laboratory pours the master cast in stone from the final impressions. The master cast will be used to construct the baseplate. The bite rim will be attached to the baseplate. Once the baseplate and bite rims are constructed, they are delivered to the dental office in time for this appointment.

Performance Objective: The student will follow a routine procedure that meets the regulations and protocol set forth by the dentist and regulatory agencies, keeping in mind that assistant duties vary from state to state. The assistant may be evaluated by performance criteria, verbal/written responses, and/or combined responses and performance criteria. During this appointment, the measurements, shape, and shade of the denture are determined. The dental assistant prepares equipment and materials and assists the dentist throughout the procedure.

	Self-Evaluation	Student Evaluation	Possible Points	Instructor Evaluation	Comments
Equipment and Supplies					
1. Basic setup: mouth mirror, explorer, and cotton pliers			3		
2. HVE tip, air-water syringe tip			3		
3. Hand mirror			2		
4. Laboratory knife, 7 wax spatula, Bunsen burner			3		
5. Shade guide			3		
6. Millimeter ruler and Boley gauge			3		
7. Baseplates and bite rims			3		
8. Face bow			3		
9. Photographs of the patient, showing shapes and shades of the teeth			3		
10. Laboratory prescription form			2		
11. Disinfectant			3		

	Self-Evaluation	Student Evaluation	Possible Points	Instructor Evaluation	Comments
Competency Steps (*follow aseptic procedures*) 1. Insert the baseplates and bite rims into the patient's mouth (the assistant may transfer them to the dentist). The dentist determines and marks the midline of the maxillary and mandibular arches.			3		
2. Determine the vertical dimension.			3		
a. Adjust the bite rims with a laboratory knife (the length of the crowns of the teeth/the distance between the upper and lower jaws).			3		
b. Determine the patient's natural lip line.			3		
c. Ensure that the correct amount of the tooth and gingiva are visible when talking and smiling and that the lips are in the resting position.			3		
d. Determine the cuspid lines at the corners of the mouth.			3		
3. Determine the centric occlusion.			3		
a. Evaluate the jaw relationship (how the mandible relates to the maxilla).			3		
b. Have the patient move the mandible to the retrusion (back).			3		
c. Have the patient move the mandible laterally (right to left/side to side).			3		
d. Once the information is determined to be correct, articulate the casts to duplicate the patient's normal motions.			3		
e. The laboratory technician constructs a complete denture in wax and with artificial teeth from these records.			3		

	Self-Evaluation	Student Evaluation	Possible Points	Instructor Evaluation	Comments
4. Select denture teeth.			3		
a. Discuss teeth arrangement with the patient.			3		
b. Select proper shade and use natural light.			3		
c. Compare shade with the patient's complexion.			3		
d. Compare shade with the remaining teeth.			3		
e. Compare shade with photographs.			3		
f. Use the patient's age to indicate the shade range. (Teeth staining sometimes darkens with age.)			3		
g. Shape the mold of the teeth by the face of the patient.			3		
5. Clearly communicate the following to the patient:					
a. Natural teeth appearance			3		
b. Duplicate arrangement of existing teeth (e.g., spacing, overlapping)			3		
c. Correct alignment of the natural teeth with the new denture			3		
d. Patient's expected outcome			3		
6. Patient is dismissed.			2		

TOTAL POINTS POSSIBLE 105

TOTAL POINTS POSSIBLE—2nd attempt 103

TOTAL POINTS EARNED ____

Points assigned reflect importance of step to meeting objective: Important = 1, Essential = 2, Critical = 3. Students will lose 2 points for repeated attempts. Failure results if any of the critical steps are omitted or performed incorrectly. If using a 100-point scale, determine score by dividing points earned by total points possible and multiplying the results by 100.

SCORE: _____

SKILL COMPETENCY ASSESSMENT

32-6 Try-In Appointment

Student's Name _____ Date _____

Instructor's Name _____

Skill: The dental assistant is responsible for preparing the equipment and supplies. Between appointments, the laboratory will prepare a "try-in" denture. The denture teeth are mounted in the wax bite rim according to the dentist's directions, but positions can be altered at the try-in appointment.

Performance Objective: The student will follow a routine procedure that meets the regulations and protocol set forth by the dentist and regulatory agencies, keeping in mind that assistant duties vary from state to state. The assistant may be evaluated by performance criteria, verbal/written responses, and/or combined responses and performance criteria. The procedure is performed by the dentist. The dental assistant prepares the patient, instruments, and materials, and coordinates with the dental laboratory.

	Self-Evaluation	Student Evaluation	Possible Points	Instructor Evaluation	Comments
Equipment and Supplies					
1. Basic setup: mouth mirror, explorer, and cotton pliers			3		
2. HVE tip, air-water syringe tip			3		
3. Hand mirror			2		
4. Laboratory knife, 7 wax spatula, Bunsen burner			3		
5. Try-in dentures mounted on articulor from laboratory			3		
6. Shade guide			3		
7. Millimeter ruler and Boley gauge			3		
8. Articulating forceps and paper			3		
9. Photographs of the patient, showing the shape and shade of the teeth			3		
10. Laboratory prescription form			2		
11. Disinfectant			3		

	Self-Evaluation	Student Evaluation	Possible Points	Instructor Evaluation	Comments
Competency Steps (*follow aseptic procedures*)					
1. Disinfect the "try-in" denture before placing in the patient's mouth.			3		
2. Seat the patient.			2		
3. Insert denture in the patient's mouth.			3		
4. Spend time talking to allow the patient to adjust to the denture.			3		
5. Evaluate the denture for aesthetics, retention, and comfort.			3		
6. Check the occlusion with articulating paper (transfer as needed).			3		
7. The dentist can adjust the position of the teeth because they are still in wax.			3		
8. The dental laboratory technician can change the shade in the dental laboratory.			3		
9. Once the dentist and patient are satisfied with the denture, disinfect it and place it back on the articulator.			3		
10. Return the denture to the laboratory.			2		
11. Dismiss the patient.			2		
TOTAL POINTS POSSIBLE			61		
TOTAL POINTS POSSIBLE—2nd attempt			59		
TOTAL POINTS EARNED			____		

Points assigned reflect importance of step to meeting objective: Important = 1, Essential = 2, Critical = 3. Students will lose 2 points for repeated attempts. Failure results if any of the critical steps are omitted or performed incorrectly. If using a 100-point scale, determine score by dividing points earned by total points possible and multiplying the results by 100.

SCORE: _____

SKILL COMPETENCY ASSESSMENT

32-7 Appointment for Delivery of Complete Denture

Student's Name _____ Date _____

Instructor's Name _____

Skill: The dental assistant is responsible for preparing the equipment and supplies. Between appointments, the laboratory will complete the final multistep processing of the denture. This converts the wax try-in denture to a denture with an acrylic resin base and plastic or porcelain teeth.

Performance Objective: The student will follow a routine procedure that meets the regulations and protocol set forth by the dentist and regulatory agencies. Therefore, the assistant may be evaluated by performance criteria, verbal/written responses, and/or combined responses and performance criteria. The procedure is performed by the dentist. The dental assistant prepares the patient and coordinates with the dental laboratory.

	Self-Evaluation	Student Evaluation	Possible Points	Instructor Evaluation	Comments
Equipment and Supplies					
1. Basic setup: mouth mirror, explorer, and cotton pliers			3		
2. HVE tip, air-water syringe tip			3		
3. Dentures from the laboratory			3		
4. Hand mirror			2		
5. Articulating forceps and paper			3		
6. High-speed handpiece and diamond and finishing burs			3		
7. Low-speed handpiece and assorted acrylic burs and disks			3		
8. Home-care instructions pamphlet, and denture brush and container			3		

	Self-Evaluation	Student Evaluation	Possible Points	Instructor Evaluation	Comments
Competency Steps (*follow aseptic procedures*)					
1. Keep dentures moist in a laboratory container until ready for the patient.			2		
2. Seat the patient.			2		
3. Patient removes the appliances and places them in a container to keep them moist.			2		
4. An immediate denture is inserted after extractions and alveoplasty. (For more than simple extractions, the patient is scheduled with a maxillofacial surgeon.) The dental laboratory sends the denture.			3		
5. Insert the new denture in the patient's mouth.			3		
6. Give the patient a few minutes to adjust to the new denture.			3		
7. The dentist will evaluate and examine.			3		
8. The occlusion is checked with articulating paper (the assistant will transfer as needed).			3		
9. The dentist can adjust as needed and will use the low-speed handpiece and acrylic burs to reduce any high spots inside of base.			3		
10. After adjustments, polish the denture in the laboratory.			3		
11. If adjustments are made, disinfect the denture before replacing it in the patient's mouth.			3		

	Self-Evaluation	Student Evaluation	Possible Points	Instructor Evaluation	Comments
12. The dentist evaluates the retention of the denture and jaw relationship by having the patient swallow, demonstrate various facial expressions, chew, and speak.			2		
13. The patient learns how to insert and remove the denture.			3		
14. The patient learns the daily maintenance of the denture.			3		
15. The patient is instructed to call the office if there are any questions or problems.			3		
16. Schedule appointment for patient in a few days.			3		
17. Dismiss the patient.			2		
18. As a courtesy, the dentist or assistant will call the patient the following day and check on the patient's progress.			2		

TOTAL POINTS POSSIBLE   71

TOTAL POINTS POSSIBLE—2nd attempt   69

TOTAL POINTS EARNED   _____

Points assigned reflect importance of step to meeting objective: Important = 1, Essential = 2, Critical = 3. Students will lose 2 points for repeated attempts. Failure results if any of the critical steps are omitted or performed incorrectly. If using a 100-point scale, determine score by dividing points earned by total points possible and multiplying the results by 100.

SCORE: _____

SKILL COMPETENCY ASSESSMENT

32-8 Chairside Denture Relining

Student's Name _____ Date _____

Instructor's Name _____

Skill: The dental assistant is responsible for preparing the equipment and supplies. Denture relining adds a new layer of acrylic to the inside of the denture. This procedure can be performed in the dental office or at the dental laboratory. The dental laboratory method is the subject of assessment 32–9.

Performance Objective: The student will follow a routine procedure that meets the regulations and protocol set forth by the dentist and regulatory agencies, keeping in mind that assistant duties vary from state to state. The assistant may be evaluated by performance criteria, verbal/written responses, and/or combined responses and performance criteria. The dental assistant prepares the patient and the materials.

	Self-Evaluation	Student Evaluation	Possible Points	Instructor Evaluation	Comments
Equipment and Supplies					
1. Basic setup: mouth mirror, explorer, and cotton pliers			3		
2. Low-speed handpiece with acrylic burs			3		
3. Chairside reline materials			3		
4. Mouth rinse			2		
Denture reline in the dental office **Competency Steps (*follow aseptic procedures*)**					
1. Prepare the denture, placing in an ultrasonic unit for a few minutes to be cleaned.			3		
2. The dentist uses acrylic burs to roughen the tissue side of the denture.			3		
3. Make hard or semisoft reline materials available for the doctor to choose.			3		
4. Mix material to the manufacturer's directions.			3		

	Self-Evaluation	Student Evaluation	Possible Points	Instructor Evaluation	Comments
5. Place the material in the clean denture, covering the entire tissue surface (materials have low thermal reaction and can cure directly in the patient's mouth).			3		
6. Have the patient rinse with mouthwash to clean saliva and debris from the tissues.			3		
7. Insert the denture in the patient's mouth and ask the patient to bite (occlude and hold) until the initial set stage. (Tell the patient there is sometimes a slight burning sensation from the acrylic material during setting time.)			3		
8. Remove the denture to complete the setting process.			3		
9. Dentist will trim away excess material. Disinfect denture and prepare to send to dental laboratory.			3		
10. After adjustments, polish the denture in the laboratory before returning to the patient.			3		
11. If adjustments are made, disinfect the denture before replacing it in the patient's mouth.			3		
Denture reline by the dental laboratory **Competency Steps (*follow aseptic procedures*)** 1. Use the denture or partial for the impression materials.			3		

	Self-Evaluation	Student Evaluation	Possible Points	Instructor Evaluation	Comments
2. Render impression materials available including polysulfides, polyethers, and silicone (be prepared to mix any of these).			3		
3. Mix the impression material of choice according to manufacturer's directions.			3		
4. Place the material in the tray. The material should cover the entire tissue surface evenly and without excess.			3		
5. Insert the denture in the patient's mouth and position it firmly. (The patient should occlude and hold until the material sets.)			3		
6. After the material sets, remove the denture from the patient's mouth.			2		
7. Disinfect the denture and prepare it for sending to the dental laboratory.			3		
8. Complete the laboratory prescription.			3		
9. Dismiss the patient.			2		
10. The dental laboratory processes the impression (fuses the acrylic resin base to the denture).			2		
11. The patient returns to the dental office when the laboratory completes processing of the denture reline (turnaround time varies from hours to days).			2		
12. When the patient returns to the dental office, seat the denture.			3		

	Self-Evaluation	Student Evaluation	Possible Points	Instructor Evaluation	Comments
13. Adjust the denture as needed.			3		
14. After adjustments, polish the denture in the laboratory before returning it to the patient.			3		
15. If adjustments are made, disinfect the denture before replacing it in the patient's mouth.			3		
16. Dismiss the patient.			2		

TOTAL POINTS POSSIBLE 87

TOTAL POINTS POSSIBLE—2nd attempt 85

TOTAL POINTS EARNED _____

Points assigned reflect importance of step to meeting objective. Important = 1, Essential = 2, Critical = 3. Students will lose 2 points for repeated attempts. Failure results if any of the critical steps are omitted or performed incorrectly. If using a 100-point scale, determine score by dividing points earned by total points possible and multiplying the results by 100.

SCORE: _____

Restorative and Laboratory Materials and Techniques

CHAPTER **33**

Dental Cements, Bases, Liners, and Bonding Agents

SPECIFIC INSTRUCTIONAL OBJECTIVES

The student should strive to meet the following objectives and demonstrate an understanding of the facts and principles presented in this chapter:

1. Differentiate between dental cements, bases, liners, and bonding agents.
2. List dental standards and organizations responsible for the standards.
3. Explain the role of the dental assistant in preparing materials.
4. List and explain the properties of dental materials.
5. Identify the types of dental cements. Explain their properties, composition, uses, and manipulation.
6. Describe bonding agents and their manipulation.
7. Describe the steps of cavity preparation.
8. Identify cavity preparation terminology.

Advanced Chairside Functions

9. Classify cavity preparations according to their relationships with the pulp.
10. Explain options for protecting the pulp with cavity liners, cavity varnish, and cement bases.
11. Describe the purpose of using cavity liners. List types of materials that can be used and explain the placement procedure.
12. Describe the purpose of using cavity varnish and explain the placement procedure.
13. Describe the purpose of using cement bases. List types of materials that can be used and explain the placement procedure.

SUMMARY

The general chairside assistant prepares and mixes the material, while the dentist places the material in the oral cavity. Some states allow the assistant to also place some of the materials in the oral cavity. Knowledge of dental material properties is necessary for the dental assistant to properly prepare and manipulate the materials. The assistant's knowledge of dental materials is beneficial for patient education and protection. Expanded-function dental assistants must understand and be competent in the placement and finishing of materials.

EXERCISES AND ACTIVITIES

Multiple Choice

1. An example of shearing stress and strain is _____, or grinding of the teeth.
   a. dimensional change
   b. corrosion
   c. tarnish
   d. bruxism

2. Which of the following is not a type of stress and strain?
   a. Tensile
   b. Dimensional
   c. Compressive
   d. Shearing

3. The ability of a material to withstand compressive stresses without fracturing is known as (a)
   a. malleability.
   b. ductility.
   c. palliative.
   d. viscosity.

4. _____ is the result of chemical or electrochemical attacks on pure metal in the oral environment, causing deep pitting and roughness.
   a. Tarnishing
   b. Corrosion
   c. Shearing
   d. Ductility

5. _____ is the physical property of being capable of distortion or deformation by an applied force, and then returning to the original shape once the force is removed.
   a. Flow
   b. Retention
   c. Elasticity
   d. Solubility

6. _____, or creep and slump, is the continuous deformation of a solid.
   a. Flow
   b. Elasticity
   c. Solubility
   d. Ductility

7. Change in a dental material may result from various causes. All of the following are causes of dimensional change except (the)
   a. tarnish.
   b. setting process.
   c. exposure to cold.
   d. exposure to heat.

8. The seepage of saliva and debris from the oral cavity between the tooth structure and the restorative materials is called
   a. flow.
   b. ductility.
   c. malleability.
   d. microleakage.

9. The ability of a material to transmit heat is called
   a. dimensional change.
   b. microleakage.
   c. thermal conductivity.
   d. stress and strain.

10. Which property of a dental material allows it to be useful as a base or liner only where it is not exposed to the oral fluids?

    a. Viscosity

    b. Solubility

    c. Wettability

    d. Galvanism

11. In dentistry, materials that are placed directly in the cavity preparation (direct restorative materials) are kept in place by

    a. chemical retention.

    b. mechanical retention.

    c. viscosity.

    d. stress and strain.

12. The thicker the material, the less it flows; therefore, it is said to be more _____ than a thinner material that flows easily.

    a. viscous

    b. wettable

    c. luting

    d. soluble

13. The ability of a material to flow over a surface is called

    a. viscosity.

    b. wettability.

    c. luting.

    d. solubility.

14. Dental cements are mixed to a precise ratio. Zinc phosphate cement has reached the _____ stage when the material follows the spatula about 1 inch above the mixing slab.

    a. luting

    b. base

    c. liner

    d. putty

15. _____ is placed as a thin layer on the walls and floor of the cavity preparation to protect the pulp from bacteria and irritants.

    a. Base

    b. Liner

    c. Cement

    d. Varnish

16. Bases are applied between the tooth and the restoration to protect the pulp. However, bases will not protect the pulp from

    a. chemical irritation.

    b. temperature change.

    c. inflammation (of the pulp itself).

    d. mechanical injury.

17. One of the oldest cements, which comes in a powder/liquid form and is a luting and base cement, is called

    a. zinc oxide eugenol.

    b. polycarboxylate.

    c. glass ionomer.

    d. zinc phosphate.

18. When zinc phosphate powder and liquid are mixed, a chemical reaction occurs and heat is released. This kind of reaction is called

    a. exothermic.

    b. viscosity.

    c. light cure.

    d. mechanical.

19. The following properties are true of glass ionomer material, except for stating that it

    a. mechanically bonds to tooth structure.

    b. chemically bonds to tooth structure.

    c. has nonirritating qualities.

    d. comes with a solvent.

20. Bonding agents bond to all of the following except

    a. varnish.

    b. enamel.

    c. dentin.

    d. porcelain.

21. Which cement is said to be "kind" to the pulp and was the first cement that could chemically bond to the tooth structure?

    a. Composite

    b. Polycarboxylate

    c. Amalgam

    d. Mechanical

22. Adhesion of dental materials to enamel is accomplished by

    a. dimensional change.

    b. acid etching.

    c. exothermic reaction.

    d. mechanical retention.

23. The _____ layer of debris prevents contact between intact dentin and the bonding agent/adhesive.

    a. smear

    b. liner

    c. microleakage

    d. sedative

24. The angle that is formed by the junction of the wall of the preparation and the untouched surface of the tooth is called the

    a. line angle.

    b. axial wall.

    c. cavosurface margin.

    d. pulpal floor.

25. Dental caries are detected by all of the following means except _____.

    a. Alginate impressions

    b. DIAGNOdent

    c. Radiographs

    d. Manual probing with explorer

26. What material is "resin-modified" for added strength?

    a. Composite

    b. Glass ionomer

    c. Bonding agents

    d. Polycarboxylate

27. Materials used to prepare the teeth for the restoration include which of the following?

    1. Amalgam
    2. Bases
    3. Composite
    4. Bonding agents
    5. Microfill composites
    6. Cements

    a. 1, 3, 5

    b. 2, 4, 5

    c. 2, 4, 6

    d. 1, 3, 6

28. _____ dental cement cures by a chemical reaction between two materials.

    a. Self-curing

    b. Light-curing

    c. Noncuring

    d. Heat-curing

29. _____ material is used with endodontic posts.

    a. Self-curing

    b. Light-curing

    c. Noncuring

    d. Heat-curing

30. A(n) _____ is used to condense the base into place on the floor of the cavity.

    a. explorer

    b. spoon excavator

    c. plastic filling instrument

    d. large spoon excavator

31. Which of the following considerations are used to evaluate base placement?

    1. Covers floor of cavity preparation
    2. Cavosurface margin
    3. Leaves enough room for restoration

4. Occlusal margin

5. Should not be on pins

6. Convenience form

7. Should not be in retentive grooves

8. Outline form

    a. 1, 2, 4, 6   c. 2, 4, 6, 8

    b. 1, 3, 5, 7   d. 4, 5, 7, 8

32. A thin layer of cavity varnish is placed on the dentin. The cavity varnish must dry _____ seconds before placing a second layer.

    a. 20   c. 30

    b. 15   d. 60

33. Cavity liners are placed on the _____ of the cavity preparation.

    a. occlusal line angle   c. axial wall

    b. deepest portion   d. gingival wall

34. Which type of cement is stronger, less water soluble, and more adhesive to the tooth structure?

    a. Resin-modified glass ionomer   c. Polycarboxylate

    b. Zinc phosphate   d. Calcium hydroxide

35. What is the name of the product that is used to treat hypersensitivity in teeth?

    a. Liner   c. Resin

    b. Varnish   d. Desensitizer

Critical Thinking

1. Describe the instruments used to place a cement base and the considerations and location of base placement.

2. When the dental assistant is placing the liners, base, or varnish, the cavity preparation should be examined and the pulpal involvement assessed. Explain the depths of the cavity preparation it relates to pulpal involvement.

3. Describe basic manipulation considerations for each of the following: ZOP, ZOE cement/type I, polycarboxylate, glass ionomer, and calcium hydroxide.

4. Mixing materials at chairside by the dental assistant as requested by the dentist will require knowledge of mixing terms and stages. List and describe mixing terms and stages.

CASE STUDY 1

Janice recently had a fairly large composite filling placed in the maxillary central incisor. When later contacting the dental office, she complained about long-lasting pain when she had a cold drink. An appointment for a consultation/exam was scheduled.

1. Describe desensitizers.

2. Identify the types of bases or liners that would be used in anterior composites.

3. Describe postoperative instructions for deep restorations.

CASE STUDY 2

Dental assistant Anna Mae wishes to improve her chairside skills, which would require her to know when and where bases and liners are placed. To accomplish her objective she needs to learn and receive training in the terminology of cavity preparation and preparation design.

1. List the terms involved in a cavity preparation.

2. List the elements of a cavity preparation design.

3. Enumerate basic requests from the dentist that the dental assistant can anticipate.

CASE STUDY 3

Sam's teeth are sensitive to sweets. One tooth in particular stings when exposed to sugary foods or drinks. Sam already had x-rays earlier in the year and really did not want more. The dentist, who had just invested in a DIAGNOdent, suggested that this instrument be used to detect whether caries were present. During the exam, use of the DIAGNOdent revealed newly formed caries.

1. Explain how a DIAGNOdent unit explores teeth.

2. Describe the function of the DIAGNOdent.

3. Explain low and high readings from this unit.

4. List five benefits in using the DIAGNOdent.

SKILL COMPETENCY ASSESSMENT

33-1 Mixing Zinc Phosphate Cement

Student's Name _____ Date _____

Instructor's Name _____

Skill: The dental assistant is responsible for preparing the equipment and supplies needed for the appointment. Zinc oxide phosphate cement is one of the oldest cements, and while it has some disadvantages, it is still a reliable choice for a luting and base cement. It comes in a powder/liquid form, and several brands are available. One objective in mixing the cement is to dissipate the heat from the exothermic reaction. If the heat is dissipated, the setting reaction is slowed and more powder can be incorporated to make the cement stronger.

Performance Objective: The student will follow a routine procedure that meets the regulations and protocol set forth by the dentist and regulatory agencies, keeping in mind that assistant duties vary from state to state. The assistant may be evaluated by performance criteria, verbal/written responses, and/or combined responses and performance criteria. This procedure is completed by the dental assistant for the dentist. The equipment and materials are prepared, and the material is mixed and transferred to the dentist. Sometimes the assistant places the cement in the cast restoration while the dentist places material on the prepared tooth.

	Self-Evaluation	Student Evaluation	Possible Points	Instructor Evaluation	Comments
Equipment and Supplies					
1. Zinc phosphate powder and liquid (dispensers, if needed)			3		
2. Cooled glass slab			3		
3. Flexible stainless steel cement spatula			3		
4. 2 × 2 gauze sponge			3		
5. Timer			2		
6. Plastic filling instrument			3		
Competency Steps (*follow aseptic procedures*)					
1. Shake the powder before removing the cap.			3		
2. Place an appropriate amount of powder on one end of the slab (the powder/liquid ratio amount is determined by the procedure—crown or bridge).			3		

	Self-Evaluation	Student Evaluation	Possible Points	Instructor Evaluation	Comments
3. Level the powder with the flat side of the spatula blade (layer about 1 mm thick).			3		
4. Divide the powder according to the manufacturer's directions (divide the powder into two equal portions with the edge of spatula, and continue to divide down to eighths).			3		
5. Gently shake the liquid. Dispense the liquid onto the glass slab; recap to prevent spilling and evaporation of the liquid (dispense the liquid to the opposite side of the slab; hold vertically to dispense uniform drops).			3		
6. Incorporate one small portion of powder into the liquid. Use the flat side of the spatula blade to wet powder (follow manufacturer's instructions; typically about 15 seconds).			3		
7. Spatulate the powder and liquid over a large area of the glass slab (hold the spatula blade flat against the slab and use a wide, sweeping motion).			3		
8. Add small amounts of powder to the liquid to achieve a smooth consistency. (Incorporate each increment of powder thoroughly before adding more powder; this helps to neutralize the acid.)			3		
9. The mix will appear watery at first. As more powder is incorporated, the mix will become creamy. (Gather all particles of powder and liquid from around the edges of the mix from time to time.)			3		
10. Turn the spatula blade on edge and gather the mass to check consistency.			3		

	Self-Evaluation	Student Evaluation	Possible Points	Instructor Evaluation	Comments
11. Continue to add increments to the mix until the desired consistency is reached, within the prescribed time period.			3		
12. Gather the entire mass into a single unit on the glass slab.			3		
13. Luting consistency (cementing) will be creamy (follows the spatula for about 1 inch as lifted off glass slab before breaking into a thin thread and flowing back into the mass).			3		
14. The base (putty-like) can be rolled into a ball or cylinder with the flat side of the spatula.			3		
15. Once the cement has the desired consistency, wipe off the spatula with a 2 × 2 gauze.			2		
16. Hold the glass slab under the patient's chin and transfer a plastic filling instrument.			3		
17. Receive the plastic filling instrument and wipe it and the glass slab off with a moistened 2 × 2 gauze.			3		
18. Clean glass slab and spatula. (Soak in water or a solution of bicarbonate of soda to loosen hardened cement, and then sterilize/disinfect accordingly.)			3		

TOTAL POINTS POSSIBLE   70

TOTAL POINTS POSSIBLE—2nd attempt   68

TOTAL POINTS EARNED   ____

Points assigned reflect importance of step to meeting objective: Important = 1, Essential = 2, Critical = 3. Students will lose 2 points for repeated attempts. Failure results if any of the critical steps are omitted or performed incorrectly. If using a 100-point scale, determine score by dividing points earned by total points possible and multiplying the results by 100.

SCORE: _____

SKILL COMPETENCY ASSESSMENT

33-2 Mixing Zinc Oxide Eugenol Cement—Powder/Liquid Form

Student's Name _____ Date _____

Instructor's Name _____

Skill: The dental assistant is responsible for preparing the equipment and supplies. Zinc oxide eugenol, often called ZOE cement, is another cement that has been used for many years. It is noted for its sedative or soothing effect on the dental pulp. The functions of this cement are diverse because of additives that enhance its properties. Zinc oxide eugenol comes in several forms including powder/liquid, two-paste systems, capsules, and syringes.

Performance Objective: The student will follow a routine procedure that meets the regulations and protocol set forth by the dentist and regulatory agencies, keeping in mind that assistant duties vary from state to state. The assistant may be evaluated by performance criteria, verbal/written responses, and/or combined responses and performance criteria. This procedure is completed by the dental assistant when the dentist requests it. The equipment and materials are prepared, and the material is mixed and transferred to the dentist. The assistant follows the manufacturer's directions for precise information on proportions, incorporation technique, and mixing and setting times.

	Self-Evaluation	Student Evaluation	Possible Points	Instructor Evaluation	Comments
Equipment and Supplies					
1. Zinc oxide eugenol cement			3		
2. Dispensers specific to material			2		
3. Paper pad or glass slab			3		
4. Cement spatula			3		
5. Timer			2		
6. Plastic filling instrument			3		
7. 2 × 2 gauze sponges			2		
8. Alcohol or orange solvent			2		
Competency Steps (*follow aseptic procedures*)					
1. Fluff the powder before removing the cap.			3		

	Self-Evaluation	Student Evaluation	Possible Points	Instructor Evaluation	Comments
2. Place the powder on the mixing pad (follow the manufacturer's directions, and replace the cap to avoid spilling and contamination).			3		
3. After swirling, place the liquid on a paper pad. (Hold the dispensing dropper perpendicular to the mixing pad and dispense drops. Dispense drops near the powder but not touching it.)			3		
4. Incorporate the powder into the liquid in divided increments or all at once (according to manufacturer's directions).			3		
5. Spatulate with the flat part of the blade, applying even pressure to "wet" all particles (some cements require firm pressure).			3		
6. Gather the powder and liquid from the edges of the mix.			3		
7. Gather the entire mass into a single unit on the slab to test consistency.			3		
8. Consistency for temporary luting will be creamy, like frosting.			3		
9. Consistency for insulating base or IRM will be putty-like and can be rolled into a ball or cylinder.			3		
10. Once the material has been mixed to desired consistency, wipe the spatula with a 2 × 2 gauze.			2		
11. Hold the pad under the patient's chin and transfer the cement on the plastic filling instrument.			3		
12. Receive the plastic filling instrument and wipe it off.			3		

	Self-Evaluation	Student Evaluation	Possible Points	Instructor Evaluation	Comments
13. Remove the top paper pad and fold to prevent accidentally contacting the cement.			2		
14. To clean material that has hardened on the spatula or glass slab, wipe it with alcohol or orange solvent.			3		

TOTAL POINTS POSSIBLE   60

TOTAL POINTS POSSIBLE—2nd attempt   58

TOTAL POINTS EARNED   ____

Points assigned reflect importance of step to meeting objective: Important = 1, Essential = 2, Critical = 3. Students will lose 2 points for repeated attempts. Failure results if any of the critical steps are omitted or performed incorrectly. If using a 100-point scale, determine score by dividing points earned by total points possible and multiplying the results by 100.

SCORE: _____

SKILL COMPETENCY ASSESSMENT

33-3 Mixing Zinc Oxide Eugenol Cement—Two-Paste System

Student's Name _____ Date _____

Instructor's Name _____

Skill: The dental assistant is responsible for preparation of equipment and supplies. The two-paste system is mixed on a small paper pad with a cement spatula or a plastic filling instrument. The base and the catalyst of the two-paste system come as a set and cannot be interchanged with other calcium hydroxide paste systems.

Performance Objective: The student will follow a routine procedure that meets the regulations and the protocol set forth by the dentist and regulatory agencies. Therefore, the assistant may be evaluated by performance criteria, verbal/written responses, and/or combined responses and performance criteria. This material is dispensed and mixed by the dental assistant. This material is often used for temporary luting of provisional coverage.

	Self-Evaluation	Student Evaluation	Possible Points	Instructor Evaluation	Comments
Equipment and Supplies 1. Two-paste zinc oxide eugenol (accelerator and base)			3		
2. Small paper pad			2		
3. Cement spatula			3		
4. 2 × 2 gauze sponge			2		
5. Plastic filling instrument			3		
Competency Steps (*follow aseptic procedures*) 1. Dispense small equal amounts of both accelerator and base onto paper pad (equal length/parallel to each other).			3		
2. Wipe off ends of tubes and replace caps.			3		
3. Mix the two materials, using circular motion (mix together to a homogenous consistency).			3		

	Self-Evaluation	Student Evaluation	Possible Points	Instructor Evaluation	Comments
4. Spread over a small area, and then gather. Repeat the process; material should be creamy mix that follows spatula up 1 inch (luting consistency).			3		
5. Wipe both sides of the spatula and then gather all material into a single area.			3		
6. Transfer plastic filling instrument to dentist and hold paper pad close to patient's chin.			3		
7. Wipe the instrument off with gauze for the dentist between applications.			2		
8. Receive the instrument; wipe off, tear, and fold the top page of paper pad and dispose. Wipe off cement spatula with moist gauze.			3		
TOTAL POINTS POSSIBLE			36		
TOTAL POINTS POSSIBLE—2nd attempt			34		
TOTAL POINTS EARNED			_____		

Points assigned reflect importance of step to meeting objective: Important = 1, Essential = 2, Critical = 3. Students will lose 2 points for repeated attempts. Failure results if any of the critical steps are omitted or performed incorrectly. If using a 100-point scale, determine score by dividing points earned by total points possible and multiplying the results by 100.

SCORE: _____

SKILL COMPETENCY ASSESSMENT

33-4 Mixing Polycarboxylate Cement

Student's Name _____ Date _____

Instructor's Name _____

Skill: The dental assistant is responsible for preparing the equipment and supplies. Polycarboxylate cement, also known as zinc polycarboxylate, is used for permanent cementation and as an insulating base. There are several brands of polycarboxylate cement, and the cement comes in a powder/liquid form.

Performance Objective: The student will follow a routine procedure that meets the regulations and protocol set forth by the dentist and regulatory agencies, keeping in mind that assistant duties vary from state to state. The assistant may be evaluated by performance criteria, verbal/written responses, and/or combined responses and performance criteria. The dental assistant prepares and mixes the polycarboxylate materials to the desired consistency. The amount of materials dispensed depends on the size of restoration and the number of units involved.

	Self-Evaluation	Student Evaluation	Possible Points	Instructor Evaluation	Comments
Equipment and Supplies					
1. Polycarboxylate powder and liquid and a dispenser for the powder			3		
2. Paper pad or glass slab			2		
3. Flexible stainless steel spatula			3		
4. 2 × 2 gauze sponge (moistened)			2		
5. Timer			2		
6. Plastic filling instrument			3		
Competency Steps (*follow aseptic procedures*)					
1. Fluff the powder before dispensing with a dispensing scoop.			3		
2. Measure the powder and dispense on one side of a paper pad or glass slab.			3		

	Self-Evaluation	Student Evaluation	Possible Points	Instructor Evaluation	Comments
3. Place uniform drops of liquid toward the opposite side of the powder. (Follow manufacturer's directions for appropriate powder/liquid ratio.)			3		
4. Incorporate from three-fourths to all of the powder into the liquid.			3		
a. Use a folding motion while applying pressure to wet all the powder.			2		
b. Mix quickly until all the powder is incorporated. (Liquid is thick, harder to incorporate into powder.)			2		
5. The mix will be slightly more viscous than zinc phosphate cement and glossy.			3		
6. Gather all cement, wiping both sides of the spatula.			2		
7. For luting consistency, the mix will follow the spatula up 1 inch.			3		
8. For base consistency, use the same amount of powder, but decrease the liquid ratio.			3		
a. The base mix should be glossy.			3		
b. Consistency is tacky and stiff.			3		
9. Mix must be used immediately before it becomes dull, stringy, and forms cobwebs.			3		

	Self-Evaluation	Student Evaluation	Possible Points	Instructor Evaluation	Comments
10. Clean immediately.			3		
a. Wipe the spatula with a wet 2 × 2 gauze.			3		
b. Or soak the spatula with dried cement in 10% sodium hydroxide solution.			3		
c. Remove, fold, and dispose of the paper pad sheet.			2		

TOTAL POINTS POSSIBLE   56

TOTAL POINTS POSSIBLE—2nd attempt   54

TOTAL POINTS EARNED   _____

Points assigned reflect importance of step to meeting objective: Important = 1, Essential = 2, Critical = 3. Students will lose 2 points for repeated attempts. Failure results if any of the critical steps are omitted or performed incorrectly. If using a 100-point scale, determine score by dividing points earned by total points possible and multiplying the results by 100.

SCORE: _____

SKILL COMPETENCY ASSESSMENT

33-5 Mixing Glass Ionomer Cement

Student's Name _____ Date _____

Instructor's Name _____

Skill: The dental assistant is responsible for preparing the equipment and supplies. Glass ionomer cement is one of the newer cement systems. This cement has many applications; therefore, there is more than one type of glass ionomer material. There are many brands of glass ionomer cement, and it is available in powder/liquid, paste systems, syringes, and capsule forms. The glass ionomers come in both self-curing and light-curing materials. The materials should be mixed quickly following manufacturer's directions because of the water content of the liquid. Water evaporation will affect the properties of the cement.

Performance Objective: The student will follow a routine procedure that meets the regulations and protocol set forth by the dentist and regulatory agencies, keeping in mind that assistant duties vary from state to state. The assistant may be evaluated by performance criteria, verbal/written responses, and/or combined responses and performance criteria. This procedure is completed by the assistant for the dentist. The equipment and materials are prepared and mixed when the dentist indicates. The material must be used immediately when the mix is completed. This material requires the tooth to be clean of debris and dry, so the dental assistant should rinse and evacuate and then isolate the area before beginning to mix the cement.

	Self-Evaluation	Student Evaluation	Possible Points	Instructor Evaluation	Comments
Equipment and Supplies 1. Glass ionomer materials and appropriate dispensers			3		
2. Paper pad or cool glass slab			3		
3. Flexible stainless steel spatula			3		
4. 2 × 2 gauze sponge (moistened)			2		
5. Timer			2		
6. Plastic filling instrument			3		
Competency Steps (*follow aseptic procedures*) 1. Fluff the powder before dispensing.			3		
2. Using a recommended scoop, place an appropriate number of scoops on a paper pad or glass slab.			3		

	Self-Evaluation	Student Evaluation	Possible Points	Instructor Evaluation	Comments
3. Swirl the liquid, and then place the specified amount of drops on the pad near the powder. (Replace the cap on the liquid immediately to prevent evaporation.)			3		
4. Divide the powder into halves or thirds, and then draw sections into the liquid one at a time.			3		
5. Mix over a small area until all powder is incorporated.			3		
a. Luting consistency—creamy and glossy			3		
b. Base consistency—tacky and stiff			3		
6. Once the cement has obtained final consistency:					
a. Wipe the spatula off with a 2 × 2 gauze.			2		
b. Hold the pad or glass slab under the patient's chin.			2		
c. Transfer the plastic filling instrument to the dentist.			3		
7. To clean up, remove, fold, and dispose of the top paper. Wipe instruments after use for easier cleanup.			3		
8. Activate glass ionomer capsules by placing them in "activator" or dispenser to break the seal (allows the powder and liquid to mix).			3		
9. Place capsules in amalgamator to mix (triturate) for a specific amount of time (usually 10 seconds; follow manufacturer's directions).			3		
10. Insert a capsule in the appropriate dispenser and transfer to the dentist for dispensing.			3		

	Self-Evaluation	Student Evaluation	Possible Points	Instructor Evaluation	Comments
11. To clean up, discard the capsule and disinfect the activator and/or the dispenser.			3		

TOTAL POINTS POSSIBLE 59

TOTAL POINTS POSSIBLE—2nd attempt 57

TOTAL POINTS EARNED ____

Points assigned reflect importance of step to meeting objective: Important = 1, Essential = 2, Critical = 3. Students will lose 2 points for repeated attempts. Failure results if any of the critical steps are omitted or performed incorrectly. If using a 100-point scale, determine score by dividing points earned by total points possible and multiplying the results by 100.

SCORE: _____

SKILL COMPETENCY ASSESSMENT

33-6 Mixing of Calcium Hydroxide Cement—Two-Paste System

Student's Name _____ Date _____

Instructor's Name _____

Skill: The dental assistant is responsible for preparing the equipment and supplies. The two-paste system is mixed on a small paper pad with a metal spatula, explorer, or small ball-ended instrument. The base and the catalyst of the two-paste system come as a set and cannot be interchanged with other calcium hydroxide paste systems.

Performance Objective: The student will follow a routine procedure that meets the regulations and protocol set forth by the dentist and regulatory agencies, keeping in mind that assistant duties vary from state to state. The assistant may be evaluated by performance criteria, verbal/written responses, and/or combined responses and performance criteria. This material is dispensed and mixed by the dental assistant. It is often the first step in restoring the cavity preparation.

	Self-Evaluation	Student Evaluation	Possible Points	Instructor Evaluation	Comments
Equipment and Supplies					
1. Calcium hydroxide two-paste system			3		
2. Small paper pad			2		
3. Small ball-ended instrument or explorer			3		
4. 2 × 2 gauze sponge			2		
Competency Steps (*follow aseptic procedures*)					
1. Dispense small, equal amounts of both catalyst and base onto a paper pad.			3		
2. Wipe off the ends of the tubes, and replace the caps.			3		
3. Mix the two materials, using a circular motion.			3		
4. Mix until the materials are of a uniform color within the 10- to 15-second mixing time.			3		

	Self-Evaluation	Student Evaluation	Possible Points	Instructor Evaluation	Comments
5. Use a 2 × 2 gauze to remove excess material from the mixing instrument.			3		
6. Transfer the instrument to the dentist, and hold the paper pad close to the patient's chin.			3		
7. Wipe off the instrument with gauze for the dentist between applications.			2		
8. Receive the instrument and wipe it off; tear and fold the top page of the paper pad and dispose of the page.			3		
TOTAL POINTS POSSIBLE			33		
TOTAL POINTS POSSIBLE—2nd attempt			31		
TOTAL POINTS EARNED			____		

Points assigned reflect importance of step to meeting objective: Important = 1, Essential = 2, Critical = 3. Students will lose 2 points for repeated attempts. Failure results if any of the critical steps are omitted or performed incorrectly. If using a 100-point scale, determine score by dividing points earned by total points possible and multiplying the results by 100.

SCORE: _____

SKILL COMPETENCY ASSESSMENT

33-7 Preparing Cavity Varnish

Student's Name _____ Date _____

Instructor's Name _____

Skill: The dental assistant is responsible for preparation of equipment and supplies. Varnishes are placed in a thin layer over the dentin tubules. Cavity varnishes are insoluble in oral fluids and reduce leakage around the margins of restorations, thereby preventing microleakage. Varnish also prevents penetration of the acids from some cements into the dentin.

Performance Objective: The student will follow a routine procedure that meets the regulations and the protocol set forth by the dentist and regulatory agencies. Therefore, the assistant may be evaluated by performance criteria, verbal/written responses, and/or combined responses and performance criteria. The material needed for application of cavity varnish is prepared by the dental assistant. Depending on state expanded-function laws, the assistant applies the varnish or assists the dentist during placement.

	Self-Evaluation	Student Evaluation	Possible Points	Instructor Evaluation	Comments
Equipment and Supplies					
1. Cavity varnish and solvent			3		
2. Two cotton pliers			3		
3. Cotton pellets, or pieces of cotton rolled into small football-shaped balls, or small brush or cotton tipped applicators			3		
4. Cotton roll			2		
Competency Steps (*follow aseptic procedures*)					
1. Clean and dry cavity preparation.			3		
2. Prepare cotton pellets for application (must be small to apply varnish on dentin surface).			3		

	Self-Evaluation	Student Evaluation	Possible Points	Instructor Evaluation	Comments
3. Remove cap from varnish bottle.			2		
a. Hold two cotton pellets in pliers (dip).			2		
b. Dip pellets into varnish until moistened.			2		
c. Remove and replace cap on varnish.			3		
4. Place cotton pellets on 2 × 2 gauze to dab off excess.			3		
5. Using one pellet, apply varnish to cavity preparation, coating the preparation surface.			3		
6. Allow first coat to dry, and then apply a second coat in same manner.			3		
7. Dispose of cotton pellets, and clean cotton pliers with solvent before sterilizing.			3		
8. If using small brushes or cotton tip applicator prepare two brushes/applicators and follow same steps as cotton pellet application			3		

TOTAL POINTS POSSIBLE 40

TOTAL POINTS POSSIBLE—2nd attempt 38

TOTAL POINTS EARNED _____

Points assigned reflect importance of step to meeting objective: Important = 1, Essential = 2, Critical = 3. Students will lose 2 points for repeated attempts. Failure results if any of the critical steps are omitted or performed incorrectly. If using a 100-point scale, determine score by dividing points earned by total points possible and multiplying the results by 100.

SCORE: _____

SKILL COMPETENCY ASSESSMENT

33-8 Placing Resin Cement—Dual-Curing Technique

Student's Name _____ Date _____

Instructor's Name _____

Skill: The dental assistant is responsible for preparing the equipment and supplies. Resin cements may be supplied in a two-paste system, powder/liquid set, or syringe. The manufacturer may supply the acid-etch gel or liquid with the material. Some of these materials may be shaded to complement the translucency of the crown or inlay.

Performance Objective: The student will follow a routine procedure that meets the regulations and protocol set forth by the dentist and regulatory agencies, keeping in mind that assistant duties vary from state to state. The assistant may be evaluated by performance criteria, verbal/written responses, and/or combined responses and performance criteria. This procedure is prepared by the assistant for the dentist. The equipment and materials are prepared, and the material is mixed and transferred to the dentist. Because this material is dual curing, a curing light and eye protection are necessary.

	Self-Evaluation	Student Evaluation	Possible Points	Instructor Evaluation	Comments
Equipment and Supplies					
1. Resin cement system			3		
2. Paper pad			2		
3. Stainless steel spatula			3		
4. Plastic filling instrument			3		
5. Curing light and protective shield or glasses			3		
6. 2 × 2 gauze sponges			2		
Competency Steps (*follow aseptic procedures*)					
1. Clean and dry the tooth, and isolate the area with cotton rolls.			3		
2. Transfer etchant to the dentist.			3		
3. Wait the time required for the etchant.			3		
4. Rinse thoroughly.			3		

	Self-Evaluation	Student Evaluation	Possible Points	Instructor Evaluation	Comments
5. Dry the tooth (light air dry). Apply adhesive.			3		
6. Dispense and mix the two components to a homogeneous, creamy mixture.			3		
7. Hold the pad close to the patient and transfer the placement instrument (the dentist places material on the tooth and restoration).			3		
8. Hold a 2 × 2 gauze to remove any excess materials.			2		
9. Receive the placement instrument, and prepare the curing light.			3		
10. Use a protective shield when curing light is activated. (The dentist or the assistant holds the light.)			3		
11. Clean up immediately; wipe any excess cement off instruments and discard disposable items.			3		

TOTAL POINTS POSSIBLE 48

TOTAL POINTS POSSIBLE—2nd attempt 46

TOTAL POINTS EARNED ____

Points assigned reflect importance of step to meeting objective: Important = 1, Essential = 2, Critical = 3. Students will lose 2 points for repeated attempts. Failure results if any of the critical steps are omitted or performed incorrectly. If using a 100-point scale, determine score by dividing points earned by total points possible and multiplying the results by 100.

SCORE: _____

SKILL COMPETENCY ASSESSMENT

33-9 Placing Etchant

Student's Name _____ Date _____

Instructor's Name _____

Skill: The dental assistant is responsible for preparing the equipment and supplies. Adhesion of dental materials to enamel is accomplished by acid etching with phosphoric acid. This solution alters the surface of the enamel and creates microscopic undercuts between the enamel rods. Unfilled resin-bonding agents penetrate these undercuts and mechanically lock into them. The restorative material then bonds to this layer and becomes a solid unit.

Performance Objective: The student will follow a routine procedure that meets the regulations and protocol set forth by the dentist and regulatory agencies, keeping in mind that assistant duties vary from state to state. The assistant may be evaluated by performance. The dentist will place the etchant. When the allotted time has passed, the assistant thoroughly rinses the tooth.

	Self-Evaluation	Student Evaluation	Possible Points	Instructor Evaluation	Comments
Equipment and Supplies					
1. Acid etchant, usually a 30% to 40% solution			3		
2. Isolation materials—rubber dam or cotton rolls			3		
3. Applicator—syringe, cotton pellets, small applicator tips			3		
4. Dappen dish			2		
5. Air-water syringe			2		
6. Timer			2		
Competency Steps (*follow aseptic procedures*)					
1. Isolate the area.			3		
2. Thoroughly clean the surface.			3		
3. Prepare the etchant applicator or syringe.			3		

	Self-Evaluation	Student Evaluation	Possible Points	Instructor Evaluation	Comments
4. Place etchant on the surface for 15 to 30 seconds (follow manufacturer's directions).			3		
5. When the time is up, rinse the tooth for 15 to 20 seconds with an air-water syringe and evacuate thoroughly for 10 to 20 seconds.			3		
6. The etched surface should have a frosty appearance.			3		
7. Until the bonding is completed, keep the surface isolated and dry. (If saliva or other fluids contact the surface, repeat the etching process.)			3		

TOTAL POINTS POSSIBLE   36

TOTAL POINTS POSSIBLE—2nd attempt   34

TOTAL POINTS EARNED   ____

Points assigned reflect importance of step to meeting objective: Important = 1, Essential = 2, Critical = 3. Students will lose 2 points for repeated attempts. Failure results if any of the critical steps are omitted or performed incorrectly. If using a 100-point scale, determine score by dividing points earned by total points possible and multiplying the results by 100.

SCORE: _____

SKILL COMPETENCY ASSESSMENT

33-10 Placing Bonding Agent

Student's Name _____ Date _____

Instructor's Name _____

Skill: The dental assistant is responsible for preparing the equipment and supplies. The current dentin-bonding materials use an etchant to remove the smear layer, because the smear layer is not firmly attached and is unreliable. When the smear layer is removed, the adhesives can achieve a mechanical bond with the dentin. Many of the bonding agents are suitable for both enamel and dentin surfaces because of the application of the acid etchant.

Performance Objective: The student will follow a routine procedure that meets the regulations and protocol set forth by the dentist and regulatory agencies, keeping in mind that assistant duties vary from state to state. The assistant may be evaluated by performance criteria, verbal/written responses, and/or combined responses and performance criteria. Steps in the application of bonding agents vary among manufacturers, so follow the directions that come with the product. The dental assistant prepares the materials for each step and keeps the area dry and free of debris.

	Self-Evaluation	Student Evaluation	Possible Points	Instructor Evaluation	Comments
Equipment and Supplies 1. Bonding system that contains acid etchant, primer or conditioner, adhesive material			3		
2. Applicators (disposable tips or brushes)			3		
3. Dappen dish			2		
4. Isolation means			3		
5. Air-water syringe			2		
6. Curing light and shield			3		
7. Timer			2		
Competency Steps (*follow aseptic procedures*) 1. Clean the cavity preparation. (Ensure that it is free of debris; if needed, use cavity cleaners.)			3		

	Self-Evaluation	Student Evaluation	Possible Points	Instructor Evaluation	Comments
2. If the cavity preparation is near the pulp, place calcium hydroxide or glass ionomer lining cement over the area.			3		
3. Place etchant on the surface (15 to 20 seconds), first on the enamel and then on the dentin.			3		
4. Rinse the tooth as soon as the time is up. Continue to rinse for 5 to 10 seconds. Move quickly to prevent bacterial contamination of dentin.			3		
5. Primer or conditioner is placed with a brush or an applicator. If bonding involves both enamel and dentin, include a primer step (this "wets" dentin and penetrates dentin tubules).			3		
6. Apply bonding resin.			3		
7. Use curing light to harden the material.			3		
8. Cleanup: dispose of applicator tips or brushes.			2		

TOTAL POINTS POSSIBLE   41

TOTAL POINTS POSSIBLE—2nd attempt   39

TOTAL POINTS EARNED   _____

Points assigned reflect importance of step to meeting objective: Important = 1, Essential = 2, Critical = 3. Students will lose 2 points for repeated attempts. Failure results if any of the critical steps are omitted or performed incorrectly. If using a 100-point scale, determine score by dividing points earned by total points possible and multiplying the results by 100.

SCORE: _____

SKILL COMPETENCY ASSESSMENT

33-11 Placing Cavity Liners—Glass Ionomer

Student's Name _____   Date _____

Instructor's Name _____

Skill: Routine steps should be followed for all treatment areas to maintain absolute clinical asepsis. The dental assistant is responsible for preparing the equipment and supplies. Dental liners are placed in the deepest portion of the cavity preparation on the axial or pulpal walls. After the liners are hardened, they form a cement layer with minimum strength.

Performance Objective: The student will follow a routine procedure that meets the regulations and protocol set forth by the dentist and regulatory agencies, keeping in mind that assistant duties vary from state to state. The assistant may be evaluated by performance criteria, verbal/written responses, and/or combined responses and performance criteria. This procedure is performed by the dentist or an expanded-functions dental assistant. The preparation of the cavity has been completed, and this procedure begins the restorative process.

	Self-Evaluation	Student Evaluation	Possible Points	Instructor Evaluation	Comments
Equipment and Supplies					
1. Cavity liner (calcium hydroxide, glass ionomer)			3		
2. Application instrument—small ball-ended instrument or explorer			3		
3. Gauze sponges and cotton rolls			3		
4. Mixing pad and spatula, if material is needed			3		
5. Curing light (if material is light cured)			3		
Competency Steps (*follow aseptic procedures*)					
1. Examine the cavity preparation. Determine the deepest portion of the cavity preparation and access to that area.			3		

	Self-Evaluation	Student Evaluation	Possible Points	Instructor Evaluation	Comments
2. Clean and dry the cavity preparation, remove debris from the cavity preparation, and wash and dry the area with an air-water syringe.			3		
3. Prepare the liner. Dispense and mix according to directions.			3		
4. Place the liner in the cavity preparation. Using a small ball-ended instrument, place the material in the deepest portion of the cavity preparation in a thin layer.			3		
5. Complete the placement, remove the instrument, wipe it clean with gauze, and repeat the procedure until the liner covers the deepest portion of the cavity preparation.			3		
6. Light cure the liner. a. If the liner is self-curing, allow the mix to harden. b. If the liner is light curing, hold the light over the tooth and activate to cure for the appropriate time (usually 10 to 20 seconds).			3 3		
7. Examine the cavity preparation. After the liner has cured, examine the preparation. If any material is on the enamel walls, remove with an explorer.			3		

TOTAL POINTS POSSIBLE   39

TOTAL POINTS POSSIBLE—2nd attempt   37

TOTAL POINTS EARNED   _____

Points assigned reflect importance of step to meeting objective: Important = 1, Essential = 2, Critical = 3. Students will lose 2 points for repeated attempts. Failure results if any of the critical steps are omitted or performed incorrectly. If using a 100-point scale, determine score by dividing points earned by total points possible and multiplying the results by 100.

SCORE: _____

SKILL COMPETENCY ASSESSMENT

33-12 Placing Cavity Varnish

Student's Name _____ Date _____

Instructor's Name _____

Skill: The dental assistant is responsible for preparation of equipment and supplies. Varnishes are placed in a thin layer over the dentin tubules. Cavity varnishes are insoluble in the oral fluids and reduce leakage around the margins of restorations, thus preventing microleakage. Varnish also prevents penetration of the acids from some cement into the dentin.

Performance Objective: The student will follow a routine procedure that meets the regulations and the protocol set forth by the dentist and regulatory agencies. Therefore, the assistant may be evaluated by performance criteria, verbal/written responses, and/or combined responses and performance criteria. The materials needed for application of cavity varnish are prepared by the dental assistant. Depending on the state expanded-function laws, the assistant applies the varnish or assists the dentist during placement. The preparation of the cavity has been completed, and this procedure is part of preparing the tooth for the restoration.

	Self-Evaluation	Student Evaluation	Possible Points	Instructor Evaluation	Comments
Equipment and Supplies					
1. Cavity varnish (varnish and solvent)			3		
2. Cotton pliers			3		
3. Cotton balls/pellets, sponge applicators, brush applicators			2		
4. Gauze sponges			2		
Competency Steps (*follow aseptic procedures*) 1. Prepare two very small cotton balls/pellets, about 2 mm in size, in the shape of small footballs or prepare two applicators and follow same steps.			3		
2. Evaluate access, visibility, and placement of liners or bases. Wash and dry tooth if not done already.			3		

	Self-Evaluation	Student Evaluation	Possible Points	Instructor Evaluation	Comments
3. Remove cap from varnish bottle.			2		
a. Hold two cotton pellets/ balls in sterile cotton pliers (dip).			2		
b. Dip pellets into varnish until moistened.			2		
c. Remove and replace cap on varnish.			3		
4. Place cotton pellets/balls on 2 × 2 gauze to dab off excess.			3		
5. Using one pellet/ball picked up with the cotton pliers, paint a thin layer of varnish to dentin in cavity preparation (sterile disposable brush or sponge may be used).			3		
6. Allow first coat to dry (30 seconds), and then apply a second coat in same manner.			3		
7. Dispose of cotton pellets/ balls/brushes, and clean cotton pliers with solvent before sterilizing.			3		
8. To prevent contamination, never place an applicator that has been used in the patient's mouth back in the bottle of varnish.			3		

TOTAL POINTS POSSIBLE   40

TOTAL POINTS POSSIBLE—2nd attempt   38

TOTAL POINTS EARNED   ____

Points assigned reflect importance of step to meeting objective: Important = 1, Essential = 2, Critical = 3. Students will lose 2 points for repeated attempts. Failure results if any of the critical steps are omitted or performed incorrectly. If using a 100-point scale, determine score by dividing points earned by total points possible and multiplying the results by 100.

SCORE: _____

SKILL COMPETENCY ASSESSMENT

33-13 Placement of Cement Bases

Student's Name _____ Date _____

Instructor's Name _____

Skill: Routine steps should be followed for all treatment areas to maintain absolute clinical asepsis. The dental assistant is responsible for preparing the equipment and supplies. Cement bases are mixed to thick putty consistency and placed in the cavity preparation to protect the pulp and to provide mechanical support for the restoration. These cement bases are placed on the floor of the cavity preparation to raise the floor of the preparation to ideal height. The preparation, sensitivity of the pulp, and type of restoration determines which cement to use.

Performance Objective: The student will follow a routine procedure that meets the regulations and protocol set forth by the dentist and regulatory agencies, keeping in mind those assistant duties vary from state to state. The assistant may be evaluated by performance criteria, verbal/written responses, and/or combined responses and performance criteria. This procedure is performed by the dentist or an expanded-functions dental assistant. The preparation of the cavity has been completed, and this procedure is part of preparing the tooth for the restoration.

	Self-Evaluation	Student Evaluation	Possible Points	Instructor Evaluation	Comments
Equipment and Supplies					
1. Cement base materials, usually powder/liquid			3		
2. Mixing pad			3		
3. Cement spatula			3		
4. Gauze sponges			3		
5. Plastic filling instrument			3		
6. Explorer or spoon excavator			3		
Competency Steps (*follow aseptic procedures*)					
1. Determine the previous treatment and decide where to place the base as well as the size of the area. Evaluate access and visibility.			3		
2. Prepare the preparation area. Remove debris with an air-water syringe and an HVE.			3		

	Self-Evaluation	Student Evaluation	Possible Points	Instructor Evaluation	Comments
3. Prepare the cement base materials according to manufacturer's instructions. Mix the cement base to thick putty consistency and gather into a small ball.			3		
4. Collect the base on the blade of a plastic filling instrument. Place the base into the cavity preparation.			3		
5. Using the small condensing end of the plastic filling instrument, condense the base into place on the floor of the cavity prep. Continue until the base layer suffices.			3		
6. Evaluate the placement. The base should cover the floor of the cavity preparation; there should be enough room left for the restorative materials, and there should be no base on the pins or retentive grooves.			3		
7. Remove any excess materials with a spoon excavator or an explorer.			3		
8. Clean up mixing materials, removing cement from the spatula as soon as possible and paper from the pad.			3		

TOTAL POINTS POSSIBLE   42

TOTAL POINTS POSSIBLE—2nd attempt   40

TOTAL POINTS EARNED   _____

Points assigned reflect importance of step to meeting objective: Important = 1, Essential = 2, Critical = 3. Students will lose 2 points for repeated attempts. Failure results if any of the critical steps are omitted or performed incorrectly. If using a 100-point scale, determine score by dividing points earned by total points possible and multiplying the results by 100.

SCORE: _____

CHAPTER 34

Restorative Materials, Dental Dam, Matrix, and Wedge

SPECIFIC INSTRUCTIONAL OBJECTIVES

The student should strive to meet the following objectives and demonstrate an understanding of the facts and principles presented in this chapter:

1. Explain the properties, composition, and manipulation of dental amalgam.

2. Identify the armamentarium and steps of an amalgam procedure.

3. Explain the composition of composite resins.

4. Explain the properties and manipulation of various composite restorations.

5. Identify the armamentarium and steps of a composite restoration.

6. Explain the use of glass ionomer, resin, resin-reinforced glass ionomer, and compomer restorative materials.

Advanced Chairside Functions

7. Explain the purpose of the dental dam and identify who places it on a patient.

8. List and explain advantages and contraindications of the dental dam.

9. Identify the armamentarium needed for the dental dam procedure and explain the function of each.

10. Explain how to prepare the patient for dental dam placement and how to determine the isolation area. Describe and demonstrate how dental dam material is prepared.

11. List and demonstrate steps of placing and removing the dental dam.

12. Explain and demonstrate the dental dam procedure for the child patient.

13. Define matrix and wedge. List the uses and types of matrices.

14. Describe the functions, parts, placement, and removal of the Tofflemire matrix.

15. Explain and demonstrate placement and removal of the strip matrix.

SUMMARY

The general chairside assistant prepares restorative materials for the dentist to place in the prepared cavity. In some states dental assistants and/or hygienists are allowed to place restorative materials. The restorative dental assistant or restorative dental hygienist completes specific education including didactic and clinical training to become licensed to perform these skills.

Knowledge of the properties of the restorative materials is necessary for the dental assistant to properly prepare and manipulate the materials and also allows the dental assistant to be a step ahead of the dentist.

Two expanded functions are included in this chapter: the placement and removal of the dental dam (sometimes referred to as rubber dam) and the placement and removal of a matrix when restoring a tooth. The dental dam has many advantages such as greater visibility, control of moisture, and protection for the patient. The dental assistant is usually responsible for preparing, placing, and removal of the dental dam. The materials and equipment needed for this procedure are discussed as they relate to their function. The procedure for placing the dental dam begins with selecting the clamp, dividing and punching the dental dam material, and then placing and securing the clamp and dental dam material. Once the procedure is completed the dental assistant removes the dental dam from the patient and cleans up the area.

Several types of matrices are discussed including the Tofflemire, the AutoMatrix system, sectional matrix systems, and the plastic strip and cervical matrices. The matrices are used to hold and contour the restorative materials in place. The dental assistant assembles and readies the matrix for placement except in states that allow the dental assistant to also place and remove the various matrices. The dental assistant gains knowledge of sequence and techniques in this chapter.

EXERCISES AND ACTIVITIES

Multiple Choice

1. Which of the following materials are a combination of and alloy and mercury?

   a. Composite
   b. Amalgam
   c. Glass ionomer
   d. Resin

2. Which dental dam instrument has a working end that is a sharp projection and is used to provide holes in the dam?

   a. Clamp
   b. Punch
   c. Forceps
   d. Pliers

3. Dental dam clamps are designed to be used on specific teeth. One of the basic parts of the clamp is the section of arched metal that joins the two jaws of the clamp together, which is called the

   a. points.
   b. wings.
   c. bow.
   d. hole.

4. All of the following are true about mercury except:

   a. Metal in a liquid state
   b. Not toxic
   c. Vaporizes at low room temperature
   d. Scraps should be kept in sealed container

5. There are many advantages to using the dental dam, but certain conditions contraindicate its use. Which of the following are contraindications?

   1. Provides greater visibility
   2. Latex allergies
   3. Respiratory congestion
   4. Herpetic lesions
   5. Retracts tongue
   6. Provides greater accessibility

   a. 1, 2, 5
   b. 2, 3, 6
   c. 2, 3, 4
   d. 1, 3, 5

6. Dental amalgam alloy is composed of:

   a. Silver, tin, copper & aluminum
   b. Silver, tin, zinc, & gold
   c. Silver, tin, copper, & zinc
   d. Tin, Zinc, mercury, and copper

7. Trituration is the _____ means of combining dental alloy and mercury.

   a. Self-cure
   b. light-cure
   c. chemical
   d. mechanical

8. Which part of the Tofflemire matrix retainer holds the ends of the matrix band in place in the diagonal slot?

   a. Spindle
   b. Vise
   c. Guide channels
   d. Inner knob

9. Which material dominates the field of aesthetic restorations?

   a. Composite
   b. Glass ionomer
   c. Bonding agents
   d. Polycarboxylate

10. Main component of composite restorations is which of the following:

    a. Organic polymer matrix
    b. Inorganic polymer particles
    c. Inorganic silane matric
    d. Resin silane particles

11. When the incisal edge on anterior teeth is involved, a Class V _____ type matrix is used to restore the tooth.

    a. stainless-steel
    b. crown-form
    c. celluloid matrix strip
    d. sectional

12. The sectional matrix system benefits tooth contour by

    a. restoring anatomic contacts.
    b. acting as a stabilizing matrix.
    c. producing a tight contact.
    d. All of the above.

13. With which material is the plastic matrix strip used?

    a. Composite
    b. Glass ionomer
    c. Compomer
    d. All of the above

14. This type of composite combines strength and esthetics and is used in the anterior and posterior areas of the mouth.

    a. Hybrid composites
    b. Microfill composites
    c. Macrofill composites
    d. Minifill composites

15. Which of the following holds the matrix strip in place?

    a. 212 clamp
    b. Tofflemire
    c. Clip retainer
    d. Wedge

16. The occlusal edge of the Tofflemire matrix band should extend no more than _____ mm above the highest cusp.

    a. 1
    b. 1.5
    c. 2
    d. All of the above

17. Composites restorative materials _____.

    a. Come in flowable and condensable forms
    b. Available in a variety of shades
    c. Can be light-cured, self-cured, or dual-cured
    d. All of the above

18. To ensure contact with the adjacent tooth, the Tofflemire matrix band

    a. needs to be contoured.

    b. requires application of pressure with a burnisher.

    c. must be concave at the contact area.

    d. All of the above.

19. The guide channels toward the operator's right would be placed in the _____ quadrant.

    a. maxillary right

    b. mandibular left

    c. a. and b.

    d. maxillary left

20. Before the composite material in placed in the cavity preparation _____.

    a. a layer of amalgam is placed

    b. the tooth is etched and rinsed

    c. an enamel sealant is placed

    d. fluoride is placed on the tooth

Critical Thinking

1. The dental assistant plays an important role in explaining to the patient the rubber dam removal procedure. Describe the interseptal step in removing the dental dam.

2. One of the purposes of dental dam placement is isolation. Describe the steps, purpose, and method of inverting the dam material.

3. Describe common errors that occur when punching the dental dam.

4. Dental dam clamps are designed for use on specific teeth. The dental assistant must be able to evaluate the tooth before making a clamp selection. Describe the purpose of these clamps and the selection process. Identify parts of the clamp in the following figure.

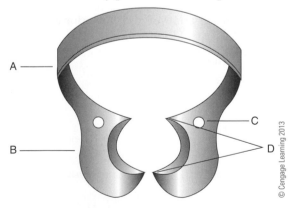

© Cengage Learning 2013

5. Once the tooth has been prepared for a composite restoration, the strip matrix is placed. List the functions, types, and uses of the plastic strip matrix.

CASE STUDY 1

Radiographs reveal that Kevin has an overhang on an MOD restoration. The dentist then defines for Kevin an overhang and describes the recommended treatment.

1. Explain when a wedge is placed.

2. Describe the pros and cons of wedge placement.

3. List the types of wedges.

4. Describe the sequence of wedge placement.

CASE STUDY 2

A young patient has little tolerance for manipulations in his mouth and cannot respond to requests about oral movement (or nonmovement). Therefore, the procedure to be performed must be isolated. A rubber dam is the best choice for the procedure and the isolation requirement.

1. Name the alternative to full dam placement.

2. Explain how regular hole alignment will be determined.

3. Describe the hole sizes that will be used.

4. Describe placement in the patient's mouth.

5. Explain how the quickdam method for the final fit of the dental dam differs from that of the full dam.

CASE STUDY 3

April has a missing molar and a rotated canine. The dental team's treatment will consist of a bridge from the first molar to the canine. The restoration will be a Class V.

1. Describe the process of evaluation in this case.

2. Describe the punching when teeth are malpositioned.

3. Describe the punching when the teeth are part of bridgework.

4. Outline the dam punching in preparation for a Class V restoration placement.

Labeling

The Tofflemire matrix is the most common matrix and retainer used for amalgam restorations. Label its parts.

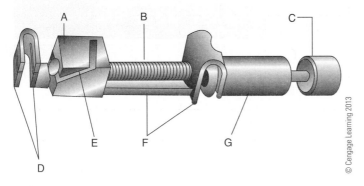

© Cengage Learning 2013

A. _____

B. _____

C. _____

D. _____

E. _____

F. _____

G. _____

SKILL COMPETENCY ASSESSMENT

34-1 Using Dental Amalgamator

Student's Name _____ Date _____

Instructor's Name _____

Skill: The dental assistant is responsible for preparing the equipment and supplies. Trituration is the mechanical means of combining the dental alloy and mercury. Specially designed machines used to triturate (amalgamate) the alloy and mercury are called dental amalgamators or triturators. These machines comprise a cradle to hold the capsules, cradle cover, timer, and variable speed control. Amalgamators must be set for the type of dental alloy used.

Performance Objective: The student will follow a routine procedure that meets the regulations and protocol set forth by the dentist and regulatory agencies. The assistant may be evaluated by performance criteria, verbal/written responses, and/or combined responses and performance criteria. This procedure is completed by the dental assistant. The materials and equipment are prepared before the procedure begins. The type of amalgamator and capsules will vary.

	Self-Evaluation	Student Evaluation	Possible Points	Instructor Evaluation	Comments
Equipment and Supplies 1. Amalgamator			3		
2. Premeasured capsule of dental alloy and mercury			3		
3. Amalgam well, dappen dish, or squeeze cloth			3		
4. Amalgam carrier/condenser			3		
5. Scrap container for excess amalgam			3		
Competency Steps (*follow aseptic procedures*) 1. Assemble materials for the procedure (select trituration, time, speed, type of alloy, and amalgamator).			3		
2. Prepare the capsule by twisting the cap, squeezing the capsule, or using an activator.			3		

	Self-Evaluation	Student Evaluation	Possible Points	Instructor Evaluation	Comments
3. Insert the capsule in the cradle (prongs) of the amalgamator; place one end first, and then slide the other end downward into place, practicing with one hand.			3		
4. Close the amalgamator cover.			3		
5. Activate the amalgamator for the prescribed time and speed.			3		
6. The timer will automatically switch off after the prescribed trituration time.			2		
7. Lift the cover and remove the capsule.			2		
8. Open the capsule and empty the amalgam into an amalgam well.			3		
9. Avoid touching amalgam with gloved hands. Use cotton pliers if necessary. The amalgam will be glossy, smooth, and velvety.			3		
10. Reassemble the capsule and place it to the side.			2		
11. Hold the carrier and load the amalgam.			3		
12. Pack the carrier tightly, wiping away excess. (Wipe excess material from the end of carrier on the sides of the amalgam well.)			3		
13. Transfer amalgam carrier to the dentist.			3		

	Self-Evaluation	Student Evaluation	Possible Points	Instructor Evaluation	Comments
14. Prepare to exchange a condenser for the carrier. (Practice dispensing amalgam from the carrier into a dappen dish and evaluate the mix.)			3		
15. Repeat loading and dispensing of all material. Toward the end, loading becomes more difficult as the material begins to set (practice to become proficient).			3		
16. To clean up, expel any excess amalgam into the appropriate container. Clean and sterilize the instruments.			3		

TOTAL POINTS POSSIBLE   60

TOTAL POINTS POSSIBLE—2nd attempt   58

TOTAL POINTS EARNED   ____

Points assigned reflect importance of step to meeting objective: Important = 1, Essential = 2, Critical = 3. Students will lose 2 points for repeated attempts. Failure results if any of the critical steps are omitted or performed incorrectly. If using a 100-point scale, determine score by dividing points earned by total points possible and multiplying the results by 100.

SCORE: _____

SKILL COMPETENCY ASSESSMENT

34-2 Complete Amalgam Restoration—Class II

Student's Name _____ Date _____

Instructor's Name _____

Skill: The dental assistant is responsible for preparing the equipment and supplies. Steps include administering anesthetic; placing the rubber dam; placing liners and bases; assembling the matrix and wedge; and mixing, placing, condensing, and finishing the amalgam restoration.

Performance Objective: The student will follow a routine procedure that meets the regulations and protocol set forth by the dentist and regulatory agencies, keeping in mind those assistant duties vary from state to state. The assistant may be evaluated by performance criteria, verbal/written responses, and/or combined responses and performance criteria. The dental assistant assists the dentist throughout the procedure.

	Self-Evaluation	Student Evaluation	Possible Points	Instructor Evaluation	Comments
Equipment and Supplies					
1. Basic setup: mouth mirror, explorer, cotton pliers			3		
2. Air-water syringe tip, HVE tip, and saliva ejector			3		
3. Cotton rolls, gauze sponges, pellets, cotton-tip applicators, and floss			3		
4. Topical and local anesthetic setup			3		
5. Rubber dam setup			3		
6. High- and low-speed handpieces			3		
7. Assortment of dental burs			3		
8. Spoon excavator			2		
9. Hand cutting instruments (hatches, chisels, hoes, gingival margin trimmers)			3		
10. Base, liner, varnish, and/or bonding agent			3		
11. Paper pad, cement spatula, and placement instrument			3		

	Self-Evaluation	Student Evaluation	Possible Points	Instructor Evaluation	Comments
12. Matrix retainer, matrix bands, and wedges			3		
13. Locking pliers or hemostat			2		
14. Amalgam capsules			3		
15. Amalgam well			2		
16. Amalgam carrier and condensers			3		
17. Amalgamator			3		
18. Carving instruments			3		
19. Articulating paper and forceps			3		
Competency Steps (*follow aseptic procedures*) 1. Greet and prepare the patient for the procedure.			3		
2. Review the patient's medical history.			3		
Anesthetic 1. Prepare topical for the local anesthetic.			2		
2. Dry the injection site and apply topical anesthetic (Expanded Function [EF]).			3		
3. Prepare a syringe and summon the dentist.			2		
4. Transfer the mirror and explorer to the dentist (examine the tooth before beginning the procedure).			3		
5. When the dentist is ready, transfer a 2 × 2 gauze in one hand, and a syringe in the other.			3		
6. The dentist replaces the needle cap and places the syringe on the tray.			3		
7. Rinse and evacuate the patient's mouth (after the injection).			3		

	Self-Evaluation	Student Evaluation	Possible Points	Instructor Evaluation	Comments
Dental Dam Placement					
8. Place the dental dam (EF) (see next step for alternative).			3		
9. Alternatively (see Step 8), prepare rubber dam materials and equipment, and assist the dentist in their placement.			3		
Cavity Preparation					
1. Transfer a mouth mirror and high-speed handpiece with a bur.			3		
2. Position the HVE tip and maintain visibility throughout the procedure.			3		
3. Maintain cheek and tongue retraction.			3		
4. Keep the mirror clear with an air-water syringe while evacuating the site.			3		
5. Transfer and receive instruments at the dentist's signals (such as an explorer, an excavator, hatches, hoes, angle formers, gingival margin trimmers, and chisels).			3		
Cavity Liner and Cement Base Placement (EF)					
1. When the preparation is finished, transfer a cotton pellet for cavity cleaning inside the preparation.			3		
2. Rinse and dry the area.			3		
3. At the dentist's direction, mix the cavity liner.			3		
4. Prepare the varnish.			2		
5. Prepare the base.			3		
6. Transfer the varnish and base to the dentist for placement. (Includes glass ionomer, polycarboxylate, zinc phosphate, modified ZOE, and bonding agent if used.)			3		

	Self-Evaluation	Student Evaluation	Possible Points	Instructor Evaluation	Comments
7. Light-cured materials: a. Hold the light tip near the material. b. Hold the protective shield. c. Activate the light to cure the material.			3 3 3		
Placement of Matrix and Wedge (EF) 1. Assemble matrix retainer and band (correct position for tooth being restored).			3		
2. Transfer the assembled matrix and band to the dentist.			3		
3. After the matrix is placed, transfer a wedge in cotton pliers or a hemostat.			3		
4. The dentist places the wedge.			3		
Amalgam Placement 1. Prepare an amalgam capsule when the dentist is ready (twist the cap, squeeze the capsule together, or place it in the activator and then place it in the amalgamator).			3		
2. Set the amalgamator for the type of amalgam and size of mix.			3		
3. Mix the amalgam material.			3		
4. Remove the capsule from the amalgamator and place the amalgam in the well or dappen dish.			3		
5. Load amalgam into the carrier (when double-ended, load both ends).			3		
6. Transfer the loaded carrier to the dentist.			3		
7. Alternately exchange carrier and condenser (in some offices, the assistant loads the carrier and places the amalgam as the dentist directs).			3		

	Self-Evaluation	Student Evaluation	Possible Points	Instructor Evaluation	Comments
8. After the last exchange, transfer the explorer (the amalgam is loosened from the matrix band).			3		
9. Clean up scrap amalgam from the carrier and well and place the debris in a sealed container.			3		
Remove Matrix and Carve Restoration 1. Receive the explorer and transfer carving and finishing instruments at the dentist's signals. Operate the HVE tip near the site to evacuate any amalgam particles.			3		
2. After the dentist completes the preliminary carving, transfer cotton pliers to remove the wedge.			3		
3. Receive the pliers and matrix retainer.			3		
4. Cotton pliers may be used again to remove the band.			3		
5. Receive the cotton pliers and band and transfer the carver.			3		
Dental Dam Removal (EF) (The rubber dam is carefully removed at this time.) 1. Transfer clamp forceps.			3		
2. Receive the forceps with a clamp.			3		
3. Transfer scissors (cut the interseptal dam).			3		
4. Receive scissors, frame, napkin, and dam material.			3		
5. Rinse and evacuate the patient's mouth.			3		

	Self-Evaluation	Student Evaluation	Possible Points	Instructor Evaluation	Comments
Evaluation of Patient's Bite					
1. Dry the area and transfer articulating paper (already assembled in forceps to transfer to the dentist).			3		
2. The dentist may instruct the assistant to place paper over the restoration.			2		
3. Instruct the patient to gently tap the teeth together.			2		
4. Additional carving may be continued until the dentist is satisfied that the patient is comfortable.			2		
Patient Dismissal					
1. Wipe off the restoration with a wet cotton roll (to remove any blue marks left by the articulating paper).			2		
2. Rinse and evacuate the patient's mouth thoroughly.			3		
3. Clean any debris from the patient's face.			2		
4. Caution the patient not to chew on the side of the restoration for a few hours.			3		
5. Dismiss the patient.			2		
TOTAL POINTS POSSIBLE			216		
TOTAL POINTS POSSIBLE—2nd attempt			214		
TOTAL POINTS EARNED			_____		

Points assigned reflect importance of step to meeting objective: Important = 1, Essential = 2, Critical = 3. Students will lose 2 points for repeated attempts. Failure results if any of the critical steps are omitted or performed incorrectly. If using a 100-point scale, determine score by dividing points earned by total points possible and multiplying the results by 100.

SCORE: _____

SKILL COMPETENCY ASSESSMENT

34-3 Composite Restoration—Class III

Student's Name _____ Date _____

Instructor's Name _____

Skill: The dental assistant is responsible for preparing the equipment and supplies. These direct restorative materials are inserted into the cavity preparation, and then self-cured, light cured, or dual cured. They are available in syringe or single-application cartridge (compule) forms, and a variety of shades or shade modifiers. The location and size of the cavity will determine the material the dentist chooses.

Performance Objective: The student will follow a routine procedure that meets the regulations and protocol set forth by the dentist and regulatory agencies, keeping in mind those assistant duties vary from state to state. The assistant may be evaluated by performance criteria, verbal/written responses, and/or combined responses and performance criteria. The dental assistant assists the dentist throughout the procedure.

	Self-Evaluation	Student Evaluation	Possible Points	Instructor Evaluation	Comments
Equipment and Supplies					
1. Basic setup: mouth mirror, explorer, cotton pliers			3		
2. Air-water syringe tip, HVE tip, and saliva ejector			3		
3. Cotton rolls, gauze sponges, cotton pellets, cotton-tip applicators, and floss			3		
4. Topical and local anesthetic setup			3		
5. Rubber dam setup			3		
6. High- and low-speed handpieces			3		
7. Assortment of dental burs (including diamond and cutting burs)			3		
8. Spoon excavator			2		
9. Hand cutting instruments (the dentist's choices may include binangle chisel and Wedelstaedt chisel.)			3		

	Self-Evaluation	Student Evaluation	Possible Points	Instructor Evaluation	Comments
10. Base and liner with mixing materials and placement instruments			3		
11. Bonding material; etchant and applicator, if necessary (usually comes with composite system)			3		
12. Primer (usually comes with composite system)			3		
13. Composite materials, including shade guide			3		
14. Composite placement instrument (plastic filling instrument)			3		
15. Curing light with protective shield			3		
16. Celluloid matrix strip and wedges			3		
17. Locking pliers or hemostat			3		
18. Finishing burs or diamonds			3		
19. # 12 scalpel (optional)			3		
20. Abrasive strips			3		
21. Polishing discs			3		
22. Lubricant			2		
23. Articulating paper and forceps			3		
Competency Steps (*follow aseptic procedures*) 1. Greet and prepare the patient for the procedure (the patient is seated).			3		
2. Review the patient's medical history.			3		

	Self-Evaluation	Student Evaluation	Possible Points	Instructor Evaluation	Comments
Anesthetic					
1. Prepare topical for the local anesthetic (have the patient rinse mouth).			3		
2. Dry the injection site and apply topical anesthetic (EF).			3		
3. Prepare the syringe and summon the dentist.			2		
4. Remove the topical anesthetic applicator, and transfer the mirror and explorer to the dentist.			3		
5. When the dentist is ready, receive the mirror and explorer, transfer the 2 × 2 gauze in one hand, and transfer the anesthetic syringe to the dentist in the other.			3		
6. The dentist replaces the needle cap and places the syringe on the tray.			3		
7. After the injection, rinse and evacuate the patient's mouth.			3		
Determine Shade					
1. Select the shade under natural light.			3		
2. A combination of shades may be selected.			3		
3. Record the shade selection on the patient's chart.			3		
Dental Dam Placement					
1. Place the dental dam or prepare the rubber dam materials and equipment for the dentist.			3		

	Self-Evaluation	Student Evaluation	Possible Points	Instructor Evaluation	Comments
Cavity Preparation					
1. Transfer a mouth mirror and high-speed handpiece with a bur.			3		
2. Position the HVE tip and maintain visibility throughout the procedure.			3		
3. Maintain cheek and tongue retraction.			3		
4. Keep the mirror clear with an air-water syringe while evacuating the site.			3		
5. At the dentist's signal, transfer and receive instruments, such as the explorer, excavator, binangle chisel, and Wedelstaedt chisel.			3		
6. Change the dentist's bur if directed to do so.			3		
Cavity Protection: Cavity Liner and Cement Base Placement (EF)					
1. When the preparation is finished, transfer a cotton pellet for cavity cleaning inside the preparation.			3		
2. Rinse and dry the area.			3		
3. At the dentist's direction, mix cavity liner (determined by the base and liner).			3		
4. Hold the mixing pad, applicator, and 2 × 2 gauze near the patient's chin (after each application, wipe the instrument).			3		
5. Transfer the items to the dentist for placement.			3		

	Self-Evaluation	Student Evaluation	Possible Points	Instructor Evaluation	Comments
6. Light-cured materials: a. Hold the light tip near the material. b. Hold the protective shield. c. Activate the light to cure the material.			3 3 3		
Application of Etchant 1. Transfer the brush or applicator tip containing acid etchant material to the dentist.			3		
2. Rinse etchant thoroughly after the recommended time.			3		
Matrix and Wedge 1. The dentist places the celluloid matrix strip.			2		
2. Transfer the matrix to the dentist.			2		
3. After the matrix is placed, transfer the wedge in cotton pliers or hemostat (use a plastic wedge, if needed).			3		
4. The dentist places the wedge.			3		
Placement of Bonding Material 1. Place the bonding material according to the manufacturer's directions.			3		
2. Place bonding resins—primer or conditioner (place before the bonding material).			3		
Placement of Composite 1. Prepare the chosen composite.			3		
2. Load a syringe with the color-selected material.			3		
3. Transfer the syringe to the dentist.			3		

	Self-Evaluation	Student Evaluation	Possible Points	Instructor Evaluation	Comments
4. Transfer the filling instrument.			3		
5. Place light-cured material in incremental layers.			3		
6. Within a few minutes, the material begins to set.			3		
Remove Matrix and Carve Restoration 1. Transfer cotton pliers to the dentist to remove the wedge and matrix strip.			3		
2. After receiving the wedge and matrix strip, transfer the explorer.			3		
Finishing and Polishing 1. Transfer the low-speed handpiece with finishing bur to the dentist.			3		
2. Use the air syringe while the dentist uses a handpiece.			3		
3. Change burs, finishing burs, diamonds, and abrasive disks as needed.			3		
4. If needed, use abrasive strips to smooth interproximal areas.			3		
5. To smooth, use polish points, disks, and cups.			3		
Dental Dam Removal (EF) 1. Transfer clamp forceps.			3		
2. Receive the forceps with a clamp.			3		
3. Transfer scissors for cutting the interseptal dam.			3		
4. Receive the scissors, frame, napkin, and dam material.			3		

	Self-Evaluation	Student Evaluation	Possible Points	Instructor Evaluation	Comments
5. Rinse and evacuate the patient's mouth.			3		
Evaluation of Patient's Bite 1. Dry the area and transfer articulating paper already assembled in the forceps.			3		
2. The dentist may instruct the assistant to place articulating paper over the restoration.			2		
3. Instruct the patient to tap the teeth together.			2		
4. Additional carving may be continued until the dentist is satisfied that the patient is comfortable.			2		
Dismiss Patient 1. Wipe off the restoration with a wet cotton roll (to remove any blue marks left by the articulating paper).			2		
2. Rinse and evacuate the patient's mouth thoroughly.			3		
3. Clean any debris from the patient's face.			2		
4. Give the patient postoperative instructions.			3		
5. Dismiss the patient.			2		

TOTAL POINTS POSSIBLE   244

TOTAL POINTS POSSIBLE—2nd attempt   242

TOTAL POINTS EARNED   _____

Points assigned reflect importance of step to meeting objective: Important = 1, Essential = 2, Critical = 3. Students will lose 2 points for repeated attempts. Failure results if any of the critical steps are omitted or performed incorrectly. If using a 100-point scale, determine score by dividing points earned by total points possible and multiplying the results by 100.

SCORE: _____

SKILL COMPETENCY ASSESSMENT

34-4 Placing and Removing Dental Dam

Student's Name _____ Date _____

Instructor's Name _____

Skill: Routine steps should be followed for all treatment areas to maintain absolute clinical asepsis. The dental assistant is responsible for preparing the equipment and supplies. There are many techniques for placing the dental dam. Through practice, the operator will find what works best for her or him.

Performance Objective: The student will follow a routine procedure that meets the regulations and protocol set forth by the dentist and regulatory agencies, keeping in mind that assistant duties vary from state to state. The assistant may be evaluated by performance criteria, verbal/written responses, and/or combined responses and performance criteria. This procedure is performed by the dentist or the dental assistant. The patient has been anesthetized before the placement of the dental dam and before the cavity preparation begins. Only the items for the dental dam are listed for this procedure.

	Self-Evaluation	Student Evaluation	Possible Points	Instructor Evaluation	Comments
Equipment and Supplies					
1. Dental dam material (6 × 6 sheets)			3		
2. Dental dam napkin			3		
3. Dental dam punch			3		
4. Assortment of clamps			3		
5. Dental dam forceps			3		
6. Dental dam frame			3		
7. Dental floss			3		
8. Lubricant			3		
9. Cotton-tip applicator			3		
10. Tucking instrument			3		
11. Scissors			3		
Competency Steps (*follow aseptic procedures*) **Placement of Dental Dam** 1. Inform the patient of the dental dam procedure.			3		

	Self-Evaluation	Student Evaluation	Possible Points	Instructor Evaluation	Comments
2. Examine the patient's oral cavity to determine the following: a. Anchor tooth b. Shape of arch c. Tooth alignment d. Missing teeth e. Presence of crowns or bridges f. Gingival tissue condition g. Tight contacts			3 3 3 3 2 3 3		
3. Prepare the dam material by dividing it into sixths, and punch the dam, carefully aligning the stylus and holes.			3		
4. Center the punch in the upper or lower middle third of the dam.			3		
5. Punch holes according to the size of the tooth. The largest key punch accommodates the anchor tooth and clamp.			3		
6. Punch holes following the pattern of the patient's arch. Lubricate the dental dam on the tissue side of the dam (water-soluble lubricant).			3		
7. Select one clamp or several to try on the tooth. (Selection: design—winged/wingless; mesiodistal width, faciolingual width— both at the CEJ of the anchor tooth; height of occlusal plane of anchor tooth.)			3		
8. Attach a safety line on all clamps to be tried.			3		
9. Secure the clamp on the forceps and spread the jaws slightly to lock the forceps.			3		

	Self-Evaluation	Student Evaluation	Possible Points	Instructor Evaluation	Comments
10. Place the clamp over the anchor tooth. (To widen the jaws, squeeze the forceps handle slightly to release the locking bar.)			3		
11. Fit the jaws of the clamp:					
a. Fit the lingual jaw of the clamp on the lingual side of the tooth first.			3		
b. Next, spread the clamp and slide the buccal jaws of the clamp over the height of the contour of the buccal surface of the tooth.			3		
c. Release pressure on the clamp forceps slightly against the tooth to evaluate the clamp, but do not release the clamp from the forceps.			3		
12. Place the clamp on the tooth:					
a. Point the jaw at the CEJ.			3		
b. Adapt the jaws to the gingival embrasures on the buccal and lingual.			3		
c. Secure the clamp.			3		
d. Pinch no gingival tissue.			3		
e. Confirm the patient's comfort.			3		
13. Place the dental dam over the clamp bow:					
a. Grasp the dam material with the index fingers on each side of the key punch hole.			3		
b. Spread the hole wide enough to slip over the clamp.			3		
c. Stretch the hole over the anchor tooth and to one side of the clamp.			3		
d. Expose the other clamp jaw—expose the entire clamp and tooth.			3		
e. Pull the safety line through the dam and drape to the side of the patient's mouth.			3		

	Self-Evaluation	Student Evaluation	Possible Points	Instructor Evaluation	Comments
14. Isolate the most forward tooth, usually opposite the canine, and secure the dam material on the distal of the tooth (with a double loop of floss, a corner cut of dam, or stabilizing cord).			3		
15. Place a dental napkin around the patient's mouth.			3		
16. Place a frame or holder to stretch the dam to cover the oral cavity. (Place the frame under or over the dental dam material depending on the type of frame and operator preference.)			3		
17. Isolate the remaining teeth: a. Work the dental dam gently between contacts. b. Use dental floss to place the dam and expose teeth. c. Use an air syringe to dry the teeth.			3 3 3		
18. Invert or tuck the dam material. (Edge of dam that surrounds tooth must be inverted or tucked into the sulcus of the gingival to seal the tooth and prevent leakage.)			3		
19. Coat all tooth-colored restorations with lubricant.			3		
20. Place and position the saliva ejector and/or bite-block under the dam for patient comfort as needed.			3		
21. Double-check the dam placement and patient comfort.			3		
Removal of Dental Dam When the operator is ready to remove the dental dam, the area is rinsed and dried using the evacuator and the three-way syringe. 1. Explain to the patient the procedure for removing the dental dam. Caution the patient not to bite down during removal.			3		

	Self-Evaluation	Student Evaluation	Possible Points	Instructor Evaluation	Comments
2. Free the interseptal dam with scissors, protecting the patient's lip. Use scissors to clip each septum.			3		
3. Remove the dental dam clamp (lift straight off the tooth).			3		
4. Remove the frame or holder of dam material.			3		
5. Remove the napkin, wiping the area around the mouth.			3		
6. Examine the dam material, spreading material out flat to make certain that all interseptal material is present. (Check for missing pieces, floss between the teeth, and dislodge the remaining dam.)			3		
7. Massage the gingiva around the anchor tooth.			3		
8. Rinse and evacuate patient's mouth thoroughly.			3		

TOTAL POINTS POSSIBLE   173

TOTAL POINTS POSSIBLE—2nd attempt   171

TOTAL POINTS EARNED   _____

Points assigned reflect importance of step to meeting objective: Important = 1, Essential = 2, Critical = 3. Students will lose 2 points for repeated attempts. Failure results if any of the critical steps are omitted or performed incorrectly. If using a 100-point scale, determine score by dividing points earned by total points possible and multiplying the results by 100.

SCORE: _____

SKILL COMPETENCY ASSESSMENT

34-5 Rubber Dam Application for Child Patient

Student's Name _____ Date _____

Instructor's Name _____

Skill: Routine steps should be followed for all treatment areas to maintain absolute clinical asepsis. The dental assistant is responsible for preparation of equipment and supplies. The dental dam is used on children as routinely as adults. The basic technique is the same for both adults and children; there are, however, several modifications. Among the many techniques for dental dam placement, with practice the operator will find what works best.

Performance Objective: The student will follow a routine procedure that meets the regulations and the protocol set forth by the dentist and regulatory agencies. The assistant may be evaluated by performance criteria, verbal/written responses, and/or combined responses and performance criteria. This procedure is performed by the dentist or the dental assistant. The patient's dentition must be evaluated to determine which teeth can be included in the isolation. Look for partially erupted teeth and loose teeth. Then quickly place the dental dam on the teeth directly involved in the procedure.

	Self-Evaluation	Student Evaluation	Possible Points	Instructor Evaluation	Comments
Equipment and Supplies					
1. Basic setup: mouth mirror, explorer, and cotton forceps			3		
2. Dark, heavy dental dam material (5 × 5 sheets)			3		
3. Dental dam napkin			3		
4. Dental dam punch			3		
5. Assortment of pedodontic clamps			3		
6. Dental dam clamp forcep			3		
7. Dental dam frame			3		
8. Dental floss			3		
9. Lubricant			3		
10. Cotton-tip applicator			3		
11. Tucking instrument (plastic instrument, T-ball, or spoon excavator)			3		
12. Scissors			3		

	Self-Evaluation	Student Evaluation	Possible Points	Instructor Evaluation	Comments
Competency Steps (*follow aseptic procedures*)					
1. Prepare child patient regarding dental dam procedure (at a level the child can understand).			3		
2. Examine patient's oral cavity to determine the following:					
a. Anchor tooth			3		
b. Shape and size of arch			3		
c. Tooth alignment			3		
d. Missing teeth and partially erupted teeth			3		
e. Loose teeth			3		
f. Condition of gingival tissue			2		
g. Tight contacts			3		
3. Prepare dam material by selecting heavy weight (5 × 5).			3		
4. Punch the predetermined dam pattern.			3		
5. Holes are punched according to size of tooth, closer than adults, the largest to accommodate anchor tooth and clamp (holes punched closer together).			3		
6. Select clamp: Winged clamps are best for retraction of heavy dam (selection: design— winged/wingless, mesio-distal width, faciolingual width—both at CEJ of anchor tooth, height of occlusal plane of anchor tooth).			3		
7. Attach safety line on all clamps to be tried.			3		
8. Secure clamp on forceps and spread jaws slightly to lock forceps.			3		
9. Place clamp over anchor tooth. (To widen jaws, squeeze forceps handle slightly to release locking bar.) *Note:* Often the clamp, dental dam, and frame are carried together (all in one) to be applied to the tooth.			3		

	Self-Evaluation	Student Evaluation	Possible Points	Instructor Evaluation	Comments
10. Fitting jaws of clamp: a. Fit lingual jaw of clamp on lingual side of tooth first. b. Next, slide buccal jaws of clamp over height of contour of buccal surface of tooth. c. Release pressure on clamp forceps slightly against the tooth to evaluate the clamp, but do not release clamp from the forceps.			3 3 3		
11. Clamp on tooth: a. Jaw points at CEJ. b. Jaws adapting to gingival embrasures buccal and lingual. c. Clamp secure. d. Clamp is not pinching any gingival tissue. e. Confirm comfort level with patient.			3 3 3 3 3		
12. Place dental dam over clamp bow: a. Grasp dam material with index fingers on each side of key punch hole. b. Spread hole wide enough to slip over clamp. c. Stretch hole over anchor tooth and on side of clamp. d. Expose other clamp jaw—entire clamp and tooth are exposed. e. Slide dam over wings of clamp to expose wings. f. Pull safety line through dam and drape to the side of patient's mouth (clamp/dental dam/frame are often carried all in one and applied).			3 3 3 3 3 3		
13. Isolate most forward tooth, usually opposite canine. Dam material is secured on distal of tooth (with double loop of floss, a corner cut of dam, stabilizing cord, or ligature of widget).			3		

	Self-Evaluation	Student Evaluation	Possible Points	Instructor Evaluation	Comments
14. Place dental napkin around patient's mouth.			3		
15. Place frame or holder to stretch dam to cover oral cavity. (Frame can be placed under or over dental dam material, depending on the type of frame and preference of operator).			3		
16. Isolate remaining teeth: a. Gently work dental dam between contacts. b. Dental floss used to place dam and expose teeth. c. Use air syringe to dry teeth.			3 3 3		
17. Invert or tuck dam material. (Edge of dam that surrounds tooth must be inverted or tucked into sulcus of gingiva to seal tooth and prevent leakage.)			3		
18. Ligatures of dental floss or ligature of stabilizing cord placed to secure dental dam in place (primary teeth).			3		

TOTAL POINTS POSSIBLE 146

TOTAL POINTS POSSIBLE—2nd attempt 144

TOTAL POINTS EARNED _____

Points assigned reflect importance of step to meeting objective important = 1, Essential = 2, Critical = 3. Students will lose 2 points for repeated attempts. Failure results if any of the critical steps are omitted or performed incorrectly. If using a 100-point scale, determine score by dividing points earned by total points possible and multiplying the results by 100.

SCORE: _____

SKILL COMPETENCY ASSESSMENT

34-6 Quickdam Placement

Student's Name _____ Date _____

Instructor's Name _____

Skill: Routine steps should be followed for all treatment areas to maintain absolute clinical asepsis. The dental assistant is responsible for preparation of equipment and supplies. There are many techniques and alternatives for placement of the dental dam, and the operator will find through practice what works best. One of these alternatives is the quickdam.

Performance Objective: The student will follow a routine procedure that meets the regulations and the protocol set forth by the dentist and regulatory agencies. The assistant may be evaluated by performance criteria, verbal/written responses, and/or combined responses and performance criteria. This procedure is performed by the dentist or the dental assistant. The patient is anesthetized and the quickdam is placed.

	Self-Evaluation	Student Evaluation	Possible Points	Instructor Evaluation	Comments
Equipment and Supplies					
1. Quickdam			3		
2. Quickdam template			3		
3. Dental dam punch			3		
4. Dental dam clamps			3		
5. Dental dam clamp forceps			3		
6. Dental floss			3		
7. Tucking instrument			3		
Competency Steps (*follow aseptic procedures*)					
1. Examine patient's oral cavity to determine:					
a. Anchor tooth			3		
b. Shape of arch			3		
c. Tooth alignment			3		
d. Missing teeth			3		
e. Presence of crowns or bridges			3		
f. Gingival tissue condition			2		
g. Tight contacts			3		

	Self-Evaluation	Student Evaluation	Possible Points	Instructor Evaluation	Comments
2. Prepare dam material. Use quickdam template and mark each tooth; allow for deviations (can be marked with felt-tip pen).			3		
3. Punch marked teeth to corresponding hold for each tooth.			3		
4. Quickdam placed with or without clamp.			3		
5. *Quickdam without a clamp:* a. Fold ends of quickdam toward each other and press sides together. b. Insert quickdam in patient's mouth and release sides. c. Quickdam fits into patient's vestibule. d. Slide dam over teeth to be isolated. e. Use dental floss to tuck dental dam. f. Secure dam with floss ligatures on distal of last isolated tooth.			3 3 3 3 3 3		
6. *Quickdam with a clamp:* a. Select a clamp to try on tooth. b. Attach safety line on all clamps to be tried. c. Place clamp in dam (one step). d. Apply clamp forceps to clamp and place over tooth. e. Once clamp is secure on tooth, remove clamp forcep. f. Place dam over teeth to be isolated. g. Tuck dam.			3 3 3 3 3 3 3		

TOTAL POINTS POSSIBLE   89

TOTAL POINTS POSSIBLE—2nd attempt   87

TOTAL POINTS EARNED   _____

Points assigned reflect importance of step to meeting objective: Important = 1, Essential = 2, Critical = 3. Students will lose 2 points for repeated attempts. Failure results if any of the critical steps are omitted or performed incorrectly. If using a 100-point scale, determine score by dividing points earned by total points possible and multiplying the results by 100.

SCORE: _____

SKILL COMPETENCY ASSESSMENT

34-7 Assembly of Tofflemire Matrix

Student's Name _____ Date _____

Instructor's Name _____

Skill: Routine steps should be followed for all treatment areas to maintain absolute clinical asepsis. The dental assistant is responsible for preparing the equipment and supplies. During the preparation of a tooth for an amalgam or a composite restoration, often one or more axial surfaces will be removed. A matrix replaces the surface and acts as an artificial wall. The Tofflemire matrix, which consists of retainer and band, is the most common one used for amalgam restorations.

Performance Objective: The student will follow a routine procedure that meets the regulations and protocol set forth by the dentist and regulatory agencies, keeping in mind that assistant duties vary from state to state. The assistant may be evaluated by performance criteria, verbal/written responses, and/or combined responses and performance criteria. This procedure is performed by the dentist or the dental assistant. The assembly can be completed before the procedure begins so that it is ready when needed. Equipment and supplies listed are for the assembly of the Tofflemire matrix.

	Self-Evaluation	Student Evaluation	Possible Points	Instructor Evaluation	Comments
Equipment and Supplies					
1. Tofflemire retainer			3		
2. Assortment of matrix bands			3		
Competency Steps (*follow aseptic procedures*)					
1. Hold the retainer so that the guide channels and diagonal slot on the vise are facing the operator.			3		
2. Holding the frame of the retainer, rotate the inner knob until the vise is within one-quarter inch of the guide channels.			3		
3. Turn the outer knob until the pointed end of the spindle is clear of the slot in the vise.			3		

	Self-Evaluation	Student Evaluation	Possible Points	Instructor Evaluation	Comments
4. Prepare the matrix band for placement in the retainer, holding the band (like a smile) with gingival edge on top and occlusal edge on bottom.			3		
5. Bring the ends together to form a teardrop-shaped loop. (Do not crease; place the larger circumference of the band, the occlusal, on the bottom, and the smaller, the gingival, on top.)			3		
6. With the gingival edge still on top, place the occlusal edge of the band in the diagonal slot of the vise. The loop will extend toward the guide channels.			3		
7. Place the matrix band into the appropriate guide channels. The direction of the matrix band depends on the tooth being restored. *Hold the matrix retainer with the guide channel up, facing the operator, and the matrix band looped. Then take the following steps:* a. In the maxillary right/ mandibular left quadrant, place the matrix in the guide channels, toward the operator's right. b. In the maxillary left/ mandibular right quadrant, place the matrix in the guide channels toward the operator's left.			3 3 3		

	Self-Evaluation	Student Evaluation	Possible Points	Instructor Evaluation	Comments
8. Once the band is placed in the slot with the guide channels, turn the outer knob until the tip of the spindle is tight against the band in the vise slot.			3		
9. Move the inner knob to increase or decrease the size of the loop to match the tooth diameter.			3		
10. Smooth the band, eliminating creasing (use handle of mouth mirror, similar to curling ribbon).			3		

TOTAL POINTS POSSIBLE   42

TOTAL POINTS POSSIBLE—2nd attempt   40

TOTAL POINTS EARNED   ____

Points assigned reflect importance of step to meeting objective: Important = 1, Essential = 2, Critical = 3. Students will lose 2 points for repeated attempts. Failure results if any of the critical steps are omitted or performed incorrectly. If using a 100-point scale, determine score by dividing points earned by total points possible and multiplying the results by 100.

SCORE: _____

SKILL COMPETENCY ASSESSMENT

34-8 Placement of Tofflemire Matrix

Student's Name _____ Date _____

Instructor's Name _____

Skill: Routine steps should be followed for all treatment areas to maintain absolute clinical asepsis. The dental assistant is responsible for preparing the equipment and supplies. During the preparation of a tooth for an amalgam or composite restoration, often one or more axial surfaces will be removed. A matrix replaces the surface and acts as an artificial wall. The Tofflemire matrix, which consists of retainer and band, is the most common one used for amalgam restorations.

Performance Objective: The student will follow a routine procedure that meets the regulations and protocol set forth by the dentist and regulatory agencies. The assistant may be evaluated by performance criteria, verbal/written responses, and/or combined responses and performance criteria. This procedure is performed by the dentist or the dental assistant. After the Tofflemire matrix is assembled, it is ready for positioning on the prepared tooth.

	Self-Evaluation	Student Evaluation	Possible Points	Instructor Evaluation	Comments
Equipment and Supplies 1. Assembled Tofflemire retainer and matrix band			3		
2. Cotton pliers or hemostat			3		
3. Ball burnisher			3		
4. 2 × 2 gauze sponges			3		
5. Assortment of wedges			3		
Competency Steps (*follow aseptic procedures*) 1. Place matrix retainer over prepared tooth. a. Place the smaller edge of the band toward the gingiva. b. Place the slot on the vise directed toward the gingiva. c. Keep the retainer parallel to the buccal as the loop is placed around the tooth.			3 3 3		
2. Move the loop through the interproximal surface. Place one finger over loop to stabilize the loop and retainer.			3		

	Self-Evaluation	Student Evaluation	Possible Points	Instructor Evaluation	Comments
3. Place the matrix around the tooth, adjusting the guide channel to center the retainer on the buccal surface of the tooth.			3		
4. Turn the inner knob to tighten the band around the tooth. a. Secure the band around the tooth. b. The retainer should be snug to the tooth. c. When the band is too tight or too loose, the contours of the restoration may change proximal contact.			3 3 3		
5. Check band margins. a. Margins should not extend more than 1.0 to 1.5 mm beyond the gingiva of the cavity preparation edge. b. The occlusal should not extend more than 2.0 mm above highest cusp.			3 3		
6. Contour the band to the adjacent tooth. a. Use a ball burnisher. b. Apply the burnisher to the inner surface of the band, applying pressure until the band becomes slightly concave at the contact area.			3 3		
7. Place the matrix band on the tooth and place wedge(s).			3		
8. Check the seal at the gingival margin of the preparation with the explorer. (There should be no gap between the band and the preparation.)			3		
TOTAL POINTS POSSIBLE			60		
TOTAL POINTS POSSIBLE—2nd attempt			58		
TOTAL POINTS EARNED			____		

Points assigned reflect importance of step to meeting objective: Important = 1, Essential = 2, Critical = 3. Students will lose 2 points for repeated attempts. Failure results if any of the critical steps are omitted or performed incorrectly. If using a 100-point scale, determine score by dividing points earned by total points possible and multiplying the results by 100.

SCORE: _____

SKILL COMPETENCY ASSESSMENT

34-9 Removal of Wedge and Tofflemire Matrix

Student's Name _____ Date _____

Instructor's Name _____

Skill: Routine steps should be followed for all treatment areas to maintain absolute clinical asepsis. The dental assistant is responsible for preparing the equipment and supplies. During the preparation of a tooth amalgam or a composite restoration, often one or more axial surfaces will be removed. A matrix replaces the surface and the artificial wall. The Tofflemire matrix, which consists of retainer and band, is the most common matrix for amalgam restorations.

Performance Objective: The student will follow a routine procedure that meets the regulations and protocol set forth by the dentist and regulatory agencies. The assistant may be evaluated by performance criteria, verbal/written responses, and/or combined responses and performance criteria. This procedure is performed by the dentist or the dental assistant. Once the tooth has been filled with restorative material, the matrix and wedge are removed to finish carving the anatomy of the tooth.

	Self-Evaluation	Student Evaluation	Possible Points	Instructor Evaluation	Comments
Equipment and Supplies					
1. Cotton pliers or hemostat			3		
2. 2 × 2 gauze sponges			3		
Competency Steps					
1. Remove the wedge.					
a. Use cotton pliers or hemostat.			3		
b. Grasp the wedge at the base.			3		
c. Pull in the opposite direction of insertion.			3		
2. Remove the retainer.					
a. Hold the matrix in place with a finger at the occlusal surface.			3		
b. Turn the outer knob of the retainer to loosen the spindle in the vise.			3		
3. Separate the retainer from the band, and lift the retainer toward the occlusal surface of the tooth.			3		

	Self-Evaluation	Student Evaluation	Possible Points	Instructor Evaluation	Comments

4. Use cotton pliers.
  a. Gently free the band from the tooth.
  b. Lift one end of the band in the lingual occlusal direction.
			3
			
			3		

5. Lift the band from the proximal surface and repeat with the other end of the band.			3		
6. The tooth is ready for final carving.			3		

TOTAL POINTS POSSIBLE	36	
TOTAL POINTS POSSIBLE—2nd attempt	34	
TOTAL POINTS EARNED	____	

Points assigned reflect importance of step to meeting objective: Important = 1, Essential = 2, Critical = 3. Students will lose 2 points for repeated attempts. Failure results if any of the critical steps are omitted or performed incorrectly. If using a 100-point scale, determine score by dividing points earned by total points possible and multiplying the results by 100.

SCORE: _____

SKILL COMPETENCY ASSESSMENT

34-10 Placement of Strip Matrix

Student's Name _____ Date _____

Instructor's Name _____

Skill: Routine steps should be followed for all treatment areas to maintain absolute clinical asepsis. The dental assistant is responsible for preparation of equipment and supplies. During the preparation of a tooth for an amalgam or composite restoration, often one or more axial surfaces will be removed. A matrix replaces the surface and acts as an artificial wall. The plastic strip matrix is used on anterior teeth with composite, glass ionomer, or compomer restorative materials. The strip can be made of nylon, acetate, celluloid, or resin, and is approximately 3 inches long and 3/8 inch wide.

Performance Objective: The student will follow a routine procedure that meets the regulations and protocol set forth by the dentist and regulatory agencies. The assistant may be evaluated by performance criteria, verbal/written responses, and/or combined responses and performance criteria. This procedure is performed by the dentist or the dental assistant. After the tooth has been prepared, the strip matrix is placed.

	Self-Evaluation	Student Evaluation	Possible Points	Instructor Evaluation	Comments
Equipment and Supplies					
1. Strip matrix			3		
2. Cotton pliers			3		
3. Mouth mirror			3		
4. Assortment of clear wedges			3		
Competency Steps (*follow aseptic procedures*)					
1. Contour strip, draw strip over mirror handle. (Like the Tofflemire matrix, band is contoured.)			3		
2. Place strip matrix between teeth, hold strip tightly, and slide toward gingiva.			3		
3. Adjust strip (entire preparation is covered by strip).			3		
4. Seat wedge to secure strip in place.			3		

	Self-Evaluation	Student Evaluation	Possible Points	Instructor Evaluation	Comments
5. With restorative materials in place, pull the strip matrix tightly around the tooth to adapt the material to the convex surface of the tooth.			3		
6. Hold the strip matrix in place by hand or with a clip retainer until material has been cured.			3		

TOTAL POINTS POSSIBLE   30

TOTAL POINTS POSSIBLE—2nd attempt   28

TOTAL POINTS EARNED   _____

Points assigned reflect importance of step to meeting objective: Important = 1, Essential = 2, Critical = 3. Students will lose 2 points for repeated attempts. Failure results if any of the critical steps are omitted or performed incorrectly. If using a 100-point scale, determine score by dividing points earned by total points possible and multiplying the results by 100.

SCORE: _____

SKILL COMPETENCY ASSESSMENT

34-11 Removal of Strip Matrix

Student's Name _____ Date _____

Instructor's Name _____

Skill: Routine steps should be followed for all treatment areas to maintain absolute clinical asepsis. The dental assistant is responsible for preparing the equipment and supplies. During the preparation of a tooth for an amalgam or composite restoration, often one or more axial surfaces will be removed. A matrix replaces the surface and acts as an artificial wall. The plastic strip matrix is used on anterior teeth with composite, glass ionomer, or compomer restorative materials. The strip can be made of nylon, acetate, celluloid, or resin, and is approximately 3 inches long and 3/8 inch wide.

Performance Objective: The student will follow a routine procedure that meets the regulations and protocol set forth by the dentist and regulatory agencies. The assistant may be evaluated by performance criteria, verbal/written responses, and/or combined responses and performance criteria. This procedure is performed by the dentist once the restorative material is placed and cured.

	Self-Evaluation	Student Evaluation	Possible Points	Instructor Evaluation	Comments
Equipment and Supplies 1. Cotton pliers			3		
2. 2 × 2 gauze sponges			3		
Competency Steps (*follow aseptic procedures*) 1. Once material has been cured, remove clip retainer, and remove wedge if one was used. Remove with cotton pliers (material is completely hardened).			3		
2. Gently strip the matrix away from the restorative material.			3		

	Self-Evaluation	Student Evaluation	Possible Points	Instructor Evaluation	Comments
3. Remove the strip by pulling the matrix strip in the lingual incisal or facial incisal direction.			3		

TOTAL POINTS POSSIBLE   15

TOTAL POINTS POSSIBLE—2nd attempt   13

TOTAL POINTS EARNED   ____

Points assigned reflect importance of step to meeting objective: Important = 1, Essential = 2, Critical = 3. Students will lose 2 points for repeated attempts. Failure results if any of the critical steps are omitted or performed incorrectly. If using a 100-point scale, determine score by dividing points earned by total points possible and multiplying the results by 100.

SCORE: _____

CHAPTER 35

Laboratory Materials and Techniques

SPECIFIC INSTRUCTIONAL OBJECTIVES

The student should strive to meet the following objectives and demonstrate an understanding of the facts and principles presented in this chapter:

1. Identify materials used in the dental laboratory and perform associated procedures.

2. Demonstrate the knowledge and skills needed to prepare, take, and remove alginate impressions and wax bites.

3. Demonstrate the knowledge and skills necessary to prepare reversible hydrocolloid impression material for the dentist.

4. Demonstrate the knowledge and skills necessary to prepare elastomeric impression materials such as polysulfide, silicone (polysiloxane and polyvinyl siloxanes), and polyether for the dentist.

5. Demonstrate the knowledge and skills necessary to use gypsum products such as Type I, impression plaster; Type II, laboratory or model plaster; Type III, laboratory stone; Type IV, die stone; and Type V, high-strength die stone.

6. Demonstrate the knowledge and skills necessary to pour and trim a patient's alginate impression (diagnostic cast).

7. Identify use of a dental articulator and facebow for dental casts or study models.

8. Demonstrate taking a facebow transfer and mounting models on an articulator.

9. Identify various classifications and uses of waxes used in dentistry.

10. Demonstrate the knowledge and skills necessary to fabricate acrylic tray resin self-curing and light-curing custom trays, vacuum-formed trays, and thermoplastic custom trays.

11. Demonstrate the knowledge and skills necessary to contour prefabricated temporary crowns and to fabricate and fit custom temporary restorations.

12. Gain an understanding of computer-aided design (CAD) equipment and computer-aided manufacturing (CAM) systems and how they are used in the dental office.

SUMMARY

A number of basic functions in the dental laboratory are routinely performed by the dental assistant, such as pouring and trimming study models, fabricating custom trays, and fabricating provisional temporaries. Many newer technologies are completed by dental assistants today such as mounting models on the articulator, taking digital impressions, and designing and fabricating crowns through computer-aided manufacturing. To accomplish these procedures, the dental assistant must understand the materials that are used, the properties of each material, the steps in each procedure, and seek ongoing education and training on new technologies introduced in the field. Any dental assistant who has skills in performing laboratory duties will be an asset to his or her employer. The better crossed-trained the dental team members are, the better the dental office functions.

EXERCISES AND ACTIVITIES

Multiple Choice

1. Alginate impressions make a _____ mold.

   a. negative
   b. positive
   c. sol
   d. agar-agar

2. Alginate is a generic name used for a group of _____ impression materials.

   a. reversible hydrocolloid
   b. irreversible hydrocolloid
   c. polysulfide
   d. gypsum

3. The disadvantages of alginates primarily derive from the loss of accuracy due to atmospheric conditions. If an impression loses water content due to heat, dryness, or exposure to air, shrinkage occurs, a condition known as

   a. imbibition.
   b. exothermic reaction.
   c. polymerization.
   d. syneresis.

4. If an impression takes on additional water that causes swelling, the impression will have a dimensional enlargement that is known as

   a. calcination.
   b. syneresis.
   c. imbibition.
   d. exothermic reaction.

5. All the elastomeric impression materials have a catalyst and base that are mixed to start the chemical self-curing process. The process by which the catalyst and accelerator begin to cure is called (an)

   a. exothermic reaction.
   b. polymerization.
   c. distortion.
   d. calcination.

6. The elastomeric impression materials have a rubber-like quality and are used for areas that require precise duplication. _____ is a dimensional change in shape.

   a. Imbibition

   b. Distortion

   c. Calcination

   d. Syneresis

7. To start the chemical self-curing process, a _____ and base are mixed.

   a. gel

   b. sol

   c. resin

   d. catalyst

8. Which of the following is not an elastomeric impression material?

   a. Silicone

   b. Agar-agar

   c. Polyether

   d. Polysulfide

9. Of the primary types of gypsum used in dentistry, which type is for model or laboratory plaster?

   a. Type I

   b. Type II

   c. Type III

   d. Type IV

10. _____ is an elastomeric impression material that is available in putty form and is used for making a custom tray.

    a. Silicone

    b. Polyether

    c. Polysulfide

    d. Methacrylate

11. The strengths of gypsum products are determined by the _____ process and the water/powder ratio needed to incorporate the mixture.

    a. thermoplastic

    b. exothermic

    c. polymerization

    d. calcination

12. A(n) _____ holds models of the patient's teeth to maintain the patient's occlusion and represent the patient's jaws.

    a. articulator

    b. vacuum former

    c. conditioner

    d. extruder

13. Utility wax is used to bead around trays to extend them. Under which of the following groups of waxes would utility wax be classified?

    a. Impression

    b. Processing

    c. Pattern

    d. Other

14. The most common material used to make custom trays is self-curing acrylic tray resin. The liquid catalyst that mixes with the powder is called the

    a. polymer.

    b. base.

    c. monomer.

    d. sol.

15. The self-curing acrylic material goes through several stages of curing. During one of the stages, the material goes through a(n) _____ reaction, giving off a great deal of heat while setting.

    a. initial set

    b. exothermic

    c. kneaded

    d. thermoplastic

16. _____ are recessed areas in a model that make it impossible to seat or remove a custom tray properly.

    a. Spacers

    b. Undercuts

    c. Matrices

    d. Stops

17. Which term means that a material becomes soft and pliable when exposed to heat?

    a. Exothermic
    b. Thermoplastic

    c. Imbibition
    d. Syneresis

18. A material that is mixed uniformly is called

    a. homogenous.
    b. exothermic.

    c. irreversible.
    d. thermoplastic.

19. Which of the following are advantages of using reversible hydrocolloid?

    1. More accurate than alginate
    2. Comparatively economical after initial equipment purchase
    3. Can be used for impressions for crown and bridge construction
    4. Less equipment needed
    5. Less setting time required
    6. Not affected by atmospheric conditions
       a. 1, 4, 5
       b. 1, 2, 6

       c. 1, 2, 3
       d. 2, 3, 4

20. Which of the following equipment and supplies would indicate the taking of a polysulfide impression?

    1. Custom tray painted with adhesive
    2. Water measure
    3. Glass slab
    4. Two pastes, base and catalyst
    5. Rubber bowl
    6. Rigid laboratory spatulas
       a. 2, 3, 5
       b. 2, 3, 6

       c. 1, 4, 6
       d. 1, 2, 3

21. The CAD/CAM system that uses the Blue light LED camera to obtain the virtual impression is:

    a. Cerec.
    b. iTero.

    c. LAVA COS.
    d. E4D.

22. Placing wax around the border of the impression tray is called the _____ process.

    a. beading
    b. sol

    c. gel
    d. pattern

23. The _____ is the ingredient that accelerates or starts the process of setting the impression material.

    a. catalyst
    b. base

    c. monomer
    d. polymer

24. _____ can be used to study malocclusion, to wax and carve teeth for crowns and bridges, and demonstrate to the patient the action that is of concern.

    a. Matrices
    b. Articulators

    c. Thermoplastic
    d. Polymerization

25. _____ wax is used to bead around trays to extend those trays.

    a. Utility
    b. Pattern

    c. Inlay
    d. Sticky

26. The _____ matrix uses alginate, impression material, and the freehand (block) technique.

   a. indirect

   b. direct

   c. thermo-forming

   d. vacuum-formed

27. The _____ matrix utilizes wax and is made on the model or cast.

   a. indirect

   b. direct

   c. impression material

   d. freehand block technique

28. The custom acrylic or composite temporary restoration must have

   a. good proximal contacts.

   b. good occlusal contacts.

   c. good marginal contours.

   d. All of the above

29. What equipment is used to duplicate the function of the temporomandibular joint?

   a. Facebow and articulator

   b. Study model and bite rims

   c. Custom tray and articulator

   d. Study model and custom tray

30. Which imaging technology is now allowing dental offices to create crowns, bridges, and veneers in the office without the need to send then out to a lab for construction?

   a. Panoramic systems

   b. Cephalometric systems

   c. Magnetic resonance imaging systems

   d. CAD/CAM systems

✗ Critical Thinking

1. The dentist has explained to the patient the need to wear a temporary restoration. The dentist directs the dental assistant to make a provisional restoration. Explain what the terms *provisional/temporary* mean and state the criteria for temporaries.

2. The dentist selected a self-cured acrylic resin custom tray for patient Charles. The dental assistant will make the tray for a crown impression. Describe the *stops* that will be a part of the tray.

3. The dental assistant may perform the task of mounting models and/or assisting the dentist. It will be important to demonstrate the knowledge and skills required to mount bases and models. Explain articulating casts and their uses.

4. Study models are used as an important teaching tool to educate the patient. They are also an integral part of the case presentation and treatment plan for the patient. List the evaluation criteria of trimmed diagnostic casts (study models).

CASE STUDY 1

Jack is a patient having a first molar prepared for a crown; the molar is the largest tooth in the mouth, and Jack's molar is no understatement. The dentist has directed the dental assistant to fabricate and place the temporary restoration for Jack.

1. List types of temporaries.

2. Explain custom temporaries.

3. Describe the direct matrix technique.

4. Describe the indirect matrix technique.

CASE STUDY 2

Rudy is a robust patient. The dental trays at try-in for the alginate impressions were barely large enough. Rudy was going to need a custom tray. The dentist will need the most accurate impression for his final impression of the premolar crown.

1. Explain how the need for a custom tray is determined.

2. Describe the benefit of a custom tray.

3. List criteria for custom trays.

4. List types of trays.

CASE STUDY 3

A patient is being seen for the first time in the dental office. As part of the examination, a study cast is required to document records and be a part of the treatment record. The dental assistant will make the study cast or primary model. The dental assistant must be accurate in taking the impression, taking materials from the treatment room to the dental laboratory, and preventing any cross-contamination.

1. Explain alginate material and what it may also be called.

2. Explain when alginate is used.

3. Describe the most common areas in which alginate is used.

4. List the purposes for which the alginate impression material is routinely used.

SKILL COMPETENCY ASSESSMENT

35-1 Mixing Alginate with Alginator II Mixing Device

Student's Name _____ Date _____

Instructor's Name _____

Skill: The dental assistant is responsible for preparation of equipment and supplies. Alginate is a generic name used for a group of irreversible hydrocolloid impression materials. Alginate is commonly used in making diagnostic casts or study models. In some states, dental assistants are allowed to take alginate impressions; in other states they can select the tray, mix the material, load the material into the tray, and transfer the tray for the dentist to place in the patient's mouth.

Performance Objective: The student will follow a routine procedure that meets the regulations and protocol set forth by the dentist and regulatory agencies. The assistant may be evaluated by performance criteria, verbal/written responses, and/or combined responses and performance criteria. This procedure is performed by the dental assistant in states where it is allowed. The materials are prepared and the Alginator II mixing device is prepared and ready.

	Self-Evaluation	Student Evaluation	Possible Points	Instructor Evaluation	Comments
Equipment and Supplies 1. Flexible spatula/broad blade or disposable spatula			**3**		
2. Flexible rubber bowl(s) or Alginator II flexible bowl only			3		
3. Alginate material with water and powder measuring devices			3		
4. Water			3		
Competency Steps (*follow aseptic procedures*) 1. Impression water (room temperature) is measured (normally two calibrations are recommended by manufacturer).			3		
2. Water is placed in the attached rubber bowl of the Alginator II.			3		
3. Alginator bowl is attached by rotating it slightly to the side—fits into grooves on bottom of bowl.			3		
4. Fluff the powder prior to opening if recommended by manufacturer.			3		

	Self-Evaluation	Student Evaluation	Possible Points	Instructor Evaluation	Comments
5. Fill measure of powder by over-filling and then level off (use flat blade, not edge of spatula). Dispense two corresponding scoops in rubber bowl/water.			3		
6. Lightly incorporate the mixture.			2		
7. Using light pressure, hold spatula to side of bowl. Turn on Alginator II; as the bowl rotates it mixes the material.			3		
8. Side of blade/spatula is used during this process (bowl rotates 300 times a minute).			2		
9. When the material is completely mixed, it can be gathered up easily, using the edge of spatula starting from the deepest area within the bowl. (Material is gathered with few bubbles if any.)			3		
10. Upon completion material should be homogenous and smooth without bubbles.			3		
11. Bowls can be wiped out with paper towels and cleaned thoroughly, and then disinfected along with edges of impression tray.			3		

TOTAL POINTS POSSIBLE   43

TOTAL POINTS POSSIBLE—2nd attempt   41

TOTAL POINTS EARNED   ____

Points assigned reflect importance of step to meeting objective: Important = 1, Essential = 2, Critical = 3. Students will lose 2 points for repeated attempts. Failure results if any of the critical steps are omitted or performed incorrectly. If using a 100-point scale, determine score by dividing points earned by total points possible and multiplying the results by 100.

SCORE: _____

SKILL COMPETENCY ASSESSMENT

35-2 Preparing for Alginate Impression

Student's Name _____ Date _____

Instructor's Name _____

Skill: The dental assistant is responsible for preparing the equipment and supplies. Alginate is a generic name used for a group of irreversible hydrocolloid impression materials. Alginate is commonly used in making diagnostic casts or study models. In some states, dental assistants are allowed to take the alginate impressions; in other states, the assistant can select the tray, mix the material, load the material into the tray, and transfer the tray for the dentist to place in the patient's mouth.

Performance Objective: The student will follow a routine procedure that meets the regulations and protocol set forth by the dentist and regulatory agencies, keeping in mind that assistant duties vary from state to state. The assistant may be evaluated by performance criteria, verbal/written responses, and/or combined responses and performance criteria. This procedure is performed by the dental assistant in states where it is allowed. The materials are prepared, and the alginate impression is taken on the maxillary and mandibular arches.

	Self-Evaluation	Student Evaluation	Possible Points	Instructor Evaluation	Comments
Equipment and Supplies					
1. Flexible spatula/broad blade or disposable spatula			3		
2. Flexible rubber bowl(s) or disposable bowl			3		
3. Alginate material with water and powder measuring devices			3		
4. Water			3		
5. Impression tray(s)			3		
6. Beading wax			1		
Competency Steps (*follow aseptic procedures*)					
Patient Preparation					
1. Review the patient's health history.			3		
2. Seat the patient upright with a protective napkin in place.			3		
3. Rinse the patient's mouth with water or mouth rinse (to remove food debris and aid with thick saliva).			3		

	Self-Evaluation	Student Evaluation	Possible Points	Instructor Evaluation	Comments
4. Explain the procedure to the patient.			3		
5. Try impression trays in the oral cavity to determine correct size.			3		
Material Preparation 1. Place wax around the borders of the impression trays, if necessary (extend the borders of the tray for patient comfort).			3		
2. Measure impression water for a mandibular model (water, room temperature, two calibrations).			3		
3. First place water into a flexible mixing bowl.			3		
4. Fluff powder before opening the canister (follow manufacturer's directions as indicated).			3		
5. Fill the measure of powder by overfilling, and then level off with a spatula (accurate measure).			3		
6. Dispense two corresponding scoops into a second flexible rubber bowl.			3		
7. When ready, place the powder in the water.			3		
8. First mix the water and powder with a stirring motion.			3		
9. Then mix by holding the bowl in one hand, rotating the bowl occasionally, using the flat side of spatula to incorporate the material through pressure against the side of the bowl: mix Type I, fast set, 30 to 45 seconds, and mix Type II, regular set, one minute.			3		

	Self-Evaluation	Student Evaluation	Possible Points	Instructor Evaluation	Comments
10. Upon completion, the mixture should be homogeneous and creamy.			3		
11. Once the material is mixed correctly, load the tray. Mandibular: load both lingual sides, and use the flat side of the blade to condense the material firmly into the tray. If necessary to smooth the surface, use gloved hand to moisten and smooth the top.			3		

TOTAL POINTS POSSIBLE   64

TOTAL POINTS POSSIBLE—2nd attempt   62

TOTAL POINTS EARNED   ____

Points assigned reflect importance of step to meeting objective: Important = 1, Essential = 2, Critical = 3. Students will lose 2 points for repeated attempts. Failure results if any of the critical steps are omitted or performed incorrectly. If using a 100-point scale, determine score by dividing points earned by total points possible and multiplying the results by 100.

SCORE: _____

SKILL COMPETENCY ASSESSMENT

35-3 Taking Alginate Impression

Student's Name _____ Date _____

Instructor's Name _____

Skill: The dental assistant is responsible for preparing the equipment and supplies. Alginate is a generic name used for a group of irreversible hydrocolloid impression materials. Alginate is commonly used in making diagnostic casts or study models. In some states, dental assistants are allowed to take the alginate impressions; in other states, the assistant can select the tray, mix the material, load the material into the tray, and transfer the tray for the dentist to place in the patient's mouth.

Performance Objective: The student will follow a routine procedure that meets the regulations and protocol set forth by the dentist and regulatory agencies, keeping in mind that assistant duties vary from state to state. The assistant may be evaluated by performance criteria, verbal/written responses, and/or combined responses and performance criteria. This procedure is performed by the dental assistant in states where it is allowed. The materials are prepared and the alginate impression is taken on the maxillary and mandibular arches.

	Self-Evaluation	Student Evaluation	Possible Points	Instructor Evaluation	Comments
Equipment and Supplies					
1. Flexible spatula/broad blade or disposable spatula			3		
2. Flexible rubber bowl(s) or disposable bowl			3		
3. Alginate material with water and powder measuring devices			3		
4. Water			3		
5. Impression tray(s)			3		
6. Beading wax			1		
Competency Steps (*follow aseptic procedures*) **Mandibular Impression** 1. Facing the patient, slightly retract the right cheek.			3		
2. Use excess alginate material to rub onto the occlusal surfaces of teeth to obtain more accurate anatomy.			3		
3. Invert the impression tray so the material is toward the teeth.			3		

	Self-Evaluation	Student Evaluation	Possible Points	Instructor Evaluation	Comments
4. Turn the tray so that it passes through the lip opening, with one side of the tray entering first. Using the other hand, retract the opposite corner of the mouth.			3		
5. When the tray is completely in the patient's mouth, center it above the teeth.			3		
6. Lower the tray onto the teeth, placing the posterior area down first, leaving the impression tray slightly anterior.			3		
7. Have the patient raise the tongue and move it side to side to ensure that the lingual aspect of the alveolar process is defined in the impression.			3		
8. Pull out the lip from the center with the other hand.			3		
9. Finish placing impression tray down and, as this is done, push slightly toward the posterior area with the tray (while pushing impression material needed in anterior vestibule area). Observe that the lip is out of the way.			3		
10. Allow the lip to cover the tray. (Position the lip close to the handle portion of the tray.)			3		
11. Hold the tray in the patient's mouth with two fingers on the back of the tray, one on the right side, one on the left side, until set. The material should feel firm and not change shape when touched. (Check excess material to determine set at sides of bowl and edges of impression tray.)			3		

	Self-Evaluation	Student Evaluation	Possible Points	Instructor Evaluation	Comments
Maxillary Impression 12. Load maxillary alginate impression from the posterior. (Allows filling the tray without voids.)			3		
13. Take a small amount of alginate from the palate area. (Prevents impression material from going down the patient's throat after insertion.)			3		
14. Standing behind or to the side of the patient, place the maxillary tray in the patient's mouth. (Turn the tray so that it passes through the lip opening with one side of the tray entering first, using the other hand to retract the opposite corner of the mouth.)			3		
15. Raise the tray to the maxillary arch and hold out the lip before seating the tray in place.			3		
16. Hold the tray in position as in the mandibular until the material is set in the bowl.			3		

TOTAL POINTS POSSIBLE   64

TOTAL POINTS POSSIBLE—2nd attempt   62

TOTAL POINTS EARNED   ____

Points assigned reflect importance of step to meeting objective: Important = 1, Essential = 2, Critical = 3. Students will lose 2 points for repeated attempts. Failure results if any of the critical steps are omitted or performed incorrectly. If using a 100-point scale, determine score by dividing points earned by total points possible and multiplying the results by 100.

SCORE: _____

SKILL COMPETENCY ASSESSMENT

35-4 Removing Alginate Impression

Student's Name _____ Date _____

Instructor's Name _____

Skill: The dental assistant is responsible for preparing the equipment and supplies. Alginate is a generic name used for a group of irreversible hydrocolloid impression materials. Alginate is commonly used in making diagnostic casts or study models. In some states, dental assistants are allowed to take the alginate impressions; in other states, the assistant can select the tray, mix the material, load the material into the tray, and transfer the tray for the dentist to place in the patient's mouth.

Performance Objective: The student will follow a routine procedure that meets the regulations and protocol set forth by the dentist and regulatory agencies, keeping in mind that assistant duties vary from state to state. The assistant may be evaluated by performance criteria, verbal/written responses, and/or combined responses and performance criteria. This procedure is performed by the dental assistant in states where it is allowed. The materials are prepared and the alginate impression is taken on the maxillary and mandibular arches.

	Self-Evaluation	Student Evaluation	Possible Points	Instructor Evaluation	Comments
Equipment and Supplies					
1. Flexible spatula/broad blade or disposable spatula			3		
2. Flexible rubber bowl(s) or disposable bowl			3		
3. Alginate material with water and powder measuring devices			3		
4. Water			3		
5. Impression tray(s)			3		
Competency Steps (*follow aseptic procedures*)					
1. When the material is completely set, remove it from the mouth. (First, loosen the tissue of the lips and cheek around the periphery with the fingers to break the suction-like seal.)			3		
2. Place the fingers of the opposing hand on the opposite arch to protect the adjacent arch as the tray is now removed.			3		

	Self-Evaluation	Student Evaluation	Possible Points	Instructor Evaluation	Comments
3. Remove the tray in an upward or a downward motion (depending on the arch) with a quick snap.			3		
4. Turn the tray to the side to allow it to be removed from the oral cavity.			3		
5. Remove any excess alginate material from the patient's mouth.			2		
6. Rinse, evacuate, and have patient rinse out.			3		
7. Check the patient's face for any excess alginate material. If present, give the patient a tissue and mirror to remove material.			2		
8. Check the impression for accuracy.			3		
9. Rinse the impression gently with water to remove saliva or blood.			3		
10. Spray with an approved surface disinfectant. If time elapses (maximum of 20 minutes) before pouring, wrap the alginate in an airtight container and label with the patient's name.			3		

TOTAL POINTS POSSIBLE   43

TOTAL POINTS POSSIBLE—2nd attempt   41

TOTAL POINTS EARNED   _____

Points assigned reflect importance of step to meeting objective: Important = 1, Essential = 2, Critical = 3. Students will lose 2 points for repeated attempts. Failure results if any of the critical steps are omitted or performed incorrectly. If using a 100-point scale, determine score by dividing points earned by total points possible and multiplying the results by 100.

SCORE: _____

SKILL COMPETENCY ASSESSMENT

35-5 Disinfecting Alginate Impressions

Student's Name _____ Date _____

Instructor's Name _____

Skill: The dental assistant is responsible for preparing the equipment and supplies. Alginate is a generic name used for a group of irreversible hydrocolloid impression materials. Alginate is commonly used in making diagnostic casts or study models. In some states, dental assistants are allowed to take the alginate impressions; in other states, the assistant can select the tray, mix the material, load the material into the tray, and transfer the tray for the dentist to place in the patient's mouth.

Performance Objective: The student will follow a routine procedure that meets the regulations and protocol set forth by the dentist and regulatory agencies, keeping in mind that assistant duties vary from state to state. The assistant may be evaluated by performance criteria, verbal/written responses, and/or combined responses and performance criteria. This procedure is performed by the dental assistant immediately after removing the alginate impressions from the patient's mouth and caring for the patient.

	Self-Evaluation	Student Evaluation	Possible Points	Instructor Evaluation	Comments
Equipment and Supplies 1. Approved disinfectant			3		
2. Covered container			3		
Competency Steps (*follow aseptic procedures*) 1. Rinse the impressions gently under tap water to remove any debris, blood, or saliva.			3		
2. Spray the impressions with an approved disinfectant.			3		

	Self-Evaluation	Student Evaluation	Possible Points	Instructor Evaluation	Comments
3. Place the impressions in a covered container if not pouring immediately.			3		
4. Label the container with the patient's name.			3		

TOTAL POINTS POSSIBLE   18

TOTAL POINTS POSSIBLE—2nd attempt   16

TOTAL POINTS EARNED   ____

Points assigned reflect importance of step to meeting objective: Important = 1, Essential = 2, Critical = 3. Students will lose 2 points for repeated attempts. Failure results if any of the critical steps are omitted or performed incorrectly. If using a 100-point scale, determine score by dividing points earned by total points possible and multiplying the results by 100.

SCORE: _____

SKILL COMPETENCY ASSESSMENT

35-6 Taking Bite Registration

Student's Name _____ Date _____

Instructor's Name _____

Skill: The dental assistant is responsible for preparing the equipment and supplies. A wax bite registration is taken to establish the relationship between the maxillary and mandibular teeth. Normally, wax that is formed in a horseshoe shape is used, but a flat sheet of utility wax can be used as well. It is softened using warm water, and then placed on the mandibular arch of the patient.

Performance Objective: The student will follow a routine procedure that meets the regulations and protocol set forth by the dentist and regulatory agencies, keeping in mind that assistant duties vary from state to state. The assistant may be evaluated by performance criteria, verbal/written responses, and/or combined responses and performance criteria. This procedure is performed by the dental assistant under the direction of the dentist or by the dentist with the dental assistant assisting.

	Self-Evaluation	Student Evaluation	Possible Points	Instructor Evaluation	Comments
Equipment and Supplies					
1. Bite registration wax or wax horseshoe or polysiloxane and extruder gun and disposable tips			3		
2. Laboratory knife			3		
3. Warm water or torch			3		
Competency Steps (*follow aseptic procedures*)					
1. The patient remains upright after the impressions are taken. (The patient napkin is in place.)			3		
2. Explain the procedure to the patient.			3		
3. Try the bite registration wax to determine the correct length. Adjust and trim as needed with a laboratory knife.			3		
4. Instruct the patient to practice biting to establish occlusion. (If needed, instruct the patient in biting in occlusion.)			3		
5. Heat the bite registration wax. (Use warm water or torch to soften.)			3		

	Self-Evaluation	Student Evaluation	Possible Points	Instructor Evaluation	Comments
6. Place wax on the mandibular occlusal surface of the patient.			3		
7. Instruct the patient to gently bite together in the correct occlusion. Ensure that the patient is in proper occlusion.			3		
8. Allow the wax to cool (1 to 2 minutes) while the patient keeps the teeth together in occlusion.			3		
9. Gently remove the wax without distortion.			3		
10. Disinfect, label the wax or polysiloxane bite registration, and store it for use during trimming of diagnostic casts (study models).			3		

TOTAL POINTS POSSIBLE   39

TOTAL POINTS POSSIBLE—2nd attempt   37

TOTAL POINTS EARNED   _____

Points assigned reflect importance of step to meeting objective: Important = 1, Essential = 2, Critical = 3. Students will lose 2 points for repeated attempts. Failure results if any of the critical steps are omitted or performed incorrectly. If using a 100-point scale, determine score by dividing points earned by total points possible and multiplying the results by 100.

SCORE: _____

SKILL COMPETENCY ASSESSMENT

35-7 Taking Polysulfide Impression

Student's Name _____ Date _____

Instructor's Name _____

Skill: The dental assistant is responsible for preparation of equipment and supplies. Polysulfide impression materials are supplied in two pastes, a base and a catalyst. These pastes can be purchased as light (syringe material), regular, heavy, and extra heavy (tray material). Ten minutes are required from the start of the mix to the setting of the material prior to removal from the patient's mouth. Knowledge of materials and factors that can slightly accelerate or shorten setting time is critical.

Performance Objective: The student will follow a routine procedure that meets the regulations and protocol set forth by the dentist and regulatory agencies. The assistant may be evaluated by performance criteria, oral/written responses, and/or responses and performance criteria. This procedure is performed by the dentist with the dental assistant assisting. Polysulfide is a material used in taking final impressions where high levels of accuracy (precision) are required. This can be a four- or six-handed procedure. All auxiliaries involved should wear protection over clothing.

	Self-Evaluation	Student Evaluation	Possible Points	Instructor Evaluation	Comments
Equipment and Supplies 1. Two rigid tapered laboratory spatulas			3		
2. Paper pad, provided by the manufacturer			3		
3. Two pastes each from same manufacturer: a. Two syringe pastes (syringe material base and accelerator) b. Tray material base and accelerator pastes.			3 3		
4. Impression syringe with tip in place and plunger out of cylinder			3		
5. Custom tray painted with corresponding adhesive and permitted to dry			3		

	Self-Evaluation	Student Evaluation	Possible Points	Instructor Evaluation	Comments
Competency Steps (*follow aseptic procedures*)					
Patient Preparation					
1. Review health history.			3		
2. Seat patient upright with the patient napkin in place and a large drape over clothes.			3		
3. Rinse mouth with water or mouth rinse. (Remove any food debris or thick saliva.)			3		
4. Explain the procedure to the patient.			3		
5. Two individuals concurrently mix the material. (Syringe material is mixed slightly ahead of tray material; determine who will mix which part.)			3		
6. Dispense accelerator onto pad in a long, even line, about 4 inches long. (More material, more lines; wipe end of tube before placing lid back on.)			3		
7. Dispense base onto pad in a long, even line, the same length as the accelerator. (Additional lines can be added. Do not touch accelerator until the operator wants polymerization process to begin.)			3		
8. Mix materials: a. First, for syringe material, mix accelerator into base material, and spatulate the pastes together with broad sweeps. b. After a minute, the individual mixing the tray material begins, using the same process.			3 3		
9. Mix until homogenous (complete and without brown or white streaks). (Takes 45 seconds to a minute.)			3		

	Self-Evaluation	Student Evaluation	Possible Points	Instructor Evaluation	Comments
10. Prepare the impression syringe: a. Load syringe material into the impression syringe. (Fill back portion of the barrel, pushing the syringe over the material repeatedly to force material into the chamber.)			3		
b. Place the plunger in the syringe. (Wipe edges quickly.)			3		
c. Extrude material slightly. (Ensure that it works.)			3		
d. Transfer to the dentist.			3		
11. Prepare the tray material: a. Mix to same consistency, in same time frame.			3		
b. Pick up material by spatula and load it into impression tray and spread evenly.			3		
c. Transfer tray to the dentist after the syringe is used.			3		
d. Complete mix and loading within 4 minutes.			3		
12. Keep impression in the patient's mouth for 6 minutes to achieve the final set (held by the operator or the dental assistant).			3		
13. Clean up after the material has reached the rubber stage, or when it peels off the spatula. (Remove the top sheet of the paper pad, throw away the paper and disposable syringe, and sterilize spatula.)			3		
14. Remove the tray as alginate is removed. Snap quickly, while releasing seal and taking care to protect the opposing teeth.			3		

TOTAL POINTS POSSIBLE   81

TOTAL POINTS POSSIBLE—2nd attempt   79

TOTAL POINTS EARNED   ____

Points assigned reflect importance of step to meeting objective: Important = 1, Essential = 2, Critical = 3. Students will lose 2 points for repeated attempts. Failure results if any of the critical steps are omitted or performed incorrectly. If using a 100-point scale, determine score by dividing points earned by total points possible and multiplying the results by 100.

SCORE: _____

SKILL COMPETENCY ASSESSMENT

35-8 Taking Silicone (Polysiloxane) Two-Step Impression

Student's Name _____ Date _____

Instructor's Name _____

Skill: The dental assistant is responsible for preparation of equipment and supplies. This impression material is available in putty form for making a custom tray, and in tubes of base and accelerator (catalyst) in injection form (with regular and heavy types for impressions). It also is available in the cartridge form to be used with the mixing tip and extruding gun (automix cartridge system).

Performance Objective: The student will follow a routine procedure that meets the regulations and protocol set forth by the dentist and regulatory agencies. The assistant may be evaluated by performance, statement, and/or combined responses and action. This procedure is performed by the dentist with the dental assistant assisting. Silicone polysiloxane is used in taking final impressions where high levels of accuracy (precision) are required.

	Self-Evaluation	Student Evaluation	Possible Points	Instructor Evaluation	Comments
Equipment and Supplies					
1. Spatula			3		
2. Paper mixing pad			3		
3. Vinyl overgloves			3		
4. Two containers of putty with color-coordinated scoops (one base, one catalyst), or one putty base and liquid dropper of catalyst			3		
5. Stock tray with adhesive on interior			3		
6. Plastic sheet for spacer			3		
7. Extruder gun, mixing tip with intraoral tip (delivery tip or injection syringe)			3		
8. Cartridges of impression material (light-body or wash material)			3		

	Self-Evaluation	Student Evaluation	Possible Points	Instructor Evaluation	Comments
Competency Steps (*follow aseptic procedures*)					
Patient Preparation					
1. Review health history.			3		
2. Seat the patient upright with patient napkin in place.			3		
3. Place retraction cord around the prepared tooth.			3		
4. Explain the procedure to the patient.			3		
Preliminary Putty Impression					
1. Don vinyl gloves.			3		
2. Prepare the putty mix. a. Mix equal scoops of putty, or mix putty base and drops of catalyst. b. Putty must be kneaded together until homogeneous (no streaks, even color). c. Mix for manufacturer's recommended time (30 seconds, normally).			3 3 3		
3. After the material is mixed, form into a patty and load it into a prepared tray. (With finger, make a slight indentation where the teeth are located.)			3		
4. Place a plastic spacer sheet over the material and insert it into the patient's mouth. (Creates 2 mm of space for final syringeable, viscous impression material.)			3		
5. Setting of putty will take about 3 minutes.			3		
6. Remove the tray from the patient's mouth.			3		
7. Remove the spacer.			3		
8. Check the putty for accuracy and leave to set further.			3		

	Self-Evaluation	Student Evaluation	Possible Points	Instructor Evaluation	Comments
Final Impression					
1. After tooth has been prepared, clean and dry the area.			3		
2. Place the retraction cord.			3		
3. The doctor indicates readiness for final impression; the assistant prepares the material.			3		
4. Ready the tray with the preliminary impression; spacer is removed.			3		
5. Prepare the extruder gun and load it (with light-body or wash material).			3		
6. Extrude syringe material through the mixing tip and place it in the preliminary impression.			3		
7. Wipe off the tip and place an intraoral delivery tip for direct injection around the prepared tooth (after the retraction cord has been removed).			3		
8. Hand the extruder gun to the dentist (intraoral delivery tip or injection syringe loaded with mixing tip).			3		
9. The dentist seats the tray immediately (held in place 3 to 5 minutes).			3		
10. After the material sets, remove the impression tray, while releasing the seal and taking care to protect the opposing teeth from quickly snapping.			3		
11. Immediately rinse the impression with water and lightly blow dry with air.			3		

	Self-Evaluation	Student Evaluation	Possible Points	Instructor Evaluation	Comments
12. Disinfect according to manufacturer's directions.			3		
13. Pour the impression immediately.			3		

TOTAL POINTS POSSIBLE   105

TOTAL POINTS POSSIBLE—2nd attempt   103

TOTAL POINTS EARNED   _____

Points assigned reflect importance of step to meeting objective: Important = 1, Essential = 2, Critical = 3. Students will lose 2 points for repeated attempts. Failure results if any of the critical steps are omitted or performed incorrectly. If using a 100-point scale, determine score by dividing points earned by total points possible and multiplying the results by 100.

SCORE: _____

SKILL COMPETENCY ASSESSMENT

35-9 Pouring Alginate Impression with Plaster

Student's Name _____ Date _____

Instructor's Name _____

Skill: The dental assistant is responsible for preparing the equipment and supplies. Identifying the appropriate gypsum material (among several types) for the application is important. Plaster is a white stone (plaster of paris).

Performance Objective: The student will follow a routine procedure that meets the regulations and protocol set forth by the dentist and regulatory agencies. The assistant may be evaluated by performance criteria, verbal/written responses, and/or combined responses and performance criteria. This procedure is performed by the dental assistant in the dental laboratory.

	Self-Evaluation	Student Evaluation	Possible Points	Instructor Evaluation	Comments
Equipment and Supplies					
1. Metal spatula with rounded end and stiff, straight sides			3		
2. Two flexible rubber mixing bowls			3		
3. Scale			3		
4. Plaster (100 g)			3		
5. Weight-measuring device			3		
6. Liquid-measuring device			3		
7. Vibrator with paper or plastic cover on platform			3		
8. Room-temperature water			3		
9. Alginate impression (disinfected)			3		
Competency Steps (*follow aseptic procedures*)					
Mixing the plaster					
1. Measure 50 mL of room-temperature water into one of the mixing bowls.			3		
2. Place the second flexible mixing bowl on the scale (set dial to 0).			2		

	Self-Evaluation	Student Evaluation	Possible Points	Instructor Evaluation	Comments
3. Weigh 100 g of plaster.			3		
4. Add powder from the second bowl to the water of the first bowl.			3		
5. Allow several seconds for the powder to dissolve.			3		
6. Use a spatula to slowly mix the particles.			3		
7. Complete the initial mixing in 20 seconds.			3		
8. Turn the vibrator to medium speed.			3		
9. Place the rubber bowl on the vibrator platform, pressing lightly.			3		
10. Rotate the bowl on the vibrator to allow air bubbles to rise to the surface.			3		
11. Complete mixing and vibrating in a couple of minutes.			3		
12. The mix will appear like whipped cream, with a smooth, creamy texture.			3		
13. The mixture is ready when the spatula can cut through it and it sticks to the sides without moving.			3		
TOTAL POINTS POSSIBLE			65		
TOTAL POINTS POSSIBLE—2nd attempt			63		
TOTAL POINTS EARNED			____		

Points assigned reflect importance of step to meeting objective: Important = 1, Essential = 2, Critical = 3. Students will lose 2 points for repeated attempts. Failure results if any of the critical steps are omitted or performed incorrectly. If using a 100-point scale, determine score by dividing points earned by total points possible and multiplying the results by 100.

SCORE: _____

SKILL COMPETENCY ASSESSMENT

35-10 Pouring Alginate Impression for Study Model

Student's Name _____ Date _____

Instructor's Name _____

Skill: The dental assistant is responsible for preparing the equipment and supplies. Identifying the appropriate gypsum material (among several types) for the application is important. Plaster is a white stone (plaster of paris).

Performance Objective: The student will follow a routine procedure that meets the regulations and protocol set forth by the dentist and regulatory agencies, keeping in mind that assistant duties vary from state to state. The assistant may be evaluated by performance criteria, verbal/written responses, and/or combined responses and performance criteria. This procedure is performed by the dental assistant in the dental laboratory immediately after mixing the plaster.

	Self-Evaluation	Student Evaluation	Possible Points	Instructor Evaluation	Comments
Equipment and Supplies 1. Metal spatula (stiff blade with rounded end) or disposable spatula			3		
2. Mixed plaster from Procedure 35–9			3		
3. Vibrator with paper towel or plastic cover on platform			3		
Competency Steps (*follow aseptic procedures*) 1. Use a vibrator at low or medium speed. (The impression is ready to pour, excess moisture is removed, and a laboratory knife is used to eliminate excess impression material so as not to hamper pouring.)			3		
2. Hold the impression by the handle, with the tray portion on the platform of the vibrator; allow a small amount of plaster to touch the most distal surface of one side of the arch in the impression.			3		

	Self-Evaluation	Student Evaluation	Possible Points	Instructor Evaluation	Comments
3. Continue to add small increments of plaster in the same area. (Plaster flows around toward the anterior teeth and to other side of the arch.)			3		
4. Continue adding plaster until it flows out the other side of the impression and fills the anatomic portion of the model. (Rotate the impression around the platform of vibrator to allow the material to travel around the arch.)			3		
5. After the anatomy portion is filled with plaster, use larger increments to fill the entire impression. Turn off the vibrator.			3		
6. When filled, place the impression lightly on the vibrator to coalesce.			3		
7. If a two-pour method is used, leave small blobs on top of the plaster.			3		

TOTAL POINTS POSSIBLE   30

TOTAL POINTS POSSIBLE—2nd attempt   28

TOTAL POINTS EARNED   _____

Points assigned reflect importance of step to meeting objective: Important = 1, Essential = 2, Critical = 3. Students will lose 2 points for repeated attempts. Failure results if any of the critical steps are omitted or performed incorrectly. If using a 100-point scale, determine score by dividing points earned by total points possible and multiplying the results by 100.

SCORE: _____

SKILL COMPETENCY ASSESSMENT

35-11 The Art of Pouring a Plaster Study Model Using the Two-Pour Method

Student's Name _____ Date _____

Instructor's Name _____

Skill: The dental assistant is responsible for preparation of equipment and supplies. Identifying the appropriate gypsum material (among several types) for the application is important. Plaster is a white stone (plaster of paris).

Performance Objective: The student will follow a routine procedure that meets the regulations and protocol set forth by the dentist and regulatory agencies. The assistant may be evaluated by performance criteria, verbal/written responses, and/or combined responses and performance criteria. This procedure is performed by the dental assistant in the dental laboratory after the anatomical portion of the study model has set.

	Self-Evaluation	Student Evaluation	Possible Points	Instructor Evaluation	Comments
Equipment and Supplies					
1. Metal spatula or disposable (stiff blade with rounded end)			3		
2. Flexible rubber bowl or disposable bowl			3		
3. Vibrator with disposable cover on platform			3		
4. Paper towels			3		
5. Plaster			3		
6. Calibration measurement device			3		
7. Room-temperature water			3		
8. Water-measuring device			3		
Competency Steps (*follow aseptic procedures*)					
1. After pouring anatomic portion of impression, allow it to set 5 to 10 minutes.			3		
2. Cleanup of mixing bowl: a. Wipe rubber bowl and spatula with paper towel and dispose of material. b. Rubber bowl and spatula are washed, cleaned, readied for second pour.			3 3		

	Self-Evaluation	Student Evaluation	Possible Points	Instructor Evaluation	Comments
3. Ratio of powder to water (100 g powder to 40 mL water for bases of art portion of both maxillary and mandibular casts).			3		
4. Mix plaster in same manner as done before (will appear much thicker).			3		
5. Plaster can be gathered up on spatula and placed on a glass slab. Allow material to mass upward.			3		
6. After all material is on the glass slab or paper towel, the poured anatomy portion can be inverted onto base material.			3		
7. Hold tray steady and situate handle so that it is parallel with paper or glass surface. (Base should be even and uniform in thickness.)			3		
8. Carefully drag excess plaster up over edges of cast, while filling in any void areas; try to avoid covering margins.			3		

TOTAL POINTS POSSIBLE   51

TOTAL POINTS POSSIBLE—2nd attempt   49

TOTAL POINTS EARNED   ____

Points assigned reflect importance of step to meeting objective: Important = 1, Essential = 2, Critical = 3. Students will lose 2 points for repeated attempts. Failure results if any of the critical steps are omitted or performed incorrectly. If using a 100-point scale, determine score by dividing points earned by total points possible and multiplying the results by 100.

SCORE: _____

SKILL COMPETENCY ASSESSMENT

35-12 Removing Plaster Model from Alginate Impression

Student's Name _____ Date _____

Instructor's Name _____

Skill: The dental assistant is responsible for preparing the equipment and supplies. Identifying the appropriate gypsum material (among several types) for the application is important. Plaster is a white stone (plaster of paris).

Performance Objective: The student will follow a routine procedure that meets the regulations and protocol set forth by the dentist and regulatory agencies. The assistant may be evaluated by performance criteria, verbal/written responses, and/or combined responses and performance criteria. This procedure is performed by the dental assistant in the dental laboratory after the study model has set.

	Self-Evaluation	Student Evaluation	Possible Points	Instructor Evaluation	Comments
Equipment and Supplies 1. Laboratory knife			3		
2. Maxillary and mandibular plaster models, set in alginate impressions			3		
Competency Steps (*follow aseptic procedures*) 1. Allow the plaster to set for 40 to 60 minutes before removing the impression material from the tray. (Absence of heat from exothermic reaction indicates that plaster has set.)			3		
2. Using a laboratory knife, gently remove any plaster on the margin of the tray.			3		
3. Holding the handle of the impression tray, lift straight up.			3		

	Self-Evaluation	Student Evaluation	Possible Points	Instructor Evaluation	Comments
4. Remove the necessary plaster to release the tray. (Identify the area that is holding back the tray.)			3		
5. Lift upward. Wiggling side to side or sideways may fracture the teeth-anatomic portion of the cast.			3		

TOTAL POINTS POSSIBLE   21

TOTAL POINTS POSSIBLE—2nd attempt   19

TOTAL POINTS EARNED   ____

Points assigned reflect importance of step to meeting objective: Important = 1, Essential = 2, Critical = 3. Students will lose 2 points for repeated attempts. Failure results if any of the critical steps are omitted or performed incorrectly. If using a 100-point scale, determine score by dividing points earned by total points possible and multiplying the results by 100.

SCORE: _____

SKILL COMPETENCY ASSESSMENT

35-13 Trimming Diagnostic Casts/Study Models

Student's Name _____ Date _____

Instructor's Name _____

Skill: The dental assistant is responsible for preparing the equipment and supplies. Diagnostic casts (study models) are used to present the case to the patient; thus, an attractive appearance is important.

Performance Objective: The student will follow a routine procedure that meets the regulations and protocol set forth by the dentist and regulatory agencies, keeping in mind that assistant duties vary from state to state. The assistant may be evaluated by performance criteria, verbal/written responses, and/or combined responses and performance criteria. This procedure is performed by the dental assistant in the dental laboratory after the study model has set and has been separated from the alginate impression and prepared for trimming.

	Self-Evaluation	Student Evaluation	Possible Points	Instructor Evaluation	Comments
Equipment and Supplies					
1. Safety glasses			3		
2. Maxillary and mandibular models			3		
3. Two flexible rubber mixing bowls			3		
4. Laboratory knife			3		
5. Pencil			3		
6. Straight edge (ruler)			3		
Competency Steps (*follow aseptic procedures*)					
1. Wet the models before trimming. (If dry, soak the bases of the models 5 minutes before trimming; the trimming wheel on the model trimmer works best with wet models.)			3		
2. Put on safety glasses, and adjust the model trimmer. (Allow water to run freely over the grinding wheel when the trimmer is turned on.)			3		

	Self-Evaluation	Student Evaluation	Possible Points	Instructor Evaluation	Comments
3. Invert the models so that the teeth are resting on the counter. Evaluate whether the base is parallel to the counter. The art portion is 1/2 inch "high" when completed.			3		
4. Turn on the model trimmer, and trim the base so it is parallel to the occlusal plane. Hold the model as level as possible. (Apply light, even pressure to the models against the grinding wheel on the model trimmer.)			3		
5. Rest a hand on the table of the model trimmer. Keep fingers away from the grinding wheel.			3		
6. If needed, return the model to the counter for reevaluation and again to the trimmer to achieve a parallel surface. Trim both models to this stage.			3		
7. Place the models together in occlusion (wax bite may be necessary), and again reevaluate. The models must be parallel. All other cuts will be off if this step is not completed.			3		
8. When cut, maxillary and mandibular models as a pair are parallel; keep in occlusion and evaluate which posterior teeth are the most distal, maxillary, or mandibular. Once determined, use a pencil to draw a line behind the retromolar area indicating where to trim.			3		
9. Place the base surface of the model on the model trimmer table guide and cut the posterior area at a right angle with the base up to indicated lines.			3		

	Self-Evaluation	Student Evaluation	Possible Points	Instructor Evaluation	Comments
10. Put the two models back into occlusion and place the cut model on top, whether it is maxillary or mandibular. Place the opposite base on the model trimmer table guide, holding the models together, and trim the posterior at a right angle to the base. (The trimmed model will act as guide to follow while trimming.)			3		
11. To evaluate, the models can be taken off the grinding wheel and placed on their backs. The occlusal plane is at a right angle to the counter. If models stay in occlusion, the objective has been met. If they fall apart, return to the grinding wheel until they stay.			3		
12. Trim heel, side, and anterior cuts: a. Mark outward from the middle of the mandibular pre-molars to the edge of the model. b. Mark the maxillary cuspids in same manner. c. Draw the line running parallel to the teeth at the greatest depth of buccal vestibule from molars to pre-molars. d. The line will be about 5 mm from the buccal surfaces of the teeth. e. Mark both sides of maxillary and mandibular models in this manner.			3 3 3 3 3		
13. Place the model base back on the model trimmer table guide, and trim the model to pencil lines on both sides. Repeat with both models.			3		
14. With a pencil, mark a dot at the midline of the maxillary model in the vestibule area. Using the straight edge of the measuring device, draw a line from dot to canine/cuspid line on each quadrant.			3		

	Self-Evaluation	Student Evaluation	Possible Points	Instructor Evaluation	Comments
15. Execute both anterior cuts, forming a pointed area at the midline and center of both cuspids.			3		
16. After the lines are drawn, make sure that the cuts will not trim away protruding teeth. If so, move the lines outward to accommodate. The model should appear symmetrical.			3		
17. The mandibular model is marked in a rounded manner from the middle of the canine/cuspid on one side to the middle of the canine/cuspid on the other side. A pencil line can be drawn at the depth of anterior vestibule as a guide for trimming.			3		
18. Make heel cuts on both maxillary and mandibular models 3/8 to 5/8 inch wide. They should appear symmetrical in length. (They can be drawn on the model by turning the base upward, and placing an imaginary diagonal line from the cuspid [maxillary] pre-molar [mandibular] to where the side and back cuts meet. Draw a 90-degree angle across the base opposite anterior area; heel cuts are small on both maxillary and mandibular models to finish trimming of models.)			3		
19. After models are trimmed symmetrically: a. With a laboratory knife, trim the tongue area flat and smooth other areas on the art portion. b. Fill air bubbles with plaster. c. Smooth the flat surface with fine wet/dry sandpaper under water.			3 3 3		

	Self-Evaluation	Student Evaluation	Possible Points	Instructor Evaluation	Comments
20. If needed, models can be placed in model gloss for 10 minutes or sprayed with gloss for a professional appearance and to add strength. (To achieve a high gloss, polish with a dry cloth.)			3		
21. Label both models with the patient's name and the date that the models were taken. In an orthodontic office, also consider identifying the patient's age on the model.			3		

TOTAL POINTS POSSIBLE   99

TOTAL POINTS POSSIBLE—2nd attempt   97

TOTAL POINTS EARNED   ____

Points assigned reflect importance of step to meeting objective: Important = 1, Essential = 2, Critical = 3. Students will lose 2 points for repeated attempts. Failure results if any of the critical steps are omitted or performed incorrectly. If using a 100-point scale, determine score by dividing points earned by total points possible and multiplying the results by 100.

SCORE: _____

SKILL COMPETENCY ASSESSMENT

35-14 Taking the Records and Performing a Facebow Transfer

Student's Name _____ Date _____

Instructor's Name _____

Skill: Dental offices will use a facebow and an articulator to duplicate the function of the temporomandibular joint. The facebow allows the operator to obtain the records about the placement of the maxillary arch and its location to the joint. From this the mandibular arch can be mounted and the biting function can be duplicated. This provides the dentist information for diagnosis or for constructing dental appliances such as crowns, bridges, veneers, partials, and dentures.

Performance Objective: The student will follow a routine procedure that meets the regulations and protocol set forth by the dentist and regulatory agencies, keeping in mind that assistant duties vary from state to state. The assistant may be evaluated by performance criteria, verbal/written responses, and/or combined responses and performance criteria. This procedure is performed by the dental assistant under the general supervision of the dentist in some states or by the dentist with the auxiliary assisting. The patient is seated and prepared for dental treatment. The operator has washed hands and donned gloves, eyewear, and mask.

	Self-Evaluation	Student Evaluation	Possible Points	Instructor Evaluation	Comments
Equipment and Supplies					
1. Earbow			3		
2. Bitefork and transfer jig assembly			3		
3. Reference plane locator			3		
4. Firm cotton roll			3		
5. Bite registration material or base-plate wax			3		
6. Straight edge (ruler)			3		
Competency Steps (*follow aseptic procedures*)					
1. Assemble equipment and supplies.			1		
2. Explain the procedure to the patient.			1		
3. Using the reference plane marker and locator, mark the anterior reference point on patient's right side.			3		

	Self-Evaluation	Student Evaluation	Possible Points	Instructor Evaluation	Comments
4. Apply the bite registration or baseplate wax to the top of the bitefork, making sure there are three points of reference.			3		
5. Insert bitefork into patient's mouth.			3		
6. Align the patient's midline to index notch, ensuring it is parallel to patient's horizontal and coronal planes: then move the bitefork into place on the maxillary arch.			3		
7. Use cotton roll under the bitefork to stabilize as the patient bites.			2		
8. Attach the vertical shaft to the measuring facebow with the clamp and tighten the screw.			3		
9. Loosen the side finger screws and center wheel so earbow assembly will open.			3		
10. Ask patient to place earpieces in ears and tighten the screws.			3		
11. Raise or lower the bow so that the pointer aligns with the anterior reference point. When aligned, tighten the clamps.			3		
12. Loosen the anterior finger grips and screw on the measuring bow. Remove the bow away from the patient's face and have patient open mouth to also remove bitefork.			3		

	Self-Evaluation	Student Evaluation	Possible Points	Instructor Evaluation	Comments
13. Disinfect bitefork.			2		
14. Dismiss patient and document procedure.			3		

TOTAL POINTS POSSIBLE   54

TOTAL POINTS POSSIBLE—2nd attempt   52

TOTAL POINTS EARNED   ————

Points assigned reflect importance of step to meeting objective: Important = 1, Essential = 2, Critical = 3. Students will lose 2 points for repeated attempts. Failure results if any of the critical steps are omitted or performed incorrectly. If using a 100-point scale, determine score by dividing points earned by total points possible and multiplying the results by 100.

SCORE: _____

SKILL COMPETENCY ASSESSMENT

35-15 Mount Models on Articulator After Facebow Records Have Been Completed

Student's Name _____ Date _____

Instructor's Name _____

Skill: Dental offices will use a facebow and an articulator to duplicate the function of the temporomandibular joint. The facebow allows the operator to obtain the records about the placement of the maxillary arch and its location to the joint. From this the mandibular arch can be mounted and the biting function can be duplicated. This provides the dentist the information for diagnosis or for constructing dental appliances such as crowns, bridges, veneers, partials, and dentures.

Performance Objective: The student will follow a routine procedure that meets the regulations and protocol set forth by the dentist and regulatory agencies, keeping in mind that assistant duties vary from state to state. The assistant may be evaluated by performance criteria, verbal/written responses, and/or combined responses and performance criteria. This procedure is performed by the dental assistant under the general supervision of the dentist in some states or by the dentist with the auxiliary assisting. It is done in the office dental laboratory or at a commercial dental laboratory. The facebow is disinfected and ready to be mounted.

	Self-Evaluation	Student Evaluation	Possible Points	Instructor Evaluation	Comments
Equipment and Supplies 1. Facebow and bitefork assembled			3		
2. Articulator			3		
3. Two mounting rings			3		
4. Trimmed models			3		
5. Class I plaster and water			3		
6. Mixing bowl and spatula			3		
Competency Steps (*follow aseptic procedures*) 1. Assemble equipment and supplies			1		
2. Trim models to fit into the two bows.			1		
3. Score the models with a knife.			3		
4. Attach the facebow to the articulator.			3		

5. Place the maxillary model into the bite registration or base-plate wax that was used on the patient.			3		
6. Lift the articulator arm up to expose the scored area on the maxillary model.			3		
7. Mix plaster to a thick consistency and place it on the model filling the entire space between top of model and articulator. Then bring the top arm of articulator down.			2		
8. After the maxillary model is set, remove the facebow and bite-fork. Mount the mandibular model using the bite registrations obtained on the patient. Mix additional plaster and mound it on the lower articulating ring and then allow the mandibular scored model to be placed on the plaster.			3		
9. After the initial set, clean up excess plaster; leave the set models in the articulator.			3		
10. Add the pin to the articulator to establish the centric relationship.			3		

TOTAL POINTS POSSIBLE   40

TOTAL POINTS POSSIBLE—2nd attempt   43

TOTAL POINTS EARNED   _____

Points assigned reflect importance of step to meeting objective: Important = 1, Essential = 2, Critical = 3. Students will lose 2 points for repeated attempts. Failure results if any of the critical steps are omitted or performed incorrectly. If using a 100-point scale, determine score by dividing points earned by total points possible and multiplying the results by 100.

SCORE: _____

SKILL COMPETENCY ASSESSMENT

35-16 Constructing Self-Cured Acrylic Resin Custom Tray

Student's Name _____ Date _____

Instructor's Name _____

Skill: The dental assistant is responsible for preparing the equipment and supplies. The dentist may ask for a custom tray to be fabricated for the patient to obtain an accurate impression, perhaps because a stock tray does not fit. Several materials are available to make custom trays. A material used for this purpose must be rigid enough so that it does not change shape as it is inserted and removed from the mouth. It is important that the material adapts well during construction so that the final tray meets the required criteria.

Performance Objective: The student will follow a routine procedure that meets the regulations and protocol set forth by the dentist and regulatory agencies, keeping in mind that assistant duties vary from state to state. The assistant may be evaluated by performance criteria, verbal/written responses, and/or combined responses and performance criteria. This procedure is performed by the dental assistant in the dental laboratory on a working cast.

	Self-Evaluation	Student Evaluation	Possible Points	Instructor Evaluation	Comments
Equipment and Supplies					
1. Maxillary and/or mandibular casts			3		
2. Laboratory knife			3		
3. Pencil (lead or red and blue)			3		
4. Wax spatula			3		
5. Base plate wax and heating source (warm water or laboratory torch)			3		
6. Tray resin with measuring devices			3		
7. Separating medium with brush			3		
8. Wooden tongue blade and wax-lined paper cup			3		
9. Petroleum jelly			3		
10. Tray adhesive			3		

	Self-Evaluation	Student Evaluation	Possible Points	Instructor Evaluation	Comments
Competency Steps (follow aseptic procedures)					
Prepare the Cast					
1. Outline the area of the cast for the spacer to be placed (2 to 3 mm below margin of prepared tooth or 2 to 3 mm above lowest point in vestibule if arch is edentulous).			3		
2. Fill any undercuts in the cast. Heat the spacer material and contour to the pencil line. (Undercuts can be covered with spacer material.)			3		
3. Using the laboratory knife, trim the wax or spacer to the line, using an angled cut instead of a blunt one.			3		
4. Cut appropriate stops in the spacer.			3		
5. Cover the spacer with aluminum foil or paint with a separating medium.			3		
Mixing Custom Tray Acrylic Self-Curing Resin					
1. Measure precise amounts of powder and liquid. (Follow manufacturer's directions.)			3		
2. Mix the powder and liquid in a wax-lined paper cup with a wooden tongue blade until homogeneous.			3		
3. Allow the mixture to go through initial polymerization for 2 or 3 minutes. (Covering material during polymerization sometimes is indicated by the manufacturer.)			3		
4. At this time, place petroleum jelly over the cast and the palms of your hands.			3		

	Self-Evaluation	Student Evaluation	Possible Points	Instructor Evaluation	Comments
Contouring Custom Tray Acrylic Self-Curing Resin 1. When the material is no longer sticky, gather into a ball, knead the material to mix further, and set a small amount aside for the handle.			3		
2. Place the dough-like putty for the maxillary cast. a. Cover the wax spacer. b. Contour and adapt 1 to 2 mm over the wax spacer. c. Complete with a rolled edge at the designated area.			3 3 3		
3. Adapt the handle to a custom tray. (Place a drop of monomer liquid on tray where handle will be placed; it will join better.)			3		
4. Place the handle in the midline area of the arch. (If edentulous, the handle should come up from the ridge, and then outward; with teeth, it can come directly outward.)			3		
5. Place and hold the handle in proper position until the material becomes firm.			3		
Finishing Custom Tray Acrylic Self-Curing Resin 1. Setting will take 8 to 10 minutes. The custom tray can be removed from the cast and the spacer material taken out.			3		
2. Clean the tray. a. If foil is used, it may take only a short time. b. If wax is used, melt and remove it using a wax spatula, hot water, and a toothbrush.			3 3		
3. After the final set (30 minutes minimum), use an acrylic bur or an arbor band to trim the edges of the tray. (Do not trim inside.)			3		

	Self-Evaluation	Student Evaluation	Possible Points	Instructor Evaluation	Comments
4. Clean and disinfect the tray, and write the patient's name on the tray. (Disinfect following manufacturer's directions.)			3		
5. Apply adhesive to the inside of the tray and along the margins. (Adhesive is provided by the manufacturer.)			3		

TOTAL POINTS POSSIBLE   96

TOTAL POINTS POSSIBLE—2nd attempt   94

TOTAL POINTS EARNED   ____

Points assigned reflect importance of step to meeting objective: Important = 1, Essential = 2, Critical = 3. Students will lose 2 points for repeated attempts. Failure results if any of the critical steps are omitted or performed incorrectly. If using a 100-point scale, determine score by dividing points earned by total points possible and multiplying the results by 100.

SCORE: _____

SKILL COMPETENCY ASSESSMENT

35-17 Constructing Vacuum-Formed Acrylic Resin Custom Tray

Student's Name _____ Date _____

Instructor's Name _____

Skill: The dental assistant is responsible for preparing the equipment and supplies. The dentist may ask for a custom tray to be fabricated for the patient to obtain an accurate impression, perhaps because a stock tray does not fit. Several materials are available to make custom trays. A material used for this purpose must be rigid enough so that it does not change shape. It is important that the material adapts well during the construction so that the final tray meets required criteria. Vacuum-formed custom trays require additional equipment; this unit has a frame that holds a sheet directly under a heating element and when the sheet is softened, the frame drops the sheet onto the cast as vacuum pressure draws the material to the model.

Performance Objective: The student will follow a routine procedure that meets the regulations and protocol set forth by the dentist and regulatory agencies, keeping in mind that assistant duties vary from state to state. The assistant may be evaluated by performance criteria, verbal/written responses, and/or combined responses and performance criteria. This procedure is performed by the dental assistant in the dental laboratory on a working cast.

	Self-Evaluation	Student Evaluation	Possible Points	Instructor Evaluation	Comments
Equipment and Supplies					
1. Maxillary and/or mandibular cast			3		
2. Laboratory knife			3		
3. Laboratory scissors			3		
4. Vacuum former with heating element			3		
5. Acrylic sheets			3		
Competency Steps (*follow aseptic procedures*) **Preparing Cast** 1. Soak the cast before forming the custom tray on it (up to 30 minutes before). (Air bubbles are eliminated during heating phase [percolating].)			3		
2. Place the spacer, if indicated. (The wax spacer will melt under heat.)			3		
3. Mark the outer margin of the custom tray.			3		

	Self-Evaluation	Student Evaluation	Possible Points	Instructor Evaluation	Comments
4. Place the cast on the platform of the vacuum-forming unit.			3		
Contouring Acrylic Resin Sheets during Vacuum-Forming Process 1. Select an appropriate acrylic resin sheet for the product.			3		
2. Place acrylic resin sheets between the heater frame and gasket frame; turn the anterior knob tight to secure the material.			3		
3. Ensure the heating element is in the correct place (above acrylic resin sheet), and then turn it on.			3		
4. As resin heats, it will begin to sag downward. Allow it to droop down to about 1 inch. (Over-heating causes air bubbles to form on the surface of the acrylic resin.)			3		
5. After the material is heated properly, take both handles on the frame and pull downward over the cast. (Touch handles only, because the entire area is extremely hot.)			3		
6. Turn on the vacuum immediately after the resin sheet is entirely over the cast.			3		
7. Turn off the heating unit.			3		
8. Allow the vacuum to continue for 1 to 2 minutes. (Allow the resin to cool and become firm again.)			3		
Finishing Vacuum-Formed Acrylic Resin Custom Tray 1. After the resin material is cooled, remove it from the vacuum-form frame.			3		
2. Separate the resin-formed custom tray from the cast and trim to the desired form with laboratory scissors.			3		

	Self-Evaluation	Student Evaluation	Possible Points	Instructor Evaluation	Comments
3. Prepare the cutout handle section to the custom tray (using torch to heat).			3		
4. Clean and disinfect the custom tray according to manufacturer's directions, and write patient's name on tray.			3		

TOTAL POINTS POSSIBLE   63

TOTAL POINTS POSSIBLE—2nd attempt   61

TOTAL POINTS EARNED   ____

Points assigned reflect importance of step to meeting objective: Important = 1, Essential = 2, Critical = 3. Students will lose 2 points for repeated attempts. Failure results if any of the critical steps are omitted or performed incorrectly. If using a 100-point scale, determine score by dividing points earned by total points possible and multiplying the results by 100.

SCORE: _____

SKILL COMPETENCY ASSESSMENT

35-18 Sizing, Adapting, and Seating Aluminum Temporary Crown

Student's Name _____ Date _____

Instructor's Name _____

Skill: The dental assistant is responsible for preparing the equipment and supplies. After a tooth has been prepared for a crown and before seating the crown, a temporary restoration must be adapted and temporarily cemented on the tooth to protect it during the interim. These temporary restorations stabilize and protect the tooth for the period required to make the crown(s) or bridge(s). Temporary restorations, also known as provisional restorations, can be made of a number of materials.

Performance Objective: The student will follow a routine procedure that meets the regulations and protocol set forth by the dentist and regulatory agencies. The assistant may be evaluated by performance criteria, verbal/written responses, and/or combined responses and performance criteria. This procedure is performed by the dentist or the dental assistant at the dental unit after a tooth has been prepared for a crown.

	Self-Evaluation	Student Evaluation	Possible Points	Instructor Evaluation	Comments
Equipment and Supplies					
1. Maxillary and/or mandibular selection of aluminum temporary crowns			3		
2. Millimeter ruler			3		
3. Basic setup: mirror, cotton pliers, and explorer			3		
4. Crown and collar scissors			3		
5. Contouring pliers			3		
6. Acrylic or composite temporary material (optional)			3		
7. Sandpaper discs, rubber wheel, and mandrel			3		
8. Temporary cement, pad, and spatula			3		
9. Articulating paper			3		
10. Dental floss			3		

	Self-Evaluation	Student Evaluation	Possible Points	Instructor Evaluation	Comments
Competency Steps (*follow aseptic procedures*)					
1. Measure the space mesial to distal with a millimeter ruler (aids in selecting the preformed crown).			3		
2. Determine the correct crown to try in. (Any crown tried must be sterilized, so watch so cross-contamination does not take place.)			3		
3. Try the selected crown on, checking the mesial distal width. (The crown will be above the occlusal plane.)			3		
4. Place the aluminum crown over the prepared tooth, using an explorer mark at gingival height. (Indicates the area to be trimmed for fit.)			3		
5. Trim the gingival margin, removing a small amount first. a. Use crown and collar scissors. b. Use rounded edges of the scissors to trim. c. Use continuous cutting action for a smoother surface. d. Avoid taking too much off. e. Take several trims for best fit. f. Avoid sharp, uneven edges.			3 3 3 3 3 3		
6. Once the desired length is achieved, use contouring pliers to invert the gingival edge (called crimping).			3		
7. Smooth rough and jagged edges with sandpaper discs and a rubber wheel. (Smooth and polish all edges.)			3		
8. Place the aluminum crown on the prepared tooth, checking the occlusion with articulating paper and contacts with dental floss. (If a contact is weak, burnish on the inside to extend the crown and get better contact.)			3		

	Self-Evaluation	Student Evaluation	Possible Points	Instructor Evaluation	Comments
9. Use the proper acrylic or composite lining. a. Fill the crown with material. b. Place the crown on the prepared tooth. (The tooth may require light lubricant to avoid material retention.) c. The patient will bite into normal occlusion. d. Allow the material to set, and then remove it. e. Polish away excess material.			3 3 3 3 3		
10. Conduct a final check for marginal fit; contour and occlude before cementation.			3		

TOTAL POINTS POSSIBLE   87

TOTAL POINTS POSSIBLE—2nd attempt   85

TOTAL POINTS EARNED   ____

Points assigned reflect importance of step to meeting objective: Important = 1, Essential = 2, Critical = 3. Students will lose 2 points for repeated attempts. Failure results if any of the critical steps are omitted or performed incorrectly. If using a 100-point scale, determine score by dividing points earned by total points possible and multiplying the results by 100.

SCORE: _____

SKILL COMPETENCY ASSESSMENT

35-19 Cementing Aluminum Crown

Student's Name _____ Date _____

Instructor's Name _____

Skill: The dental assistant is responsible for preparing the equipment and supplies. After a tooth has been prepared for a crown and before seating the crown, a temporary restoration must be adapted and temporarily cemented on the tooth to protect it in the interim. These temporary restorations stabilize and protect the tooth for the period it takes to make the crown(s) or bridge(s). Temporary restorations, also known as provisional restorations, can be made of a number of materials.

Performance Objective: The student will follow a routine procedure that meets the regulations and protocol set forth by the dentist and regulatory agencies. The assistant may be evaluated by performance criteria, verbal/ written responses, and/or combined responses and performance criteria. This procedure is performed by the dentist or the dental assistant at the dental unit after the aluminum crown provisional has been prepared, sized, and contoured to the prepared tooth.

  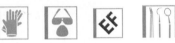

	Self-Evaluation	Student Evaluation	Possible Points	Instructor Evaluation	Comments
Equipment and Supplies					
1. Fitted aluminum temporary			3		
2. Cotton rolls			3		
3. Temporary cementation material			3		
4. Mixing pad			3		
5. Plastic filling instrument			3		
6. Basic setup: mouth mirror, explorer, and cotton pliers			3		
Competency Steps (*follow aseptic procedures*)					
1. Rinse and dry prepared tooth with cotton rolls in place.			3		
2. Mix temporary cementation material with a spatula and place it in the aluminum crown (e.g., zinc oxide eugenol).			3		
3. Place the aluminum crown over the prepared tooth, asking the patient to bite in the occlusion until the cement sets.			3		

	Self-Evaluation	Student Evaluation	Possible Points	Instructor Evaluation	Comments
4. After the cement sets, remove the excess with an explorer.			3		
5. Check contacts with floss, inspect margins, and determine that all excess cement has been removed and that the crown fits correctly.			3		
6. Conduct a final check for an occlusion with articulating paper.			3		
7. Instruct the patient in temporary aluminum crown care.			3		
TOTAL POINTS POSSIBLE			39		
TOTAL POINTS POSSIBLE—2nd attempt			37		
TOTAL POINTS EARNED			____		

Points assigned reflect importance of step to meeting objective: Important = 1, Essential = 2, Critical = 3. Students will lose 2 points for repeated attempts. Failure results if any of the critical steps are omitted or performed incorrectly. If using a 100-point scale, determine score by dividing points earned by total points possible and multiplying the results by 100.

SCORE: _____

SKILL COMPETENCY ASSESSMENT

35-20 Sizing, Adapting, and Seating Preformed Acrylic Crown

Student's Name _____ Date _____

Instructor's Name _____

Skill: The dental assistant is responsible for preparing the equipment and supplies. After a tooth has been prepared for a crown and before the seating of the crown, a temporary restoration must be adapted and temporarily cemented on the tooth to protect it in the interim. These temporary restorations stabilize and protect the tooth for the period required to make the crown(s) or bridge(s). Temporary restorations, also known as provisional restorations, can be made of a number of materials. Preformed acrylic or plastic temporary crowns are available in various sizes, shapes, and shades. The advantage to this type of temporary is that it is more aesthetically pleasing for anterior use. Preformed acrylic crowns are more easily used because they require little adjustment and can be immediately seated.

Performance Objective: The student will follow a routine procedure that meets the regulations and protocol set forth by the dentist and regulatory agencies, keeping in mind that assistant duties vary from state to state. The assistant may be evaluated by performance criteria, verbal/written responses, and/or combined responses and performance criteria. This procedure is performed by the dentist or the dental assistant at the dental unit after the preformed acrylic provisional has been prepared, sized, and contoured to the prepared tooth.

	Self-Evaluation	Student Evaluation	Possible Points	Instructor Evaluation	Comments
Equipment and Supplies					
1. Maxillary and/or mandibular selection of acrylic temporary crowns			3		
2. Basic setup: mouth mirror, cotton pliers, and explorer			3		
3. Acrylic or composite temporary material (optional)			3		
4. Acrylic bur			3		
5. Temporary cement, pad, and spatula			3		
6. Articulating paper			3		
7. Dental floss			3		

	Self-Evaluation	Student Evaluation	Possible Points	Instructor Evaluation	Comments
Competency Steps (*follow aseptic procedures*) **Preparing Preformed Acrylic Temporary Restoration** 1. After the tooth is prepared for the crown, select and adapt a preformed acrylic temporary.			3		
2. Choose a crown for the tooth, ensuring that it is: a. Wide enough to contact adjacent teeth b. Long enough for proper occlusion c. The correct shade			3 3 3		
3. Retrieve the crown without cross-contaminating the other acrylic crowns. (The tab on the incisal edge allows the operator to try the crown over the prepared tooth.)			3		
4. Make adjustments with an acrylic bur, and polish with a rag wheel and pumice. (Adjust as needed for fit.)			3		
5. Take off the tag, place the crown, and check the occlusion with articulating paper.			3		
6. If further adjustments are necessary, make them. Again, polish the adjustment areas for a smooth surface for patient comfort.			3		
Cementing Acrylic Provisional Crown 1. Rinse and dry the prepared tooth with cotton rolls in place.			3		
2. Mix temporary cementation material with a spatula, placing it in the preformed acrylic crown.			3		
3. Place preformed acrylic crown over prepared tooth. Ask the patient to bite in the occlusion until the cement sets (or the operator will hold it in place).			3		

	Self-Evaluation	Student Evaluation	Possible Points	Instructor Evaluation	Comments
4. After the cement sets, remove the excess with an explorer.			3		
5. Check contacts with floss.			3		
a. Inspect all margins to determine whether all excess cement was removed.			3		
b. Ensure that the crown fits correctly.			3		
6. Conduct a final check for occlusion with articulating paper.			3		
7. Instruct the patient in care of the temporary preformed acrylic crown.			3		

TOTAL POINTS POSSIBLE   72

TOTAL POINTS POSSIBLE—2nd attempt   70

TOTAL POINTS EARNED   ____

Points assigned reflect importance of step to meeting objective: Important = 1, Essential = 2, Critical = 3. Students will lose 2 points for repeated attempts. Failure results if any of the critical steps are omitted or performed incorrectly. If using a 100-point scale, determine score by dividing points earned by total points possible and multiplying the results by 100.

SCORE: _____

SKILL COMPETENCY ASSESSMENT

35-21 Adapting, Trimming, and Seating Matrix and Custom Temporary Restoration

Student's Name _____ Date _____

Instructor's Name _____

Skill: The dental assistant is responsible for preparing the equipment and supplies. After a tooth has been prepared for a crown and prior to the seating of the crown, a temporary restoration must be adapted and temporarily cemented on the tooth to protect it in the interim. These temporary restorations stabilize and protect the tooth for the period required to make the crown(s) or bridge(s). Temporary restorations, also known as provisional restorations, can be made of a number of materials. In making custom acrylic or composite temporary restorations, a matrix is used. A custom acrylic or composite temporary restoration must have good proximal contacts, occlusal contacts, food deflection, and marginal contours.

Performance Objective: The student will follow a routine procedure that meets the regulations and protocol set forth by the dentist and regulatory agencies, keeping in mind that assistant duties vary from state to state. The assistant may be evaluated by performance criteria, verbal/written responses, and/or combined responses and performance criteria. This procedure is performed by the dentist or the dental assistant at the dental unit after the tooth has been prepared for a crown.

	Self-Evaluation	Student Evaluation	Possible Points	Instructor Evaluation	Comments
Equipment and Supplies					
1. Basic setup: mouth mirror, cotton pliers, and explorer			3		
2. Thermoplastic buttons/hot water (one option to make matrix)			3		
3. Composite temporary material			3		
4. Diamond bur			3		
5. Temporary cement, pad, and spatula			3		
6. Articulating paper			3		
7. Dental floss			3		

	Self-Evaluation	Student Evaluation	Possible Points	Instructor Evaluation	Comments
Competency Steps (*follow aseptic procedures*)					
Making Thermo-Forming Matrix before Tooth Preparation					
1. Place thermo-forming matrix buttons in hot water (one per tooth).			3		
2. Allow the white color of the button to clear. (Transparency indicates that the material is pliable and can be adapted.)			3		
3. Adapt the material over the tooth to be prepared and tightly conform it to the tooth area and slightly below gingival.			3		
4. When the material cools, the matrix will appear white and firm. (Use air to make this more rapid if needed.)			3		
5. Remove the matrix from the area and set it aside.			3		
Preparing Custom Temporary Restoration					
1. After the tooth has been prepared for the crown, coat the teeth lightly with petroleum jelly.			3		
2. Dispense self-curing material onto a paper pad by holding tubes at a 45-degree angle. (This applies to composite self-curing temporary material in two tubes.)			3		

	Self-Evaluation	Student Evaluation	Possible Points	Instructor Evaluation	Comments
3. Method of dispensing: a. The larger of the two tubes is the base; rotate the end-dispensing handle until a click is heard.			3		
b. The smaller of the two holds the catalyst and has two dispensing ends; rotate the end-dispensing handle and two small amounts will be expelled.			3		
c. Dispense both tubes. (One tube has two small tips that will each click enough material for one temporary.)			3		
4. If shade is being used, mix it with the base before bringing materials together. (If a mottled effect is desired, mix shade after base and catalyst are mixed together.)			3		
5. Mix the material to obtain a creamy substance (about 30 seconds).			3		
6. Place the material into the matrix.			3		
7. Place the matrix over the prepared tooth (manipulation time is 1 1/2 minutes).			3		
8. Hold in place for 2 minutes in the mouth.			3		
9. Remove from the mouth and set aside for 2 minutes.			3		
10. Remove material from the matrix (crown or bridge).			3		

	Self-Evaluation	Student Evaluation	Possible Points	Instructor Evaluation	Comments
11. Additional curing time will take 1 minute.			3		
12. Allow 7 minutes total from start to finish of set.			3		
13. Remove the greasy layer with alcohol or any other solvent.			3		
14. Trim with a diamond or an acrylic bur.			3		
15. Check contacts with floss.			3		
16. Check the occlusion with articulating paper and by having patient bite the same.			3		
17. Check the margins with an explorer and a mirror.			3		

TOTAL POINTS POSSIBLE   93

TOTAL POINTS POSSIBLE—2nd attempt   91

TOTAL POINTS EARNED   _____

Points assigned reflect importance of step to meeting objective: Important = 1, Essential = 2, Critical = 3. Students will lose 2 points for repeated attempts. Failure results if any of the critical steps are omitted or performed incorrectly. If using a 100-point scale, determine score by dividing points earned by total points possible and multiplying the results by 100.

SCORE: _____

SKILL COMPETENCY ASSESSMENT

35-22 Preparing a Full Crown Provisional on a Lower Left Molar

Student's Name _____ Date _____

Instructor's Name _____

Skill: The dental assistant is responsible for preparing the equipment and supplies. After a tooth has been prepared for a crown and prior to the seating of the crown, a temporary restoration must be adapted and temporarily cemented on the tooth to protect it in the interim. These temporary restorations stabilize and protect the tooth for the period required to make the crown(s) or bridge(s). Temporary restorations, also known as provisional restorations, can be made of a number of materials. In making custom acrylic or composite temporary restorations, a matrix is used. A custom acrylic or composite temporary restoration must have good proximal contacts, occlusal contacts, food deflection, and marginal contours.

Performance Objective: The student will follow a routine procedure that meets the regulations and protocol set forth by the dentist and regulatory agencies, keeping in mind that assistant duties vary from state to state. The assistant may be evaluated by performance criteria, verbal/written responses, and/or combined responses and performance criteria. This procedure is performed by the dental assistant under the general supervision of the dentist most often. It also can be done by the dentist with the auxiliary assisting.

	Self-Evaluation	Student Evaluation	Possible Points	Instructor Evaluation	Comments
Equipment and Supplies					
1. Basic setup: mouth mirror, cotton pliers, and explorer			3		
2. Impression material for matrix			3		
3. Triple tray for matrix			3		
4. Composite temporary material			3		
5. Diamond bur			3		
6. Articulating paper			3		
7. Dental floss			3		
Competency Steps (*follow aseptic procedures*)					
1. Assemble equipment and supplies and explain the procedure to the patient.			3		
2. Examine the tooth.			3		

3. Use the impression material and triple tray to make a matrix for the temporary. Place the material in the patient's mouth and instruct to close lightly until it sets.			3	
4. Remove from mouth when it is set.			3	
5. Fill the impression matrix 2/3rds full with the composite material.			3	
6. Place the matrix with the impression material back in the patient's mouth over the prepared tooth and allow to set.				
7. Once set remove the matrix.			3	
8. Mark the contact point and trim with a diamond bur.			3	
9. Check contacts and occlusion			3	

TOTAL POINTS POSSIBLE   45

TOTAL POINTS POSSIBLE—2nd attempt   43

TOTAL POINTS EARNED   ____

Points assigned reflect importance of step to meeting objective: Important = 1, Essential = 2, Critical = 3. Students will lose 2 points for repeated attempts. Failure results if any of the critical steps are omitted or performed incorrectly. If using a 100-point scale, determine score by dividing points earned by total points possible and multiplying the results by 100.

SCORE: _____

SKILL COMPETENCY ASSESSMENT

35-23 Cementing Custom Self-Curing Composite Temporary Crown

Student's Name _____ Date _____

Instructor's Name _____

Skill: The dental assistant is responsible for preparing the equipment and supplies. After a tooth has been prepared for a crown and prior to the seating of the crown, a temporary restoration must be adapted and temporarily cemented on the tooth to protect it in the interim. These temporary restorations stabilize and protect the tooth for the period required to make the crown(s) or bridge(s). Temporary restorations, also known as provisional restorations, can be made of a number of materials.

Performance Objective: The student will follow a routine procedure that meets the regulations and protocol set forth by the dentist and regulatory agencies, keeping in mind that assistant duties vary from state to state. The assistant may be evaluated by performance criteria, verbal/written responses, and/or combined responses and performance criteria. This procedure is performed by the dentist or the dental assistant at the dental unit after the temporary restoration has been prepared and is ready to be cemented.

	Self-Evaluation	Student Evaluation	Possible Points	Instructor Evaluation	Comments
Equipment and Supplies					
1. Basic setup: mouth mirror, cotton pliers, and explorer			3		
2. Cotton rolls			3		
3. Temporary luting cement			3		
4. Paper pad			3		
5. Mixing spatula			3		
6. Plastic filling instrument			3		
7. Dental floss			3		
Competency Steps (*follow aseptic procedures*)					
1. Rinse and dry the prepared tooth with cotton rolls in place.			3		
2. Mix temporary cement material with a spatula and place into custom composite temporary crown.			3		
3. Place the temporary crown over the prepared tooth. Ask the patient to bite in the occlusion until the cement sets.			3		

	Self-Evaluation	Student Evaluation	Possible Points	Instructor Evaluation	Comments
4. After the cement sets, remove excess with an explorer.			3		
5. Check contacts with floss, inspect margins, and determine that all excess cement has been removed and that the crown fits correctly.			3		
6. Conduct a final check for occlusion with articulating paper.			3		
7. Instruct the patient in care of the custom composite temporary crown.			3		

TOTAL POINTS POSSIBLE   42

TOTAL POINTS POSSIBLE—2nd attempt   40

TOTAL POINTS EARNED   ____

Points assigned reflect importance of step-to meeting objective: Important = 1, Essential = 2, Critical = 3. Students will lose 2 points for repeated attempts. Failure results if any of the critical steps are omitted or performed incorrectly. If using a 100-point scale, determine score by dividing points earned by total points possible and multiplying the results by 100.

SCORE: _____

Dental Practice Management

Dental Office Management

SPECIFIC INSTRUCTIONAL OBJECTIVES

The student should strive to meet the following objectives and demonstrate an understanding of the facts and principles presented in this chapter:

1. Identify the dental office staff and their areas of responsibility.

2. Identify marketing ideas for dentistry.

3. Outline the proper procedure for answering an incoming call.

4. Describe the information every message should contain.

5. Describe telephone and business office technology and its uses.

6. Give examples of the ways in which computers are used in the dental office.

7. Explain how database management concepts can be used in the dental office.

8. Explain why ergonomics is important at a computer workstation.

9. Explain ways in which effective patient scheduling can be accomplished in the dental office.

10. Identify the equipment needed for record management.

11. Define key terms related to accounts receivable.

12. Identify computerized and manual systems for management of patient accounts.

13. Identify accounts payable expenses that the dental practice is responsible for.

SUMMARY

The dental reception area must be an environment in which all patients feel welcome and comfortable. Today, dentistry can be a positive experience, and dental treatment can be pain free. That image is developed when the patient first steps into the reception area.

Patients may not consciously realize the message that is being received, but the dental office should present an atmosphere that relieves anxiety.

Front office staff has changed dramatically in recent years. All individuals in the front office require

718

knowledge of business machines such as computers, fax machines, and copy machines. These individuals must be organized, have knowledge of dental treatments, and have good communication and problem-solving skills.

Marketing is also an important part of the dental practice. A dental office is a business as well as a health care facility. Dental assistants, along with all members of the dental team, need to be involved in marketing the practice.

EXERCISES AND ACTIVITIES

Multiple Choice

1. This act that Congress passed mandates that health care facilities with more than 15 employees must be accessible to individuals with disabilities.

   a. External Marketing Act
   b. Ergonomics Consultant Act
   c. On-sight Technology Education Services Act
   d. Americans with Disabilities Act

2. Which accounting term indicates the money owed to a practice?

   a. Accounts payable
   b. Accounts receivable
   c. Inventory
   d. Nonexpendable

3. Which accounting term indicates the amount a practice owes to others?

   a. Gross income
   b. Accounts payable
   c. Accounts receivable
   d. Petty cash

4. Which of the following items is not part of a computer function?

   a. Spreadsheet
   b. Word processing
   c. Cellular phone
   d. Database management

5. The computer program or set of instructions that tells the hardware what to do is called the

   a. hardware.
   b. software.
   c. facsimile.
   d. tickler file.

6. The goal of the receptionist is to fill the appointment book with patient care. Any time in the appointment book that is not scheduled is called

   a. downtime.
   b. overtime.
   c. overlap time.
   d. tickler file.

7. In scheduling, when patient treatment time goes beyond the estimated time frame, it is called

   a. downtime.
   b. overtime.
   c. overlap time.
   d. tickler file.

8. _____ occurs when the dentist or auxiliary is required to be in two places at the same time.

   a. Downtime
   b. Overtime
   c. Time overlap
   d. Tickler time

9. In a well-organized office, the _____ file serves as a reminder of future actions that need to be taken.

   a. recall
   b. facsimile
   c. tickler
   d. archival

10. A fee schedule is used to define what patients will be charged for a particular service. It is called the

    a. professional courtesy.
    b. usual, reasonable, and customary fee.
    c. insurance.
    d. record management.

11. When you subtract the accounts payable from gross income, the result is the

    a. overhead.
    b. net income.

    c. gross income.
    d. petty cash.

12. There are several inventory record systems that can be used to track supplies. Supplies that are retained in the office for long periods of time are called

    a. nonexpendable.
    b. expendable.

    c. shelf life.
    d. variable.

13. When supplies are shipped, the supplier encloses a list of included items. When receiving supplies, you will check this list and note any discrepancies. This list is called a

    a. statement.
    b. credit slip.

    c. back-order slip.
    d. packing slip.

14. As a part of accounts payable, this record reflects all deposits and checks made from the account and is called the

    a. bank statement.
    b. check register.

    c. payroll.
    d. credit slip.

15. Which of the following are basic telephone techniques?

    1. Enunciate, speak clearly, and articulate carefully.
    2. State who the message is for.
    3. Speak at a normal rate of speed.
    4. Ask what action is required.
    5. Use telephone etiquette (good manners).
    6. Record the date and time of the call.
       a. 1, 2, 6
       b. 1, 3, 6

       c. 1, 3, 5
       d. 1, 4, 6

16. As part of the office's business equipment, answering systems may include which of the following features?

    1. Voice mail
    2. E-mail
    3. Word processing
    4. Fax
    5. Graphics
    6. Database management
       a. 3, 4, 6
       b. 1, 2, 6

       c. 2, 3, 4
       d. 1, 2, 4

17. Total accounts receivable are calculated as _____ income.

    a. gross
    b. net

    c. deductible
    d. expendable

18. _____ requires that the sender receives a confirmation of delivery.

    a. Collect on delivery
    b. Delivery confirmation

    c. Insured mail
    d. Certified mail

19. The _____ codes, which are used for dental insurance purposes, are published under the jurisdiction of the American Dental Association.

    a. COD
    b. USPS

    c. CDT
    d. TDI

20. The individual who has dental insurance through his or her employment is called the

    a. subscriber.
    b. beneficiary.

    c. carrier.
    d. dependent.

21. The employer prepares a W-2 form for each employee by _____ of every year.

    a. December 31
    b. January 1

    c. January 31
    d. None of the above

22. Which of the following are included in the W-2 statement?

    a. Number of sick days
    b. Total wages earned

    c. Taxes deducted for the year
    d. b. and c.

23. Reconciling a bank statement includes all of the following *except*

    a. checking off each check listed on the bank statement against the checkbook.
    b. checking off each deposit.

    c. names written on each check deposited.
    d. listing all checks from the checkbook that have not cleared.

24. The Federal Insurance Contribution Act is commonly known as

    a. benefit-less-benefit.
    b. HIPPA.

    c. TILA.
    d. Social Security.

25. What newer technology is being used with more frequency to keep employees updated on training and trends in the dental field?

    a. Dentrix
    b. CAD/CAM systems

    c. Computed Tomography
    d. Web conferencing

Matching

Inventory control is effective when using an expendable and nonexpendable inventory supply system. Match each term with its description.

Term	Description
1. _d_ Price break	a. Length of time that product can be stored
2. _c_ Rate of use	b. Ensures that adequate supply is available
3. _b_ Reorder point	c. How much product is used in a specific period
4. _a_ Shelf life	d. Minimum quantity of supply at which the per unit cost is reduced

Critical Thinking

1. Advances in telecommunications have had a tremendous impact on dental office communication systems. List telecommunication technologies that are likely to be used in the dental office.

2. Computers reduce the time involved in many routine office procedures. Once the dental assistant becomes familiar with the computer and its software and applications, she or he will find more and more uses for the computer. Describe computer safety, ergonomics, and eye care.

3. Dental coverage and benefits available to patients become more complex over time. Describe managed care plans and capitation programs.

4. An understanding of dental insurance terminology is critical when filing claims. Explain the birthday rule, benefit-less-benefit, and coordination of benefits (COB).

CASE STUDY 1

Sally is a new patient who was referred to the office by a friend. Her friend was impressed by the warm and friendly (physical and interpersonal) environment.

1. Describe how dental office environments have changed over the past 30 years.

2. Explain such environmental changes.

3. List the front office staff members, and describe how their roles have changed.

4. Describe dentistry marketing strategies used to attract patients.

CASE STUDY 2

Accurate dental record management is essential for quality patient care in any dental office. Patients have the right to expect confidential treatment and record-keeping.

1. Describe equipment and supplies needed for record management.

2. Describe the patient chart filing system.

3. Explain the record confidentiality policy.

4. Describe archival storage of records.

CASE STUDY 3

Some patients will experience financial difficulties. The dentist must provide guidelines for business office employees on when and how to contact patients with past-due accounts.

1. Describe the Fair Debt Collection Practice Act.

2. Describe effective ways to contact debtors.

3. List types of dental service payments.

4. Explain when collection letters are initiated.

SKILL COMPETENCY ASSESSMENT

36-1 Preparing for the Day's Patients

Student's Name _____ Date _____

Instructor's Name _____

Skill: The dental receptionist is responsible for preparing the schedule. This schedule allows for the clinical staff to be able to plan and set up for upcoming patients. Any changes throughout the day are recorded on the daily schedule.

Performance Objective: The student will follow a routine procedure that meets the protocol set forth by the dentist and office staff. The assistant may be evaluated by performance criteria, verbal/written responses, and/or combined responses and performance criteria. This procedure is performed by the receptionist in preparation for the upcoming day.

	Self-Evaluation	Student Evaluation	Possible Points	Instructor Evaluation	Comments
Equipment and Supplies					
1. Files			3		
2. Patient charts			3		
3. Computer with word processor			3		
4. Telephone			3		
Competency Steps **Day Before** 1. The dental receptionist pulls charts for patients for the next day.			3		
2. Needed laboratory work is checked to ensure that it is ready.			3		
3. All patient appointments will be confirmed via a telephone call.			3		
4. Records will be revieed for any special concerns.			3		
5. Patient account balances can be reviewed, and notations made on charts.			3		
6. Any premedications will be identified and noted.			3		
7. A daily schedule is typed.			3		

	Self-Evaluation	Student Evaluation	Possible Points	Instructor Evaluation	Comments
8. Copies of daily schedule made (enough for entire back treatment area).			2		
9. Daily schedule posted in appropriate areas after current schedule is completed for the day.			2		
Day of Appointment 1. Meet briefly with staff in morning to examine schedule (5 minutes or less).			3		
2. Meeting allows staff to dialog about any treatment or patient concerns that may transpire during the day.			3		
3. Charts are ready for dental assistants as they seat patients.			2		
4. Patients are greeted and seated in dental treatment rooms by dental team.			3		

TOTAL POINTS POSSIBLE   48

TOTAL POINTS POSSIBLE—2nd attempt   46

TOTAL POINTS EARNED   ____

Points assigned reflect importance of step to meeting objective: Important = 1, Essential = 2, Critical = 3. Students will lose 2 points for repeated attempts. Failure results if any of the critical steps are omitted or performed incorrectly. If using a 100-point scale, determine score by dividing points earned by total points possible and multiplying the results by 100.

SCORE: _____

SKILL COMPETENCY ASSESSMENT

36-2 Day Sheet Preparation for Posting

Student's Name _____ Date _____

Instructor's Name _____

Skill: The dental receptionist or the office business assistant is responsible for all transactions and maintaining accurate records. The day sheets record every charge, payment, and adjustment for the day. All transactions must be written legibly and accurately. The day sheets consist of five sections with the first three for posting and the last two for balancing.

Performance Objective: The student will follow a routine procedure that meets the protocol set forth by the dentist and office staff. The assistance may be evaluated by performance criteria, verbal/written responses, and/or combined responses and performance criteria. The dental receptionist or office business assistant performs this task and prepares the day sheet prior to arrival of the first patient.

	Self-Evaluation	Student Evaluation	Possible Points	Instructor Evaluation	Comments
Equipment and Supplies 1. Pegboard			3		
2. New day sheet			3		
3. Block of new charge slips and receipt forms			3		
4. Ledger cards for all patients scheduled that day (or ledger card file placed close by)			3		
Competency Steps 1. Place day sheet on pegboard.			3		
2. Attach charge and receipt slips on first corresponding line.			3		
3. At top of day sheet fill in date and page number.			3		
4. Transfer information from previous page: fill in previous day's totals from columns A–D and write in place at bottom of day sheet under "previous page."			3		

	Self-Evaluation	Student Evaluation	Possible Points	Instructor Evaluation	Comments
5. Prepare ledger cards for patients scheduled that day by pulling or tabbing them, or having the storage file close by.			3		

TOTAL POINTS POSSIBLE 27

TOTAL POINTS POSSIBLE—2nd attempt 25

TOTAL POINTS EARNED ____

Points assigned reflect importance of step to meeting objective: Important = 1, Essential = 2, Critical = 3. Students will lose 2 points for repeated attempts. Failure results if any of the critical steps are omitted or performed incorrectly. If using a 100-point scale, determine score by dividing points earned by total points possible and multiplying the results by 100.

SCORE: _____

SKILL COMPETENCY ASSESSMENT

36-3 Posting Charges and Payments on Pegboard

Student's Name _____ Date _____

Instructor's Name _____

Skill: Accounts receivable encompass money owed to the practice. The bookkeeping in this area must be accurate and carries with it a great responsibility. This position may be occupied by the receptionist or the business assistant. All transactions, payments, adjustments, and charges must be handled in a safe and professional manner.

Performance Objective: The student will follow a routine procedure that meets the protocol set forth by the dentist and office staff. The assistant may be evaluated by performance criteria, verbal/written responses, and/or combined responses and performance criteria. The dental receptionist or office business assistant performs this task during or at the end of each day.

	Self-Evaluation	Student Evaluation	Possible Points	Instructor Evaluation	Comments
Equipment and Supplies					
1. Pegboard			3		
2. New day sheet			3		
3. Block of new charge slips and receipt forms			3		
4. Ledger cards for all patients scheduled that day (or ledger card file placed close by)			3		
Competency Steps **When the patient enters the dental office for a scheduled appointment:** 1. Place patient's ledger under the next charge sheet and corresponding line on pegboard.			3		
2. Write in date, responsible party's name, patient's name, and previous balance, if any, in spaces provided for each charge and receipt sheet (information will automatically copy onto ledger card and pegboard day sheet).			3		
3. Remove charge sheet from pegboard and clip it to outside of patient's chart. (Chart is ready for dental auxiliary and dentist to use during treatment.)			3		

	Self-Evaluation	Student Evaluation	Possible Points	Instructor Evaluation	Comments
4. Chart is given to patient to take to reception area or brought to reception area by auxiliary. (The dentist or auxiliary will complete chart and charge sheet prior to dismissing patient.)			3		
After the patient is dismissed and returned to the reception area: 1. Replace charge slip on pegboard aligned with patient's name, and insert patient's ledger card back into place under charge slip on pegboard.			3		
2. Enter charges and payments in designated spaces in section one.			3		
3. The final balance for patient is totaled by adding previous balance with new charges and subtracting any payment patient made.			3		
4. Place final charge in column "C." *Note:* column "D" previous balance, "A" charges, "B-1" payments, "B-2" adjustments.			3		
5. Proof of posting at bottom on day sheet indicates procedure to be used for each entry as well as entire day sheet. a. Column D total b. Plus Column A total c. Subtotal d. Less (subtract) Columns B-1 and B-2 e. Must equal Column C			3 3 3 3 3		
6. When posting is completed, first copy of charge slip goes in patient's chart.			2		
7. Second copy can be given to patient for purpose of payment and patient's records.			3		

	Self-Evaluation	Student Evaluation	Possible Points	Instructor Evaluation	Comments
8. Final copy can be used for submission for insurance reimbursement.			3		

TOTAL POINTS POSSIBLE   59

TOTAL POINTS POSSIBLE—2nd attempt   57

TOTAL POINTS EARNED   ____

Points assigned reflect importance of step to meeting objective: Important = 1, Essential = 2, Critical = 3. Students will lose 2 points for repeated attempts. Failure results if any of the critical steps are omitted or performed incorrectly. If using a 100-point scale, determine score by dividing points earned by total points possible and multiplying the results by 100.

SCORE: _____

SKILL COMPETENCY ASSESSMENT

36-4 Balancing Day Sheets and End-of-the-Month Figures

Student's Name _____ Date _____

Instructor's Name _____

Skill: The accounts receivable of the dental office encompasses the money owed to the practice. Bookkeeping in this area must be accurate and carries with it a great responsibility. This position may be occupied by the receptionist or the business assistant. All transactions, payments, adjustments, and charges must be handled safely and professionally.

Performance Objective: The student will follow a routine procedure that meets the protocol set forth by the dentist and office staff. The assistant may be evaluated by performance criteria, verbal/written responses, and/or combined responses and performance criteria. The dental receptionist or office business assistant balances the day sheets daily and totals the day sheets at the end of the month or before patient statements are sent out.

	Self-Evaluation	Student Evaluation	Possible Points	Instructor Evaluation	Comments
Equipment and Supplies					
1. Pegboard			3		
2. Day sheets totaled for month			3		
3. Ledger cards for all patients in storage file			3		
4. Calculator with tape that records entries			3		
Competency Steps					
1. Total each column and place the total in the spaces at bottom of the page in "Totals this page" (this section is identified as Section 4).			3		
2. Add column totals to "Previous page" totals and place number in "Month to Date" total spaces.			3		
3. Verify totals in the "Proof of Posting" box in Section 5 (where the total of Column D is added to the total of Column A and subtotaled). Final amount must equal Column C.			3		

	Self-Evaluation	Student Evaluation	Possible Points	Instructor Evaluation	Comments
4. Once proof of posting is complete, total accounts receivable column.					
a. Add the total of Column A to the previous day's total.			3		
b. Subtract Columns Bl and B2 from the subtotaled amount of A + D.			3		
c. Identify the true balance of accounts receivable.			3		
			3		
5. Total the amounts owed on the ledger cards (use tape for verification).			3		
6. If the total of the ledger cards balances with the total on the day sheet, accounts receivable is balanced. If it is not balanced, recheck figures and find any missing or inaccurate amount.			3		
7. Send out statements, after accounts receivable balance.			3		

TOTAL POINTS POSSIBLE   42

TOTAL POINTS POSSIBLE—2nd attempt   40

TOTAL POINTS EARNED   ____

Points assigned reflect importance of step to meeting the objective. Important = 1, Essential = 2, Critical = 3. Students will lose 2 points for repeated attempts. Failure results if any of the critical steps are omitted or performed incorrectly. If using a 100-point scale, determine score by dividing points earned by total points possible and multiplying the results by 100.

SCORE: _____

SKILL COMPETENCY ASSESSMENT

36-5 Preparing a Deposit Slip

Student's Name _____ Date _____

Instructor's Name _____

Skill: The dental receptionist or the office business assistant is responsible for promptly recording payments on the ledgers and in the bookkeeping system. Totals are deposited in the bank daily.

Performance Objective: The student will follow a routine procedure that meets the protocol set forth by the dentist and office staff. The assistant may be evaluated by performance criteria, verbal/written responses, and/or combined responses and performance criteria. The dental receptionist or office business assistant fills out the deposit slip and either takes it to the bank or the dentist takes it to the bank to be deposited. Deposits are normally made in person or placed in the night deposit box/slot.

	Self-Evaluation	Student Evaluation	Possible Points	Instructor Evaluation	Comments
Equipment and Supplies					
1. Deposit slip			3		
2. Cash and checks received for that day			3		
3. Office stamp for endorsing checks			3		
4. Envelope in which to place the deposit slip, checks, and cash			3		
Competency Steps					
1. Place the date on the deposit slip.			3		
2. Separate currency (coins, paper money) from checks.			3		
3. Tally the coins, placing the sum in the designated space on the deposit slip.			3		
4. Tally the paper money, placing the sum in the designated space on the deposit slip.			3		
5. On the back of the deposit slip, list each check separately, with the patient's last name and the amount of the check in the space provided in the right-hand column.			3		

	Self-Evaluation	Student Evaluation	Possible Points	Instructor Evaluation	Comments
6. Total the list amounts from the checks on the back of the deposit slip and place this sum in the area on the front of the check slip in the space identified for checks.			3		
7. Total the currency (coins and paper money) and check the amount. Place this sum at the bottom of the deposit slip under the total (the amount should total the total identified on the payments column on the day sheet; one other way to further check that the total is accurate is to add the coins, paper money, and each check—this verifies the sum).			3		
8. Enter the date and the amount of the deposit on the checkbook stub.			3		

TOTAL POINTS POSSIBLE   36

TOTAL POINTS POSSIBLE—2nd attempt   34

TOTAL POINTS EARNED   ____

Points assigned reflect importance of step to meeting the objective: Important = 1, Essential = 2, Critical = 3. Students will lose 2 points for repeated attempts. Failure results if any of the critical steps are omitted or performed incorrectly. If using a 100-point scale, determine score by dividing points earned by total points possible and multiplying the results by 100.

SCORE: _____

SKILL COMPETENCY ASSESSMENT

36-6 Reordering Supplies

Student's Name _____ Date _____

Instructor's Name _____

Skill: The reordering point ensures that an adequate supply is available taking into consideration the lead time and the rate of product use. Several inventory records systems can be used in the dental office to track supplies. The goal of any system is that supplies are available when needed.

Performance Objective: The student will follow a routine procedure that meets the protocol set forth by the dentist and office staff. The assistant may be evaluated by performance criteria, verbal/written responses, and/ or combined responses and performance criteria. The dental assistant may be assigned specifically to order supplies, or this task may be shared by several auxiliaries.

	Self-Evaluation	Student Evaluation	Possible Points	Instructor Evaluation	Comments
Equipment and Supplies **Red Flag Reorder Tag System** 1. Red flag reorder tags that have surfaced for reordering			3		
2. Telephone			3		
3. Index card with order information			3		
Electronic Barcode System 1. Barcode wand			3		
2. Telephone			3		
Competency Steps **Red Flag Reorder Tag System** 1. Gather red flags that indicate which items require reordering.			3		
2. Check the index card to obtain ordering information for each item.			3		
3. Place an indicator in the upper-right corner to indicate that this item is to be ordered immediately.			3		
4. After the item is ordered, place an indicator in the upper-left corner until the product arrives.			3		

	Self-Evaluation	Student Evaluation	Possible Points	Instructor Evaluation	Comments
5. When the item arrives, remove the indicator from the tag.			3		
6. Place the most recently received items to back of supply (use older materials first).			3		
7. Place the red flag ordering tag on the minimum quantity needed in stock before reordering.			3		
Electronic Bar Code System 1. Identify items that require reordering. (This system is used for commonly ordered items.)			3		
2. Obtain the book with product information and barcodes.			3		
3. Use a barcode wand to input needed items. Run the wand over the barcodes of needed items.			3		
4. Indicate on the transmitter the number of items needed. (The order is then transmitted directly to the dental supply company for ordering.)			3		
5. Place date on listed items and indicate the number that has been ordered.			3		

TOTAL POINTS POSSIBLE   51

TOTAL POINTS POSSIBLE—2nd attempt   49

TOTAL POINTS EARNED   _____

Points assigned reflect importance of step to meeting objective: Important = 1, Essential = 2, Critical = 3. Students will lose 2 points for repeated attempts. Failure results if any of the critical steps are omitted or performed incorrectly. If using a 100-point scale, determine score by dividing points earned by total points possible and multiplying the results by 100.

SCORE: _____

SKILL COMPETENCY ASSESSMENT

36-7 Reconciling a Bank Statement

Student's Name _____ Date _____

Instructor's Name _____

Skill: Each month the bank sends a statement showing transactions that took place on the account during the month. It lists all checks that have cleared the bank, deposits received by the bank, and service charges deducted from the account. It should be reconciled against entries made in the dental office check register.

Performance Objective: The student will follow a routine procedure that meets the protocol set forth by the dentist and office staff. The assistant may be evaluated by performance criteria, verbal/written responses, and/or combined responses and performance criteria. The dental receptionist or business assistant will reconcile the bank statement each month.

	Self-Evaluation	Student Evaluation	Possible Points	Instructor Evaluation	Comments
Equipment and Supplies					
1. Bank statement			3		
2. Checkbook			3		
3. Calculator			3		
Competency Steps					
1. Make sure that all checks and deposits have been added or subtracted from the checkbook.			3		
2. Subtract bank service charges from the last balance listed in checkbook.			3		
3. Check each check in the bank statement against the checkbook and verify the listed amount.			3		
4. Check each deposit in the bank statement against the checkbook and verify the listed amount.			3		
5. On the back of the bank statement, place the ending balance from the front of the statement in the ending balance space on the worksheet.			3		
6. List all checks from the checkbook that have not cleared the bank in the section on the back of the worksheet.			3		

	Self-Evaluation	Student Evaluation	Possible Points	Instructor Evaluation	Comments
7. List all deposits from the checkbook that have not been received by the bank on the space on the worksheet on the back of the statement.			3		
8. Total checks not cleared and deposits not received.			3		
9. Subtract checks not received from the ending balance on the bank statement.			3		
10. Add deposits not received to the ending balance on the bank statement.			3		
11. The balance should agree with the checkbook balance. (If bank charges are on statement, make corresponding adjustments to the checkbook balance.)			3		

TOTAL POINTS POSSIBLE   42

TOTAL POINTS POSSIBLE—2nd attempt   40

TOTAL POINTS EARNED   ____

Points assigned reflect importance of step to meeting objective: Important = 1, Essential = 2, Critical = 3. Students will lose 2 points for repeated attempts. Failure results if any of the critical steps are omitted or performed incorrectly. If using a 100-point scale, determine score by dividing points earned by total points possible and multiplying the results by 100.

SCORE: _____

SKILL COMPETENCY ASSESSMENT

36-8 Writing a Business Check

Student's Name _____ Date _____

Instructor's Name _____

Skill: Accounts payable is the amount of money that the practice owes others, including necessary expenses.

Performance Objective: The student will follow a routine procedure that meets the protocol set forth by the dentist and office staff. The assistant may be evaluated by performance criteria, oral/written responses, and/or combined responses and performance criteria. The dental receptionist or business assistant writes a check out of the office accounts payable for the dentist to review and sign.

	Self-Evaluation	Student Evaluation	Possible Points	Instructor Evaluation	Comments
Equipment and Supplies 1. Checkbook with check and stub			3		
2. Calculator			3		
Competency Steps 1. Write or type in date, making sure that the date is current.			3		
2. Write or type in the name of the payee, verifying that this is the correct payee.			3		
3. Write in correct numbers for correct amount.			3		
4. Write amount in designated area.			3		
5. Check that numerical and written amounts agree and are correct.			3		
6. Fill out memo, indicating what check is for.			3		
7. Fill out date, payee, memo information, and amount on the check stub.			3		
8. Verify that everything is accurate and spelling is correct.			3		

	Self-Evaluation	Student Evaluation	Possible Points	Instructor Evaluation	Comments
9. Have the dentist sign on the signature line after reviewing accounts payable.			3		

TOTAL POINTS POSSIBLE   33

TOTAL POINTS POSSIBLE—2nd attempt   31

TOTAL POINTS EARNED   ____

Points assigned reflect importance of step to meeting objective: Important = 1, Essential = 2, Critical = 3. Students will lose 2 points for repeated attempts. Failure results if any of the critical steps are omitted or performed incorrectly. If using a 100-point scale, determine score by dividing points earned by total points possible and multiplying the results by 100.

SCORE: _____

Employment Strategies

SPECIFIC INSTRUCTIONAL OBJECTIVES

The student should strive to meet the following objectives and demonstrate an understanding of the facts and principles presented in this chapter:

1. Identify three pathways to obtain DANB certification.

2. Explain how to obtain employment and identify types of practices.

3. Set goals and identify sources to obtain employment in the dental field.

4. Identify the steps in preparing a cover letter and résumé.

5. Define how to prepare for the interview.

6. Explain the interview process and identify skills and preparation techniques that will aid in obtaining the job.

7. Identify the skills that a successful dental assistant possesses.

8. Explain how to terminate employment.

SUMMARY

It is important to find employment that will best suit individual needs and that allows for the best possible situation for the dental assistant, employer, and patients. Before taking the first position available, plan ahead. It may be essential to obtain dental assisting national certification for the state in which employment is sought. National certification for dental assistants is not mandatory in every state, but it assures the patients and the dentist that the assistant has the basic knowledge and background to perform as a professional on the dental team. Make sure that the expectations of the job are identified and then try to meet and exceed them if planning to advance. Each dental assistant is responsible for maintaining a positive attitude at work. Set goals to learn new skills and stay abreast of changes in technology and materials. A dental assisting career is very rewarding, both professionally and personally. Be the best dental assistant possible.

EXERCISES AND ACTIVITIES

Multiple Choice

1. A dentist may hire another dentist under a contractual agreement. This hired dentist is called a dental

   a. partner.

   b. solo.

   c. associate.

   d. group.

2. Any number of dentists (both general and specialty) can share a building and still remain independent. This type of dental office is called a

   a. specialty practice.

   b. partnership.

   c. group practice.

   d. solo practice.

3. In (a/an) _____, the dental assistant treats patients who are eligible to receive dental care at a reduced rate.

   a. group practice

   b. government clinics

   c. solo practice

   d. insurance programmer

4. To obtain employment in a _____ facility, the dental assistant must obtain employment through the civil service.

   a. federal

   b. state

   c. dental school

   d. veterans' hospital

5. The dental assistant will need to access _____ to locate employment and open positions.

   a. dental supply houses

   b. the classified sections of daily newspapers

   c. the local dental society

   d. All of the above

6. The goal of the job search is to seek and obtain successful employment. Which of the following would indicate an office that would be enjoyable to work in?

   a. Goods and supplies on hand are adequate.

   b. The employer has a good advertisement in the local newspaper.

   c. The practice seems to be very interesting.

   d. Employees would not talk to job seekers.

7. A portfolio can be prepared for the interview. Which of the following items would it include?

   a. Letters of recommendation

   b. Copies of certification

   c. Radiographs taken

   d. All of the above

8. Qualities that a dentist looks for in a dental assistant include which of the following?

   a. Good clinical skills

   b. Team player

   c. Good interpersonal skills

   d. All of the above

9. To terminate employment in your office, provide your employer notice.

   a. no

   b. two weeks'

   c. one week's

   d. two days'

10. Eligibility for national certification can be obtained by which of the following criteria for Pathway I?

    1. High school graduation or equivalent

    2. Current CPR card from a DANB-accepted CPR provider

    3. Verification of dentist employer

4. Graduate of an accredited dental assistant or dental hygiene program
5. Six months full-time employment
6. 3,500 hours of employment

   a. 1, 6   c. 2, 4
   b. 2, 5   d. 1, 5

11. In developing a cover letter, there is a standard format that follows a specific order. Place the following items in the order in which they would appear in a cover letter.

1. Closing ("Sincerely")
2. Date
3. Return address
4. Second paragraph
5. First paragraph
6. Inside address
7. Third paragraph
8. Salutation ("To whom it may concern")
9. Enclosure

   a. 3, 2, 6, 8, 5, 4, 7, 1, 9   c. 2, 3, 8, 5, 4, 7, 1, 6, 9
   b. 8, 2, 3, 5, 4, 7, 1, 6, 9   d. 6, 2, 3, 8, 4, 5, 7, 1, 9

12. The résumé should fit on a single page and follow the standard format. Place the following items in the order in which they would appear in a résumé.

1. Education
2. Employment history
3. Career objective
4. Personal data
5. References

   a. 3, 4, 2, 1, 5   c. 3, 4, 1, 2, 5
   b. 4, 1, 3, 2, 5   d. 4, 3, 1, 2, 5

13. When preparing for the interview, there are several things to think about. Which of the following items make for a successful interview?

1. Arrive 5 minutes early.
2. Wear jeans.
3. Smile.
4. Demonstrate good hygiene.
5. Control the interview.
6. Being a good speller is not critical.

   a. 1, 3, 5   c. 2, 5, 6
   b. 1, 3, 4   d. 1, 2, 4

14. A dental _____ is developed through a legal agreement and makes both dentists responsible for any accounts payable.

   a. associate   c. external
   b. partnership   d. internal

15. National certification for dental assistants is not mandatory in every state. The _____ assumes the responsibility for credentialing dental assistants.

   a. ADAA
   b. DANB

   c. ADA
   d. AMA

16. If job performance expectations and/or responsibilities are unclear, the dental assistant should seek clarification from all of the following except the

   a. office manager.
   b. employer.

   c. neighbor.
   d. a. and b.

17. As an employee in a health profession, maintaining high standards includes

   a. personal hygiene.
   b. clean uniforms.

   c. clean shoes.
   d. All of the above

18. All of the following are requirements for keeping a job except:

   a. Always look professional.
   b. Be well prepared for the job.

   c. Always be on time.
   d. Arrange for one of the staff members to be responsible for driving you to work.

19. If the dentist requires a working interview, which of the following questions should you ask to prepare for it?

   a. Ask about the time.
   b. Ask about uniform needs.

   c. Ask where to park.
   d. All of the above

20. When salary has not been mentioned throughout the interviewing process, when should it be discussed?

   a. When setting up the interview
   b. After receiving the employment offer

   c. During the interview
   d. a. and b.

21. Which of the following elements should be covered in a practice interview?

   a. Firm handshake
   b. Eye contact

   c. Speaking distinctly
   d. All of the above

22. Personal appearance influences perceptions during the interviewing process. All of the following are recommended except:

   a. Demonstrate good hygiene.
   b. Dress appropriately.

   c. Bring your own coffee cup.
   d. No jeans.

 Critical Thinking

1. Rosa was the ideal dental assistant. She was healthy, certified, always on time, and wore a clean and pressed uniform. Rosa became frustrated over time, mainly because her dental assistant coworkers did not adhere to comparable standards. Upon seeking her supervisor's help and understanding that the situation was unlikely to improve, Rosa decided to seek other employment. Describe the procedure for terminating employment.

2. June is very excited about her job in a new practice. Her current goals are to keep this position and to become the ideal employee. List the basic requirements for keeping a job and explain how the employee may seek to excel.

3. After his interview, Sam feels that the feedback he received from the dentist and staff was positive. If the employer should offer him the position, what questions should Sam be prepared to ask that may not have been asked during the interview?

CASE STUDY 1

When patients ask the dental assistant about his or her education, the dental assistant must respond. Certification is recommended for all dental assistants so that they can assure patients they are receiving the best care possible.

1. Name the credentialing organization for dental assistants.

2. After passing the recognized credentialing exam, how is the dental assistant recognized?

3. Name three ways that the dental assistant can obtain certification.

4. Describe the methods to continue one's education as a dental assistant.

5. Explain how obtaining the credential enhances the dental practice and patient care.

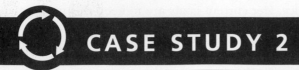

CASE STUDY 2

Carrie's husband's employer transferred him from the East Coast to the Midwest region. Because housing was an issue, she decided that beginning her search for dental assistant employment would wait until after they were settled.

1. List the types of dental practices.

2. List employment choices other than the typical dental office.

3. Describe the steps taken in an employment search.

4. Explain how to go about an employment search on the Internet.

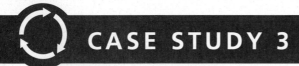

CASE STUDY 3

Phoebe is excited but anxious about an upcoming interview. In preparation for the interview, she began listing things to do.

1. List items to consider when preparing for an interview.

2. Explain the types of questions that can be asked by the applicant during an interview and those that should be avoided.

3. Describe the mock interview.

4. Describe appropriate appearance for an interview.

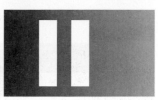

Practice Management Software

Installing Your DENTRIX®
G4 Learning Edition CD

The DENTRIX® Learning Edition CD is packaged in the back of this workbook. Before installing the software there are several important steps to follow. Following these instructions carefully will result in successful installation of the software and will minimize problems.

1. Please read all instructions before inserting the CD and beginning the installation.

2. Confirm that the computer system meets the system requirements for the software that is being installed.

3. Make sure there is adequate disk space available on the computer before starting the installation.

4. Make sure all other applications are closed when installing the CD.

5. Complete the entire installation process.

After reading this section, load the CD. The screen, *Welcome to DENTRIX® G4*, should appear. There are several important items on this screen including installation instructions for the G4 Learning CD. Review the *Important Installation Tips*, which appear second from the left at the top of the Welcome Screen.

During the installation process, the DENTRIX® software will evaluate the computer system for compatibility. If all the check marks are green, installation can proceed. Any component marked with a red "X" indicates a potential problem that could cause the installation to fail or make the DENTRIX® software run less efficiently. Correcting those items before proceeding will increase the potential for a successful installation and satisfaction with the software.

While installing DENTRIX®, there are several points at which the user will be prompted to continue the installation by selecting Next at the bottom of the screen. For example, DENTRIX® requires confirmation that the installation instructions and licensing agreements are read before continuing. For the easiest setup, hit Next to continue with the recommended installation. It is recommended to also install the *Guru Limited Edition Server*, so follow the instructions to do so. Last, it is necessary to allow access through the computer's firewall; this can be done automatically by selecting Yes, or can be modified manually if preferred.

1. Insert the CD into the disk drive.

2. Review "Important Installation Tips."

3. Go to "Install Software" on the right side of the screen under the G4 logo and begin the installation.

4. Remember, let the software install completely! The installation process takes time, so make sure to plan accordingly.

REGISTERING THE SOFTWARE

Registering the DENTRIX® Learning CD is optional. It is easy to register and registration will allow access to the *On Demand Training* resources. An email address and a password of your choice are required. The registration code will arrive via email. The DENTRIX® Learning CD can still be used with this workbook whether or not the software is registered.

USER'S GUIDE

When the DENTRIX® installation is complete, new icons or short cuts will appear on the desktop that will make it easy to access patient records and information. Among these icons will be a *User's Guide* icon. The User's Guide can be referenced to answer questions that arise while working through these exercises or if questions arise in the future. Even daily DENTRIX® users refer to the User's Guide when doing tasks that occur only occasionally or when making changes to the DENTRIX® setup. The User's Guide is also available from the Start menu and from drop-down menus throughout the software.

> **Helpful Hint:** *Sullivan-Schein technical support does not assist users of the DENTRIX® Learning Software—so if you have a problem you will need to consult the User's Guide for an answer.*

- Double Click on the User's Guide icon now

The User's Guide has more than 1000 pages, so users will want to refer to the computer copy instead of printing it. At this time, read through the table of contents to see the variety of topics covered with DENTRIX®. There is a page counter to allow easy access to any topic of interest. For practice:

- Find page 6 in your User's Guide by typing 6 in the page count box and then clicking on Enter.

This brings you to a page that begins to introduce some of the important icons that DENTRIX® uses to make navigation easy. The User's Guide will show two examples of the icon. The icon on the left is used in earlier versions of DENTRIX® that may still be in use at many dental offices, and the icon to the right is the newer version. Most of the icons are descriptive in their graphics, but reading through these notes will help while progressing through the exercises.

- Continue exploring the User's Guide until you feel comfortable finding information quickly.

SAMPLE PRACTICE

The DENTRIX® G4 Learning CD is preloaded with a practice or tutorial database complete with staff and 71 patients. It is also possible to add patients up to a total of 100. It is not possible to change the staff of tutorial; however, it is possible to work with the patient charts to practice and learn.

ACCESSING DENTRIX®

There are several easy ways to start the DENTRIX® software after installing the program.

1. From the *Start* menu, go to *Programs*, find *DENTRIX® Learning Edition,* and then select the function you would like to use.

2. DENTRIX® has installed a Quick Start button on the toolbar. Right clicking on the icon allows selection of the function you would like to use. It also allows you to choose the clock setup as well as clocking in and out as an employee.

3. You can also select the icon for the function you would like to use from the desktop.

WEB SYNC AND ESYNC OVERRIDE

DENTRIX® uses an automatic Web sync that is set to run every day at the same time of day. While this is great in an office, it is not required while using the learning system. WEBSYNC and eSYNC notifications are sent daily if this feature is not disabled.

Disabling WebSync

1. Go to DX Web on your lower toolbar (notifications area) and right click.

2. Select *Open the DX Web Toolbar.* Then click on the *Settings* icon and click on *WebSync Wizard.*

3. In the *Schedule WebSync* box, click on the button for *Do not run WebSync automatically.*

Disabling eSYNC

1. You can find the eSYNC button at the lower right toolbar (Notifications area). Look for a red circle containing a white **e**. (If it does not appear go to the Windows Start button and select it from the menu.)

2. Right click and then choose *Open eSYNC setup*. From the dialog box select *Run eSYNC manually*. Do not change any other settings in the dialog box.

3. Click OK when you are asked to confirm.

4. Click OK to close the box. eSYNC is now disabled.

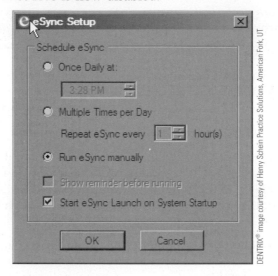

Let's get started using the software!

Patient Management

The student should strive to meet the following objectives and demonstrate an understanding of the facts and principles of patient management:

1. Using the Internet, identify at least two practice management software programs in addition to DENTRIX®.

2. Discuss three reasons the clinical dental team should be able to create and edit a patient chart.

3. Using DENTRIX®, demonstrate retrieving patient information with different search methods.

4. Explain why multiple search methods would be beneficial.

5. Demonstrate entering a family group into DENTRIX®.

6. Demonstrate how to add charting for a patient in the DENTRIX® sample practice database.

7. Demonstrate how to add periodontal charting for a patient in the DENTRIX® sample practice database.

8. Using DENTRIX®, demonstrate adding a photo to an existing patient's chart.

9. Using DENTRIX®, create an appointment for a new patient and an existing patient; then demonstrate moving those appointments to other days and times.

INTRODUCTION

Making all medical records electronic by 2014 was a goal put into place in 2004 by former President George W. Bush. While the 2014 date is not mandated and did not specifically include dental records, many dental offices are moving toward paperless electronic charting and record keeping.

For over 20 years, DENTRIX® has been a leader in dental practice management software. Developed to make managing a dental practice more efficient and profitable, it increases productivity while being user friendly. DENTRIX® allows dental offices to organize patient information, saving valuable time and eliminating time-consuming activities such as completing and submitting insurance claims forms, sending appointment reminders, and handling patient correspondence. DENTRIX® makes patient data readily available so the focus can be placed on patient treatment.

This section of the workbook simulates how a dental practice uses the software so that students can be immediately productive in the office environment. Dental offices from all across the country use DENTRIX® for practice management, so chances are excellent you will use it sometime during your career. Once you become confident using DENTRIX®, you will be able as well to transfer your skills to the other dental software available in the market.

There are several things to keep in minds that will improve your success while learning and working with DENTRIX®:

1. Relax.

This is an opportunity to *learn* DENTRIX®—any mistakes made can be easily reversed, so don't be hesitant to explore the system. Even in an office environment, errors can be edited.

753

2. Improve your keyboarding skills.

You will enjoy working with dental software more if you can add information quickly and accurately.

3. Practice, practice, practice.

Practicing with the software will build confidence and speed.

ACCESSING PATIENT INFORMATION

To access patient information, start DENTRIX® by going to the *Start* menu, first selecting *Programs*, then selecting *DENTRIX® Learning Edition*, and finally selecting *Family File* (see Figure D-1). You can also use one of the following methods to open the Patient Information screen:

- The *Family File* icon can also be accessed directly from the desktop.

- Right clicking on the *Dentrix Quick Launch* icon from the lower right toolbar and then selecting *Family File* will also open the patient information screen.

Review the toolbar icons along the top of the screen. Slowly hover and move the cursor along the icons to identify the functions of the various buttons. Currently the information on the screen is blank, so the next step is to *Select a Patient*.

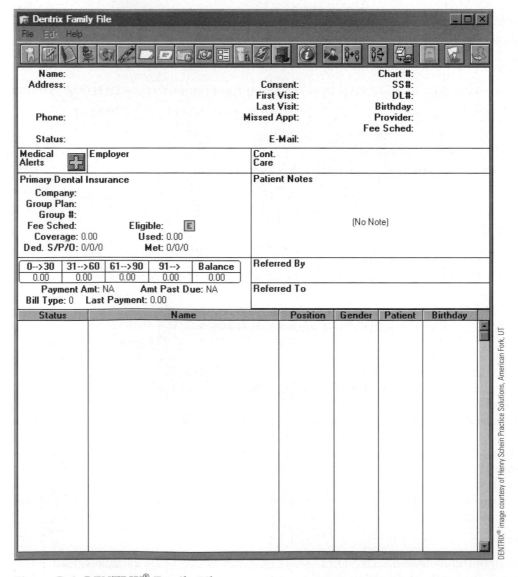

Figure D-1 DENTRIX® Family File

Selecting a Patient

The *Select a Patient* icon is found toward the right side of the toolbar. Locating patient information is a task that every member of the dental team does throughout the day, so it is important to be able to do this quickly. This icon is available throughout the program; therefore, a patient can be selected from most DENTRIX® screens.

DENTRIX® allows you to search for a patient in six different ways:

1. By name: last/first

2. By name: first/last

3. By a preferred name such as a nickname

4. By home phone number

5. By chart number

6. By social security number

Once you choose how you would like to search for a patient, DENTRIX® will continue to search this way until you reset the selection method. When there are multiple computer users, generally an office will leave the system set to one search method, but it's always nice to have an alternative.

Helpful Hint: *You will make yourself an unpopular employee if you reset the search criteria and forget to change it back.*

Using the toolbar, find the *Select Patient/New Family* icon and click on it, bringing up the *Select Patient* dialog box as seen in Figure D-2.

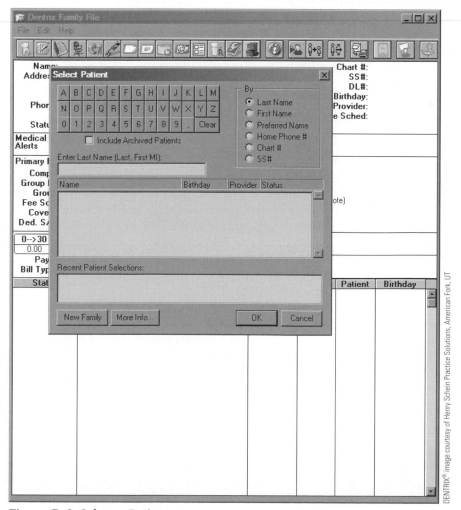

Figure D-2 Select a Patient

In the upper right of the screen are the search "By" choices, this is set to Last Name. To select a patient, simply start typing the last name; as you add letters the number of patients to choose from is reduced until the selection is easy.

>   **Helpful Hint:** *This function is helpful if you aren't sure how to spell the name. In a small family practice, patients expect you to know them. While this is their only dental practice or dentist, you see lots of patients. If you can remember how the name begins, DENTRIX® can help you identify the patient with only a small amount of information.*

The cursor is set automatically in the selection field. Begin using the patient Henry Myers from the DENTRIX® practice/tutorial database for this exercise. Start typing his name; do this slowly so you can see how it reduces the number of patients available for selection with each letter you type. Experiment with typing his name incorrectly to see what happens.

When you have identified Henry as the patient you are looking for, double click on the highlighted line or on OK and his information, along with anyone in his family group, will be displayed.

As you look at the family file, you will see information at the top including address and personal information as well as insurance information and a list of family members. You can switch between family members by double clicking on the patient's name from the list. The patient information can be edited by double clicking on any of the informational squares. For example, double click on *Patient Notes.*

>   **Helpful Hint:** *In practice, you will have patients updating their personal information and this is one point to make that change. It will change the information for everyone in that family file.*

Practice navigating around the family file until you can do it easily and with confidence.

Adding a New Patient

New patients are added from the same *Family File* screen. To add a new patient you do not have to move from the current *Family File* screen. Just choose the icon for selecting a patient that we used in the previous exercise.

You will see the same dialog box you used to type in the patient's name to select a patient. At the lower left edge of that box is a *New Family* button for patients not already in the database.

>   **Helpful Hint:** *Occasionally you will encounter a patient that insists they saw the doctor a long time ago, and they probably aren't in your computer system. Before entering them as a new patient and accidentally creating a duplicate chart, try marking the Include Archived Patients box directly under the number/letter pad at the top left of the dialog box. This will allow you to see whether their patient information is available and stored in your system. If you retrieve a patient from archive, don't forget to update their information.*

DENTRIX® groups patients into family units, so you will want to begin creating the family group with the head of household. Usually this person is the person financially responsible for the account or the person that carries dental insurance for the family. After determining that the patient or family is indeed new and who the head of household is, just enter the information in the fields provided. A nonpatient can be the head of household; just choose the appropriate *patient* or *nonpatient* status from the drop-down menu. Accuracy is important. It is better to leave a field blank than to fill it with wrong information. Go ahead and enter information for a fictitious patient, or you can enter yourself as a patient.

You can increase your speed entering patients by using the tab key to jump to the next field.

If the patient has a preferred name, such as a nickname, make sure you include it. By knowing what a patient likes being called you help create a more personal practice, but by using a formal/legal name in the *Name* field your insurance forms or future referrals will be accurate. The salutation field can be used to indicate a name you would like to use for written correspondence.

At this point you can assign a status to the patient such as patient, inactive, or nonpatient from the drop-down menu.

>   **Helpful Hint:** *Remember that Preferred Name is also a patient search category, so if a patient identifies themselves by a preferred name you can also search by that name.*

There is a field for an e-mail address. This is helpful if your office sends reminders, confirmations, or any correspondence electronically. Several fields are available for phone numbers. If you are using an auto-dialing system for confirmation calls, it will use the home number field as the number it calls. You do not need to include dashes or hyphens when entering a phone number.

At the right of the new patient information screen there are additional fields, such as provider, which is helpful in multiple-doctor offices. There is also an area for privacy requests. If your office has multiple hygienists you can use *Provider 2* as a hygienist preference field.

When you have completed the necessary information, click on Enter and you now have a new family file.

Entering the next family member is easy. On the toolbar above the *Select Patient* screen you will see a button with a stick figure and a plus sign pointing to another stick figure to its right; this is the *Add new family member* button. When you click on the icon, a window will open that allows you to add another patient as part of this family. Notice that DENTRIX® has already completed the address and other details for you. Go ahead and add a fictitious (or real) family member to your group.

Adding Medical Alerts

It is the responsibility of every member of the dental team to keep patients safe, and a part of doing that is adding medical alerts to a chart. Staff members can't assume someone else will add important changes in medical history. It is fast and easy to make these updates.

The *Medical Alert* area is clearly marked in the area just below the patient's name. When the cross is red there is an alert on the patient chart; when it is uncolored no alert exists.

When you click on the cross icon the medical alert dialog box will open. If an alert already exists you will see what it is; you can either edit this alert or add a new one.

Pat Abbott has an excellent example of an alert that will need editing; she won't be pregnant forever. When the office becomes aware of her delivery, that medical alert will be removed.

By clicking on Edit a list of medical conditions will open; highlighting the appropriate condition and clicking OK will add the alert, or highlighting the condition you would like to eliminate and clicking Clear will remove it.

Please note this is different from the *Patient Alert* icon on the toolbar that is illustrated by a patient with a white or yellow flag.

For practice, add the condition of fainting to Pat Abbott's chart. Confirm it is part of the chart, and then remove it and the pregnancy alert. Confirm that they are gone.

Congratulations. You know how to enter a patient into DENTRIX® and create a new family group. With practice you will become fast and the process will become effortless.

Helpful Hint: *"Whoops, I made a mistake." While that is not a statement you want to make chairside with a patient, updating information, editing, or correcting an error that was made while entering patient information is easy. On the Family File information screen, double click in the area you would like to change, and a dialog box will appear; then you simply make the change and click on OK.*

EXERCISES AND ACTIVITIES

Find the following patients and indicate on the line next to each name their date of birth, date of last visit, and whether the patient has medical alerts.

1. Tina Young _____

2. Mark Taylor _____

3. Rachelle Johnson _____

4. Brent Crosby _____

5. Martin Winters _____

Add the following patients:

6. Thomas Aspen
   D.O.B. 1/30/1940
   1200 Waters Street
   Tampa, Florida 33720
   813-589-4422
   Allergies: NKA
   Smoker: No

7. Wanda James
   D.O.B. 04/15/1980
   4010 Coastal Way
   St. Petersburg, Florida
   33770
   727-584-2351
   Allergies: NKA
   Smoker: No

8. Bonnie Harris
   D.O.B. 09/20/1985
   6610 Woodlawn Street
   St. Petersburg, Florida
   33770
   727-546-9871
   Allergies: Latex
   Smoker: Yes

9. Ken Summer
   D.O.B. 05/18/1970
   765 Watson Road
   Tarpon Springs, Florida
   33720
   727-546-9512
   Allergies: Peanuts
   Smoker: No

10. Arnold Winston
    D.O.B. 04/10/1930
    1020 Turner Street
    St. Petersburg, Florida 33712
    Allergies: PCN, Latex
    Smoker: Yes

PATIENT CLINICAL CHART

Before attempting the following exercise using DENTRIX®, an understanding of Chapter 14: Dental Charting in your textbook will be necessary.

While still on the *Family File* screen, the toolbar will show a single tooth icon on the far left representing the patient charts. Patient charts containing clinical information are accessed by clicking on this icon. Click on the icon now and start by examining the toolbar for this screen. It has some additional choices when compared to the last toolbar used. Once again, take a moment to move the cursor over each icon without clicking on them for a description.

> **Helpful Hint:** *Dental offices can make changes to this toolbar to create one that works efficiently for them. If you are working in a new office, take a minute to look at the toolbar and familiarize yourself with their commonly used icons and their positions on the toolbar. However, don't make changes to the toolbar without discussing with other team members.*

After accessing the clinical chart, notice the familiar *Select a Patient* icon and start by clicking there and selecting Patricia Abbott.

The patient chart contains the patient clinical charting and a Clinical Notes page where, in addition to the procedure, the doctor, hygienist, or assistant can add comments regarding treatment. You can see the *Progress Notes* field at the bottom of Figure D-3.

With paper charting you need to do the charting illustration and add treatment notes separately; this system, however, allows you to do both at the same time as well as create a treatment plan. Patricia is an excellent candidate for practice because her chart is blank, so we will add some existing treatment for her. This could be treatment already done either in the office or by a previous dentist. We will use *EO* for "existing other" and

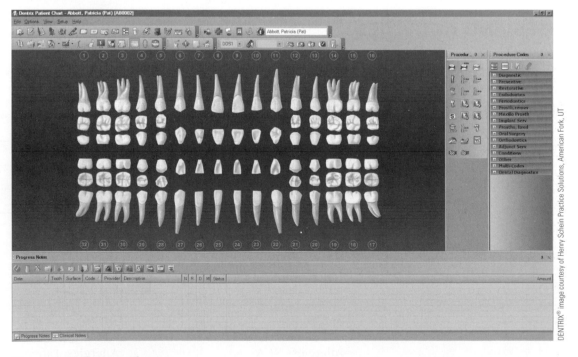

Figure D-3 Patient Chart

Ex for "existing treatment done by this office." The other status choices are *Tx* for "treatment planned" (which would be assigned to any treatment needed), and the check mark is for completed treatment.

Charting with DENTRIX® is just like traditional charting, except that instead of using a red and blue pencil you are using a keyboard.

Note: *Because of copyright laws, this learning edition of DENTRIX® does not use the standard CDT codes—they have been replaced with substitute codes.*

Begin by indicating that all her wisdom teeth or third molars were previously extracted by an oral surgeon not in this office, so we want them coded *EO*. Using the mouse, with the cursor now looking like an explorer, highlight teeth numbers 1, 16, 17, and 32. When highlighting multiple teeth, hold down the control key on the keyboard while clicking on the teeth in the illustration. If you are successful, those teeth will appear with a lighter aura around them. To unselect, click again. Practice navigating the chart with the explorer cursor.

Now that the teeth are selected, choose a code or procedure. Since they were extracted in another office, we do know that they are gone but not the exact type of extraction. At the far right of the tooth chart graphic, there are procedure codes to use. To the immediate right are the shortcuts to use. The symbol for extraction is a tooth with 2 lines down it vertically, which is found on the second row on the left. —On the far right of the toolbar are the status codes. Use the explorer to choose *EO* for "existing other" and click on it. Now the tooth chart will show the third molars—1, 16, 17 and 32—gone. If you look at the *Progress Notes* section by clicking in the lower left corner, you will notice that the treatment was automatically added to the notes.

Helpful Hint: *Correcting an error is easy. In the Progress Notes, double click on the line containing the incorrect procedure (or one you want to practice with for now). A dialog box will automatically appear allowing you to make changes. You can change the status of the procedure, the fee charged for the procedure, and even the procedure code itself.*

Practice charting a restoration that is needed. Pat has caries on tooth #14 and will need an MOD restoration.

- First choose tooth #14 and highlight it just as in the previous exercise.

- Choose *MOD Amalgam* from the procedure shortcuts followed by the *Tx* status.

- The tooth chart should now have an MOD colored in red.

- Now make an adjustment to the fee. Remember to double click in the *Procedure Notes* to select which procedure to change. What if Pat changed her mind and wanted a resin/composite filling instead? Make that change. Check for the accuracy of the change by looking at the progress notes or on the graphic charting. On the graphic, it should now be outlined in red and filled with cross hatching (Figure D-4).

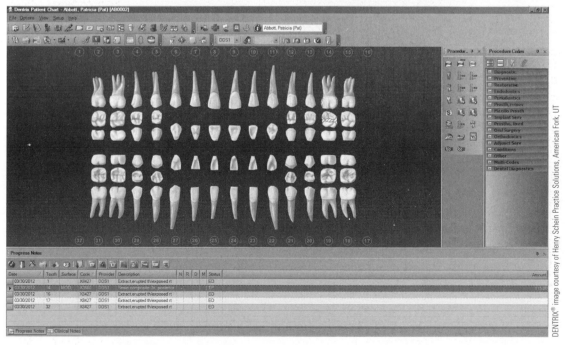

Figure D-4 Completed Patient Chart

Helpful Hint: *If you don't understand a step while working in DENTRIX®, go back and repeat the process until you do. This is your opportunity to learn; you will be able to build up speed after you know the basics.*

Periodontal Charting

Just like periodontal disease itself, charting periodontal conditions can be complicated. We are going to begin with the basics to build a strong foundation so you can add skills later. With traditional charting on paper, every tooth gets six measurements: three on the buccal or facial and three on the lingual. DENTRIX® is the same. First a patient chart must be selected, then the periodontal charting is accessed from the toolbar with the *Perio Probe* icon that is found along the second row.

- Select Pat Abbott as your patient.

- Click on the *Perio* icon that looks like a perio probe; the chart that opens should look like Figure D-5. Look at the toolbar, it has changed again. Take time now to run the mouse over the icons for their descriptions. There are 5 icons important for perio charting: *New Exam, Open Exam, Save Exam, Print Exam,* and *Delete Exam.*

- Clicking *New Exam* will presents a dialog box to choose the date for the exam; click on OK.

- *Open Exam* opens a dialog box to allow selection of a past exam date.

- The icons for *Save, Print,* and *Delete* are self-explanatory.

Recall from Pat's tooth chart that the third molars are marked as extracted, they will appear on the periodontal chart as shown by the red **M**s. Continue looking over the perio chart, and note that the tooth numbers running along the top and bottom are much like a noncomputer chart. Along the far left column, beginning at the top, are some abbreviations:

- F = Facial (this includes the buccal surfaces of posterior teeth)

- PD = Probing depth measured in millimeters using a perio probe

- GM = Gingival Margin indicates recession and is measured in millimeters

- CAL = Clinical Attachment Level, which is measured in millimeters

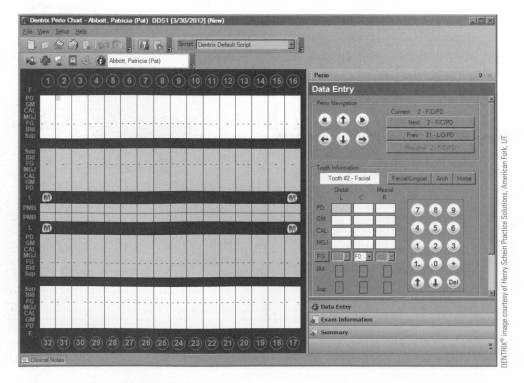

Figure D-5 Periodontal Chart

- MGJ = Mucogingival Junction measured in millimeters

- FG = Functional Grade with indication of any furcation involvement for the tooth

- Bld = Bleeding that is represented with a red oval at the point of bleeding

- Sup = Suppuration or an infection point is indicated by a yellow oval

Continuing to follow the column down on the left, and note that the abbreviations are listed in reverse as they relate to the lingual side of the tooth. In the center of the chart, the abbreviation PMB (Plaque, Mobility, and Bone Loss) is noted. This is a measurement specific to each tooth. The blank for the maxillary tooth is on the top and the mandibular is on the bottom. The chart repeats for the mandibular teeth beginning on the lingual and continuing with the previous abbreviations until reaching the facial. The chart will look like a graph (Figure D-6). Find the abbreviations, teeth locations, and area for clinical notes on the chart. It is important to understand the chart before continuing with the exercise.

Moving to the right side of the screen, note the perio information sections including *Data Entry, Exam Information,* and *Summary* (Figure D-7).

Click on each of the sections to get used to navigating between them. Click on *Data Entry* for this exercise. To enter periodontal probing for Pat, begin with the distal facial of Tooth #2. You can verify your position on the *Data Entry* box at the top with Current position or under Tooth Information. If you are not on Tooth #2, use the navigation arrows until you get to the correct place. In the *Tooth Information* box, you should see Tooth #2 and the top left PD (perio depth) highlighted in yellow. Begin charting using the key pad at the right by using the depths 3 2 3 as your distal, facial, and mesial readings. You will not need to select the next tooth, just use the key pad or the PD on Tooth #3 and the charting system will automatically advance. If you want to jump to another tooth, use the navigation system or simply use the mouse to move the cursor to the tooth you want to chart. Go to Tooth #14; notice the mesial measurement is now first. On Tooth #14, chart the PD 6 5 6 and click the Bld (bleeding) box to indicate bleeding. Notice that because these depths are outside of the normal range they are red. Add more PDs for practice.

When you have practiced entering as much data as you would like, look at the *Exam Information* screen to add some descriptions for Pat. Use the DENTRIX® default template under *Perio Notes*. As the term on the left is highlighted, descriptive choices are available in a drop-down menu on the right (Figure D-8). For practice, visualize how Pat's soft tissue might look and choose the appearance on the small drop-down menu at the right.

The *Summary* shows an overview of the patient and the information entered, as shown in Figure D-9.

Make sure to hit the *Save Exam* before moving from the periodontal charting; however, DENTRIX® will remind you if you forget.

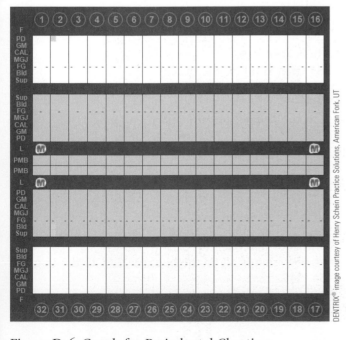

Figure D-6 Graph for Periodontal Charting

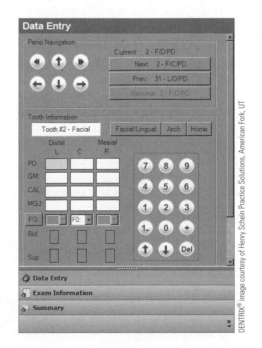

Figure D-7 Data Entry and Navigation

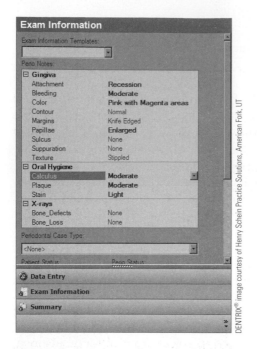

Figure D-8 Exam Information

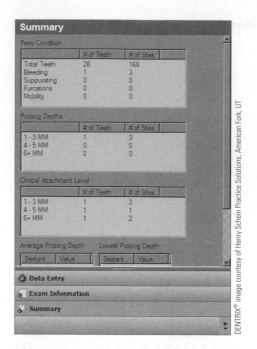

Figure D-9 Peridontal Summary

You now have the basics of DENTRIX®-assisted perio charting; by practicing you will build speed and efficiency.

Helpful Hint: *Charting is a great skill to practice with a partner because it simulates a dental office. The numbers and conditions being charted for practice are not as important as the pace. So your practice partner can be anyone.*

EXERCISES AND ACTIVITIES

1. Chart the following for Ken Summer.

All third molars, #8, and #9 are missing; these anteriors have been replaced with a fixed prosthesis that is a Maryland bridge.
Begin charting at the buccal of #2 and continue to the buccal of #15:
544; 444; 444; 445; 444; 444; 444; 444; 444; 455; 555; 455 (that is all on the buccal).
Continue to the lingual on #15 and go back to the lingual on #2:
545; 444; 354; 344; 353; 333; 333; 333; 334; 545; 454; 554.
On the lower begin on the lingual of #31 and proceed to the lingual on #18, and then from the buccal of #18 back to the buccal of #31:
455; 544; 544; 444; 343; 333; 333; 434; 444; 445; 545; 445; 455; 555 (that is all on the buccal).
Now proceed from #18 back to #31 on the lingual:
555; 554; 544; 545; 554; 444; 443; 333; 333; 333; 344; 444; 455; 555.

2. Chart the following for Pamela Schow.

The following teeth are missing: all four molars and #14, #19, and #30. Begin charting on the buccal of #2 and go to the buccal of #15; then go to the lingual of #15 and continue back to #2.
654, 444, 445, 544, 432, 333, 332, 333, 334, 445, 555, 444, 656 (that is all on the buccal). Now to the lingual:
555, 545, 433, 333, 333, 333, 333, 443, 455, 444, 544, 454, 545.
Next we will begin on the lingual of #31.
655, 755, 654, 444, 343, 333, 333, 434, 444, 545, 566, 545. That is all for the lingual. Move on to the buccal beginning at #18 and continuing back to #31:
655, 555, 443, 333, 333, 344, 444, 455, 545, 555, 555, 566.

APPOINTMENT BOOK

To start the appointment-making process, click on the *Appointment Book* icon from the desktop or toolbar; explore the *Appointment Book* toolbar by allowing the mouse to move over the icons, revealing the labels (Figure D-10).

At the far right of the screen notice the navigation arrows that allow you to move forward and backward through the days of the week. Beneath those, there are icons to allow you a view of the week and a view of the month. The graph at the left of the appointment book is color coded at the top for each provider so you can see who is scheduled with a patient and in what treatment room.

Helpful Hint: *Either directly or indirectly, every member of the dental team plays a role in scheduling appointments. By knowing when times are available, even clinical staff can guide patients into making appointments for available times.*

Find an Appointment Time

To find a space with enough time, it is necessary to determine what type of appointment is planned. As the patient charting was done, anything that was coded in red (treatment needed) automatically goes into the patient's appointment history as *Tx* so a future appointment can be made. Average time requirements for the each procedure are predetermined but can be adjusted if necessary. Double click on the *Appointment Book* page and select Pat Abbott as your patient.

The *Appointment Information* screen will show the appointment information for Pat Abbott (Figure D-11). Click *Tx* to find out what she needs to schedule. It lists her provider and shows that the reason for her visit is a 3-surface amalgam (or resin if you changed the charting). To become acquainted with this dialog box and its functions, explore the dialog box now by using the drop-down menus and other buttons. Next to the appointment description is the appointment length. By using the arrow you can increase or decrease the time needed. To find an appointment for Pat, increase the appointment length to 60 minutes, highlight her treatment, and click Pinboard on the right side of the dialog box. Now her appointment will be easy to find when we're ready for it.

If the patient you are scheduling needs several appointments, you can choose each appointment separately by highlighting it, or you can choose multiple treatments by highlighting more than one. The dialog box as shown in Figure D-11, *Appointment Information,* has more scheduling options. At the bottom of the dialog box you can check other information that will be useful. At the right you can place this appointment on a will call or wait list if the patient is not ready to schedule, you can find an appointment, or you can attach it to a pinboard while you look for a time that works to schedule the appointment.

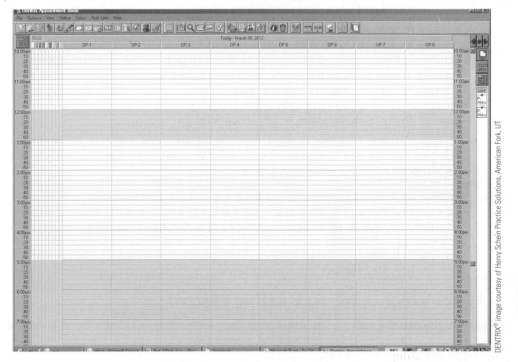

Figure D-10 Appointment Book

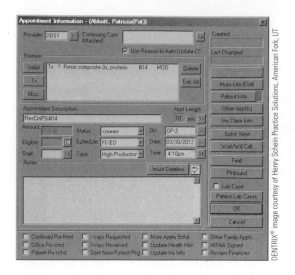

Figure D-11 Appointment Information

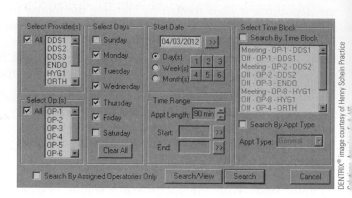

Figure D-12 Find New Appointment Time

Repeat this process selecting Carol Little as the patient. You will see under *Tx* she needs a Crown on #19 that will take 90 minutes. When you are ready to move on, highlight the treatment, and this time click on *Find*. The *Find an Appointment* dialogue box will appear with criteria to help find an appointment time (Figure D-12). When you are ready to schedule, hit Search/View and make your selection. To double check your work, look on that day in your appointment book to see her appointment.

> **Helpful Hint:** *Presetting appointment times takes the guesswork out of making appointments. The doctor and staff estimate how long procedures take them to complete and this is set as a default in the computer. However, for example, if you have a patient with back problems who must take a break during longer procedures, there has to be a way to factor that into the appointment time. This can be done at the front desk or by an assistant that is familiar with the patient.*

> *Why not just make every appointment longer so everyone can take a break? Even down time of 10–15 minutes throughout the day adds up and affects production.*

One way to find an appointment time is to search manually. This is efficient in cases where a patient has a very specific time requirement such as "I have the day off on September 20, do you have any time available?" When this happens the fastest way to look is to go directly to the day; she isn't interested in other dates. To initiate a wider search, select the looking glass icon on your *Appointment Book* screen. It will open the *New Appointment* dialog box below.

The dialog box has information regarding times and availability to look for on the schedule. It is possible to choose the dentist, treatment room, days of the week, or where in the appointment book to start looking. The appointment length will be set but you can also adjust it here.

As you look at your *Appointment Book* page you will see Pat's appointment waiting for you "pinned" on the right side under the buttons to toggle from the day to the week to the month.

Click and drag the appointment into the desired position. If after making the appointment you want to move it, you can do that by clicking and dragging. If you want to search the appointment book, double click on it to bring up the *Appointment Information* dialog box.

> **Helpful Hint:** *The "click and drag" feature is one that is often used. It is common to have a patient need to move an appointment and you will be able to do that easily. You can move it around on the same page visually or "pin" it in the upper right of the Appointment Book page and search further.*

Don't become discouraged if you have to practice to become comfortable making appointments. Good appointment scheduling takes time and patience.

Scheduling Appointments for an Existing Patient

Repeat the process using another patient by going to the *Appointment Book* icon from your current location.

- Please schedule an extraction appointment for Brent Crosby.

- Click the *Schedule Appointment* icon and access Brent's information. Look under *Tx* for what needs to be done. Highlight the extraction and move it to the Pinboard.

- Go to *Find New Appointment*. Brent would like to schedule on June 29 in the morning with DDS3. Use your tools for speed (examples: calendar and drop-down menus).

- Search/view possible options. Your appointment book should show that either Treatment Room 1 or 2 is available at that time with the doctor. Select Treatment Room 1.

- On the appointment page you will see the time available indicated by an outline.

- Click and drag Brent from the Pinboard upper right into the space available.

- Just for practice, move Brent's appointment around on the page. Notice that you are unable to move the appointment accidently because DENTRIX® asks for confirmation.

Want more practice? Choose other patients out of your database to schedule.

Scheduling Appointments for New Patients

Scheduling new patients is important because it is how the practice grows. When a new patient calls, it is their first impression of what the experience will be like in the practice. Everything needs to be perfect.

Depending on the practice, exactly how new patients are scheduled can vary, but for this exercise we are going to make the appointment with the hygienist for 1 hour and include a cleaning.

New patient, Susan Keller, calls and would like to set up an appointment for June 27 at 8 a.m.

Go to the *Appointment Book* icon and click on it. Go the requested date of June 27, and please use Treatment Room 5 as your hygiene room. Double click on 8 a.m.

The *Select a Patient* dialog box will open and you need to complete it as accurately as possible. You will need to fill in a referral source, which can be another patient or another doctor. This is important information to get because you will want to thank the source of the referral.

The *Select a Patient* dialog box will be followed by *Patient Information*. This time you will want to select DDS 1 and indicate that it is an initial visit. Highlighting the procedures will add them to the appointment. Choose Adult Prophy, Pano, 4 BW, and Periodic Exam for this example.

Click the OK button to add this appointment.

The letters "NP" next to the appointment will identify the patient as new to the practice. This patient does not have a family file and you will not be able to locate them in *Select a Patient*. New patient appointments are found by using the Locate Appointment button.

> **Helpful Hint:** *Perhaps you find you have made an error with your appointment, for example, she will need more time. From the Appointment Book page, double click on the appointment. The Patient Information dialog box will appear and you can make corrections. DENTRIX® has made scheduling a new patient very easy. Most patients have some idea of when they like to make appointments before they call. Systems that require large amounts of information before even looking for a day and time can be frustrating, especially if at the end of information gathering, your patient's day off is also your doctor's, and they decide they don't want to schedule after all.*

Rescheduling an Appointment

One thing that happens to every scheduler is managing a patient who would like to change or reschedule an appointment. When this occurs you want to make sure the appointment is not overlooked and that if it isn't scheduled again quickly, the patient receives follow-up calls. It is vital to maintain production in the office, but more importantly there is an obligation of the practice to make sure patients are adequately informed regarding the consequences of not pursuing treatment.

With DENTRIX®, when an appointment is cancelled and not rescheduled at the same time, it goes into a holding file so it can be followed up on (Figure D-13).

To save the appointment, double click on the appointment in the book to bring up the patient information, highlight the appointment in question, and then move it to the Wait/Will Call file.

The list of patients that need appointments can be retrieved by going to *Appt Lists* in the top toolbar and clicking on *Unscheduled List* (Figure D-14). This will bring up a list of unscheduled or broken appointments that may require follow-up.

Broken appointments or appointments that patients do not show up for are another problem that dental offices deal with too often. At the end of the day, all the appointments need to be accounted for:

- Marked as completed so they can be billed out

- Rescheduled and moved to a new position

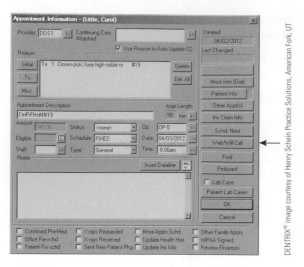

DENTRIX® image courtesy of Henry Schein Practice Solutions, American Fork, UT

Figure D-13 Putting Patient Appointment on Hold

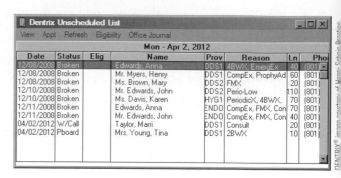

Figure D-14 Unscheduled List

- Moved to a list that can be followed up if not rescheduled

- Marked as broken so they appear on a follow-up list

To break an appointment, double click on the appointment in the appointment book and indicate it was broken using the *Broken Appointment* icon.

EXERCISES AND ACTIVITIES

Schedule the following patients for appointments:

1. Thomas Aspen
   D.O.B. 1/30/1940
   1200 Waters Street
   Tampa, Florida 33720
   813-589-4422
   Allergies: NKA
   Smoker: No

2. Wanda James
   D.O.B. 04/15/1980
   4010 Coastal Way
   St. Petersburg, Florida
   33770
   727-584-2351

   Allergies: NKA
   Smoker: No

3. Bonnie Harris
   D.O.B. 09/20/1985
   6610 Woodlawn Street
   St. Petersburg, Florida
   33770
   727-546-9871
   Allergies: Latex
   Smoker: Yes

4. Ken Summer
   D.O.B. 05/18/1970
   765 Watson Road

   Tarpon Springs, Florida
   33720
   727-546-9512
   Allergies: Peanuts
   Smoker: No

5. Arnold Winston
   D.O.B. 04/10/1930
   1020 Turner Street
   St. Petersburg, Florida
   33712
   Allergies: PCN, Latex
   Smoker: Yes

ADDING PATIENT PHOTOS

Having photos of patients in the chart is becoming a valuable part of treatment planning. It can also be helpful to put a name with a face as you are taking a phone call or to identify patients as they arrive for appointments. Adding a photo takes just a few minutes. If you are just looking for nontechnical facial recognition photos it will only require a simple digital camera. Detailed intraoral photos require a special camera and lighting.

Take photos and download them into a file where they can be edited. Even if the photo is good, you'll probably want to be able to crop it and adjust the lighting.

From the *Patient Chart, Select a Patient,* either by selecting the patient with the arrow icon or by using the file drop-down menu at the upper left.

Look for the icon of the patient in a picture frame on the toolbar.

Selecting that icon will open the DENTRIX® *Patient Photo* dialog box (Figure D-15).

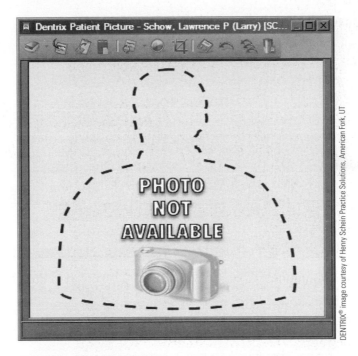

Figure D-15 Patient Photo

If your patient photo was hard copy you could access it from a scanner and the far left *Scanner* icon, but it is easier to click *Import From File* (second from the left), choose the photo, and download it.

After you have added a photo you will see it displayed on the toolbar when you open the patient chart; on the family file the picture frame will appear darkened to indicate a photo is available.

TRACKING PATIENT STATUS

You can use your appointment book to convey the status of patients on the schedule.

From the *Appointment Book* page, use the *Status* drop-down menu from the top toolbar to see the options.

If you have already created an appointment book page, use it; if not create one now to use for this exercise.

To create a patient status, single click on the patient's appointment in the book and then go to *Status* and choose from the drop-down menu. On the appointment a color code will appear on the left border of the appointment. Try indicating that one of your patients was confirmed with a message left on an answering machine.

Status is how offices that have computer monitors in multiple areas track which patients have arrived in the office but may be completing paperwork, or indicate which patients are actually ready to be seated in a treatment room.

Click on a patient in the book and to change the status. For example, you left a message for this patient so that is the status; now that they have arrived in the office you will click on the name and update the status.

By using *Status,* you will immediately see when patients are late for an appointment so you can call and verify if they are on their way.

PRESCRIPTIONS

As patients are dismissed, the doctor may also request that they receive a prescription for the treatment they received or to have before their next appointment. Even though DENTRIX® makes prescriptions easy, they still need the doctor's approval.

- Begin by *Selecting a Patient* from the *Patient Chart* or the *Family File*.

- Select the icon for *Prescriptions,* which looks like a pill bottle on the toolbar.

- Click on the *New* button at the bottom of the dialog box and you will see a blank prescription.

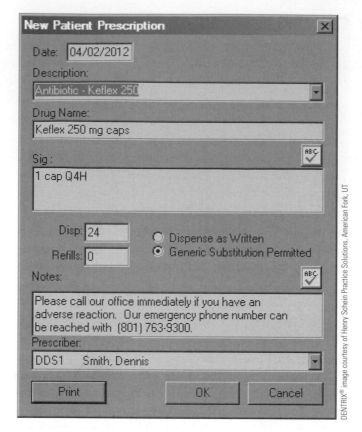

Figure D-16 Adding a Prescription

- Use the *Description* drop-down menu to see some of the most common prescriptions by this doctor. In Figure D-16, "Keflex" was selected from the drop-down menu and the remainder of the prescription was completed automatically.

- Explore the different prescriptions that could be selected by clicking on others from the drop-down menu.

In an office you would click the print button and have it ready and available for the doctor to sign. The prescription is also printed with instructions for the patient to call immediately if there is an adverse reaction. The prescription is automatically added to the patient's chart.

EXERCISES AND ACTIVITIES

Add prescriptions for the following patients:

1. Thomas Aspen
   D.O.B. 1/30/1940
   1200 Waters Street
   Tampa, Florida 33720
   813-589-4422
   Allergies: NKA
   Smoker: No

2. Wanda James
   D.O.B. 04/15/1980
   4010 Coastal Way
   St. Petersburg, Florida
   33770
   727-584-2351

   Allergies: NKA
   Smoker: No

3. Bonnie Harris
   D.O.B. 09/20/1985
   6610 Woodlawn Street
   St. Petersburg, Florida
   33770
   727-546-9871
   Allergies: Latex
   Smoker: Yes

4. Ken Summer
   D.O.B. 05/18/1970

   765 Watson Road
   Tarpon Springs, Florida
   33720
   727-546-9512
   Allergies: Peanuts
   Smoker: No

5. Arnold Winston
   D.O.B. 04/10/1930
   1020 Turner Street
   St. Petersburg, Florida
   33712
   Allergies: PCN, Latex
   Smoker: Yes

SUPPLEMENTARY ONLINE INSTRUCTION

To view *On Demand Training* you will need Internet access; use the *Help* drop-down menu from any DENTRIX®
screen and select *On Demand Training*. A variety of tutorials and tips are available for use.

MULTIPLE CHOICE

Use your sample DENTRIX practice to answer the following questions:

1. Select patient Samuel Perkins. When is his birthday?

   a. 12/4/1998   c. 08/05/1962
   b. 07/05/1960   d. 09/05/1954

2. For patient Ms. Karen Davis, who is listed as the Head of Household?

   a. Karen   c. Harmon
   b. Lyle   d. Bob

3. For patient Paul Olsen, which teeth have been extracted?

   a. All four wisdom teeth: 1, 16, 17, and 32.   c. Paul is not a patient.
   b. There are no missing teeth.   d. Due to orthodontic treatment all four
                                                      premolars.

4. John Edwards has a medical alert on his chart. What is it for?

   a. Diabetes   c. Heart Murmur
   b. Epilepsy   d. High Blood Pressure

5. When charting with DENTRIX®, missing teeth are designated by:

   a. A blue "X."   c. A lighter blue aura.
   b. A red "X."   d. They are missing from chart.

6. Which of the following is not already on Paula Pearson's prescription list?

   a. Amoxicillin 250 mg   c. Tylenol #3
   b. Keflex 300 mg   d. Clindamycin

7. Cheryl enters and makes an appointment for a new patient. After she is done she realizes she has scheduled a hygiene appointment in the doctor's favorite treatment room. Which of these solutions would work
   best to correct the situation?

   a. Go to *Appointment Information* and change the provider.
   b. Click and drag it to another treatment room.
   c. Contact the patient and discuss changing the appointment.
   d. Leave it; something will work out.

8. John forgets his appointment. What should be done with the appointment?

   a. Nothing, by leaving it in the appointment book it creates a reminder.
   b. Double click and put it in the Will Call list.
   c. Single click and move it to broken appointments.
   d. Move the appointment to another day and send him a postcard.

9. Mary Brown has a broken appointment that was not rescheduled. What was it for?

   a. MOD amalgam filling
   b. Root canal therapy #18

   c. Full Mouth Survey
   d. Mary has no additional appointment requirements.

10. Brent Crosby wants to move his appointment to next week. Where can you click and drag it to move it?

   a. To the Appointment List.
   b. To Broken Appointments.

   c. Click and drag it to the day and time requested.
   d. Use the Pinboard to park it.

11. Appointment Status options include:

   a. Broken Appointment
   b. Ready for Operatory

   c. Rescheduled Appointment
   d. Appointment Confirmed by Mail

12. For technical support with your DENTRIX® Learning CD:

   a. Call DENTRIX® directly.
   b. Consult your User's Guide.

   c. Order the support manual from DENTRIX®.
   d. None of the above

13. Dean Little's chart shows he has:

   a. An existing root canal on #30
   b. An existing crown on #30

   c. An existing root canal on #31
   d. An existing crown on #19

14. To create a custom appointment schedule from the Appointment Book:

   a. Go to *Appointment Lists*
   b. Go to *Setup*

   c. Go to *Options*
   d. Go to *Help*

15. Which of these patients has a photo attached to his chart?

   a. Harmon Davis
   b. Lyle Jones

   c. John Edwards
   d. Brent Crosby

16. Gary Gleason was referred by:

   a. Dr. Tyler
   b. Dr. Martin

   c. Susan Jones
   d. Dr. Crawford

17. Rachelle Johnson's employer is:

   a. AT & T
   b. Walmart

   c. Solutions Group
   d. IBM

18. The patient information for Doris Kenner indicates she is:

   a. Inactive
   b. Wife of Spencer

   c. Child of Bill Kenner
   d. Active

Critical Thinking

1. Learning to use a computerized appointment book can take time and patience. Describe the benefits of this type of scheduling.

2. Using a completely paperless system in the dental office increases the security of dental office documents. Explain why the information is more secure.

3. With dental management software, the requirements of HIPAA must be considered. List precautions the dental office can take to insure personal health information is not compromised.

 CASE STUDY 1

Debby has worked as a chairside assistant with Dr. Jones for almost 18 years. She isn't really interested in dealing with the new paperless patient records system that the office installed recently.

1. Describe the reasons it is important for Debby to learn to use the new system.

2. What can team members do to help Debby become more comfortable using the computer?

3. List the benefits that Debby might gain from improving her computer skills.

CASE STUDY 2

Jim calls to make an appointment. Immediately, you have access to a significant amount of information.

1. List information you can expect to find when you open Jim's records.

2. List questions you might want to ask Jim.

3. Describe how you can use Jim's information to schedule other members of his family.

SKILLS ASSESSMENT

	Successful	Needs Assistance
Accesses DENTRIX®.		
Demonstrates multiple ways to select a patient.		
Ability to add a new patient.		
Adds employer to patient information.		
Ability to add additional family members.		
Explains or shows how to add a photo.		
Charts new treatment.		
Charts existing treatment.		
Deletes incorrect chart entry.		
Ability to add perio charting.		
Makes patient appointment.		
Cancels appointment.		
Moves appointment to alternate date.		
Successfully writes a prescription for a patient.		
Updates the status of a patient.		

Practice Management

The student should strive to meet the following objectives and demonstrate an understanding of the facts and principles for practice management:

1. Demonstrate adding an employer to the DENTRIX® software.

2. Link a patient to the new employer.

3. Demonstrate adding an insurance company into the DENTRIX® software.

4. Link a patient to the new insurance company.

5. Write a patient letter using Quick Note.

6. Write a letter using the letter templates.

7. Post treatment to a patient's account.

8. Submit an insurance claim for completed patient treatment.

9. Submit a preauthorization.

10. Create a report showing patient referrals.

INTRODUCTION

As you move into practice management with DENTRIX®, you will immediately be aware of how patient management and practice management are interconnected. The accuracy of information added to the patient charts becomes important in financial transactions such as statements and insurance claims. Patient information can also assist with patient correspondence or in generating accurate reports.

Everything in practice management software attaches to the patient chart, enabling you to access information quickly and easily—but uncorrected errors compound themselves.

ADD AN INSURANCE CARRIER

The first step in assuring the accuracy of your insurance claims is when adding insurance information to the *Family File*. If family members have insurance with different carriers, make sure you include that information.

Begin by going to the *Family File* and selecting Arthur Blank as your patient.

You will want to enter the employer information because often this provides helpful information regarding the patient's dental insurance. Double click on the *Employer* box; a new box will open to complete the employment information. If the employer is already in the system, you can use the arrow next to employer to choose it. For Art, choose AT&T by clicking on it from the listed selections and select OK.

Helpful Hint: *Changing the address information for the head of household changes that information for the entire family. Adding something like an employer only adds it for the individual family member whose file you are working in when you make the addition.*

773

Double click on the *Primary Dental Insurance* box (Figure D-17). A new box opens that allows you to input the *Insurance Information*. By using the arrow to the right of the carrier information, you will be directed to a dialog box where AT&T is already highlighted. Select *Primary Insurance* (Figure D-18). If AT&T is not highlighted, find it in the list of employers and highlight it. Always double check the information for accuracy—it will take a few seconds, but finding a problem now will save time later. You can see from the list that other employers have coverage with Blue Cross/Blue Shield; that coverage may be different. If the information is correct, click on OK and return to the *Insurance Information* dialog box. Make sure to update the subscriber number. The default is set as the social security number, but most patients will have another identifier on their insurance card to comply with privacy laws.

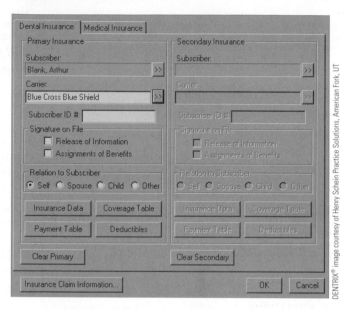

Figure D-17 Insurance Information

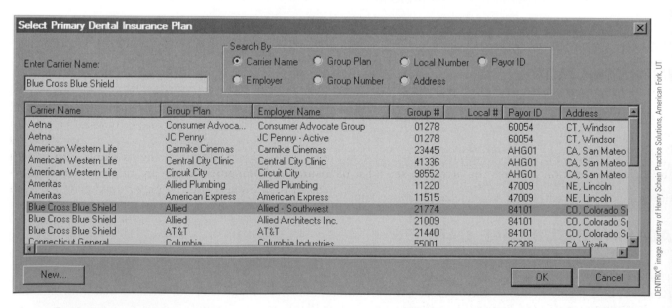

Figure D-18 Primary Insurance Selection

If your patient has signed a form for:

Release of Information, allowing the dental office to submit the claim on the patient's behalf or to speak to the insurance company if there are questions regarding treatment, make sure that box was checked when the patient information was entered.

Or

Assignment of Benefits, which means that the insurance payment is sent directly to the dentist, make sure that box was checked unless the patient has already paid you directly.

Helpful Hint: *Always remember that the contract with the insurance company is between the insurance company and the patient. You are filing the claim as a courtesy to the patient, but the policy and responsibility for payment belong to the patient. This is different if you are working on a claim for a patient on public assistance.*

To add the children to this carrier: Go to the *Family File* screen and highlight the child's name (use Kendra for this exercise), and double click. You will see that the name at the top of the file is now Kendra. To add the insurance for her, double click the *Primary Insurance* box (it is currently empty) to bring up the Insurance Information. By using the arrows to the right of subscriber, you will see Arthur's name highlighted. If you click OK, Kendra now has Blue Cross/Blue Shield insurance as part of her record.

Double check your work by highlighting each family member for accuracy.

Helpful Hint: *To the right of Insurance Information is the Patient Note area. You can add reminders for yourself about things that are important to this patient or that you will find useful in the future. One thing you might want to note is whether a college-age child is still a full-time student. Within the Patient Note area you can insert a dateline and select Hide or View.*

Adding Secondary Insurance

Adding a secondary insurance company follows the same pattern as adding a primary company. For this exercise, we'll add Melanie Blank's insurance as a secondary insurer for Art. Start by bringing up Art Blank from the *Family File* because his information is what we are changing. Double click the Primary Dental Insurance box on the *Family File* sheet to access the Insurance Information dialog box. You will see the primary insurance information completed on the left and an area for secondary insurance information on the right.

On the secondary insurance side, use the subscriber arrow to see the choices for coverage. Both Melanie and Art are listed. For secondary coverage, we are using Melanie's policy, so highlight her name and click on OK. When you return to the Insurance Information dialog box for Art Blank, you will see Melanie's Aetna policy added as the secondary carrier. Notice, DENTRIX® has automatically added the relationship to subscriber for you.

Entering a New Insurance Carrier

Even if you have a large number of insurance companies to choose from, eventually you will need to add a new company.

Choose Shawna Nelson as your next patient in the database. Currently she doesn't have insurance so you will be able to add a company for her. Under her employer, add Self-employed. Shawna has an insurance card with her for Assurant Dental. Access the insurance information by double clicking the *Primary Insurance* area of the *Family File*.

Click on the carrier search arrows. Take a moment to look down the list to make sure Assurant is not already listed before adding it. The easiest way to search is by Carrier Name, so choose that as the "Search By" feature. Once you are sure you want to add a company, click the *New* button at the bottom of the dialog box.

At this point, assuming that Shawna was your patient, you would have her insurance card available to add the information. For this exercise just use Assurant as the carrier and leave the other fields blank. Drop down to Payer Information and use the arrow to see a list of Insurance Companies. There are three Assurant Insurance companies, so find the one that matches the patient's information and add the payer number to the Plan Information. For this exercise choose Assurant Employee Benefits. Leave the options unchecked, click OK, return to the *Insurance Information* dialog box, and follow the steps to add an existing carrier until you see Assurant in the Carrier Information field.

You can practice adding insurance to the other patients you have added to your database or to the existing patients.

EXERCISES AND ACTIVITIES

Add insurance information for the following patients:

1. Thomas Aspen
   D.O.B. 1/30/1940
   1200 Waters Street
   Tampa, Florida 33720
   813-589-4422

   Allergies: NKA
   Smoker: No

2. Wanda James
   D.O.B. 04/15/1980
   4010 Coastal Way

   St. Petersburg, Florida
   33770
   727-584-2351
   Allergies: NKA
   Smoker: No

3. Bonnie Harris
   D.O.B. 09/20/1985
   6610 Woodlawn Street
   St. Petersburg, Florida 33770
   727-546-9871
   Allergies: Latex
   Smoker: Yes

4. Ken Summer
   D.O.B. 05/18/1970
   765 Watson Road
   Tarpon Springs, Florida 33720
   727-546-9512
   Allergies: Peanuts
   Smoker: No

5. Arnold Winston
   D.O.B. 04/10/1930
   1020 Turner Street
   St. Petersburg, Florida 33712
   Allergies: PCN, Latex
   Smoker: Yes

MANAGING THE PATIENT LEDGER

It doesn't matter that your office produces beautiful dentistry—if you don't keep track of fees and payments, you'll find yourself in a different line of work. Often the dentist relies completely on the staff to make sure this is being done. Clinical and administrative staff need to make sure that fees charged out reflect the work that was done. Any adjustments or discounts that the patient received as a professional courtesy or because of pre-payment must be categorized so that the management reports used to make decisions for the practice reflect the treatment completed. The ledger is the financial foundation for the practice.

From the ledger you can control everything involving the financial relationship between the office and the patient. Treatment is charged out and payments posted, fees can be changed or discounted, and statements and insurance claims are sent.

For offices using the DENTRIX® charting system, when treatment is completed and moves from the treatment plan to complete status, the charges will automatically appear on the ledger. If an office is using a paper chart, DENTRIX® can still provide account management but it must be done manually.

Go to the *Patient Ledger,* find the icon on the toolbar that looks like a pen and paper, and click on it (Figure D-19). Explore the toolbar at the top of the ledger to see the labels for each icon. The ledger contains

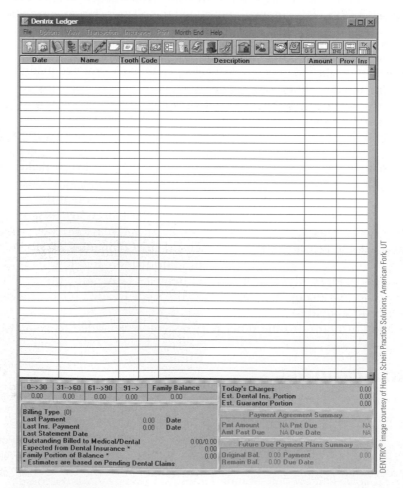

Figure D-19 Ledger

valuable information. Once a treatment is added, the ledger provides the total the patient owes for treatment and an estimate of the insurance portion as well as an estimate of the patient's portion.

Helpful Hint: *As a dental office employee you can only <u>estimate</u> the insurance portion based on information provided by the patient and the insurance company.*

The ledger gives you information about past account history including any past-due charges and when insurance claims were filed.

On the ledger page, use the icon on the toolbar to *Select a Patient*; choose Joshua Reeves for this exercise. Examine the ledger; you will notice that Joshua has an outstanding balance of $133 with no insurance claim filed.

You will be adding some additional treatment for Joshua. Click on the icon on the top for *Enter Procedure(s)*; a new dialog box opens (Figure D-20). This can also be done by clicking on *Transactions* from the top toolbar and using the drop-down menu.

The date is set as today's date by default. If you know the procedure code already, enter it in the procedure code area; if not, use the arrows to open *Procedures*. Choose the appropriate category for the treatment; this will give you specific choices on the procedure code list to the right. For Joshua, choose Restorative and X3447 Amalgam-3 surf prim/perm. Add a number for the tooth treated (let's use Tooth #30) and then add MOD as the surfaces. To save time, use the arrows to the right of the surfaces to select which surfaces to include in the restoration. The office fee will automatically display; if you want to change it, you can make those changes here.

If you are discounting the fee because of prepayment or professional courtesy, don't do it while posting the fee, you will want to account for the types of discounts separately for tracking purposes.

When the information is correct, click Add to see the treatment on the procedure list.

When your procedure list is correct, click on OK/Post to add it to the ledger. Go back to the ledger for Joshua Reeves to see the new posting. Notice the new balance and the estimated insurance portion; this is what you would want to collect from the patient today if there are no other financial arrangements.

ADJUSTING AN ACCOUNT

For practice, let's give Joshua a courtesy discount of $25

Go to the *Ledger* screen; make sure you have selected Joshua Reeves as your patient. Highlight the transaction(s) you are going to adjust, then select *Transaction* from above the icon toolbar. When you click on *Transaction,* the drop-down menu will include *Enter Adjustment*; click on it. When you select the adjustment option a dialogue box opens (Figure D-21).

Enter Adjustment has options to select the amount and reason for the discount. There is also a place to leave an additional note for clarification. By categorizing what the discount was for, you'll be able to track how much the practice has written off for each type of discount.

To complete the adjustment, click OK.

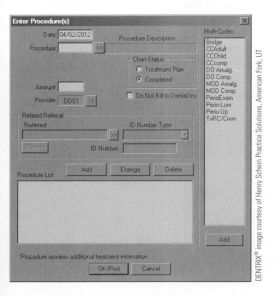

Figure D-20 Enter Procedure

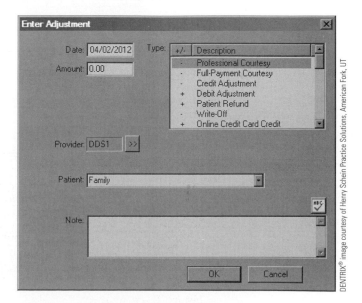

Figure D-21 Enter Adjustment

EDITING OR DELETING A TRANSACTION

It happens sometimes; you make an error you need to correct. Clicking on the transaction that is incorrect will bring up an *Edit or Delete* dialog box.

Make the correction or delete the transaction by changing the incorrect field(s) or choosing Delete in the lower left hand corner of the dialog box. If you have made an adjustment to the transaction, don't forget to remove it too.

ENTERING A PATIENT PAYMENT

The first step in entering a payment is to make certain it is accounted for correctly, that way you will be able to balance your accounts at the end of the day. To enter a payment, go to the *Ledger* and select the correct patient.

Get to the *Enter a Payment* box by choosing the icon that looks like a check with G $ under it or go to *Transactions* and choose *Enter Payment* from the drop-down menu.

Add the information to the fields and when you are satisfied that the information is correct, click OK to enter the payment. To check the accuracy of your entry, look at the ledger for the patient.

Let's say it's wrong. Correct it by double clicking on the ledger entry and DENTRIX® will bring up a correction screen.

Repeat steps to enter the payment again.

Helpful Hint: *When you make an error anywhere in DENTRIX®, first try double clicking on the incorrect entry, whether it is clinical, financial, or insurance; often you can make the correction right there.*

ENTERING AN INSURANCE PAYMENT

You will want to keep payments from patients and payments from the insurance companies separate so you immediately know which is which.

Insurance checks come two ways:

- With a total payment for the claim submitted

- With an itemized list of payments for each procedure

To enter an insurance payment, open the *Ledger* screen and select your patient, then double click on the insurance claim being paid (Figure D-22). For this example open the patient information or Joshua Reeves. At the top, under *Enter Payment,* are the drop-down choices of *Itemize by Procedure* or *Total Payment Only.*

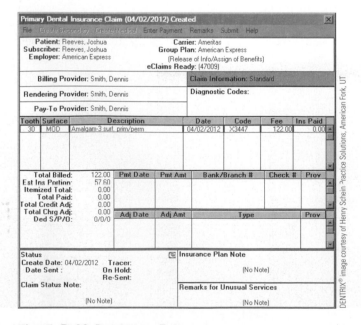

Figure D-22 Insurance Payment

Joshua had an insurance estimate of $57.60 as seen on the *Insurance Payment* screen. A coverage dialog box appears after you select *Itemize by Procedure* or *Total Payment Only* from the drop-down menu.

When you click OK to enter the amount paid, another dialog box will open for you to provide details about that payment, as seen in Figure D-23.

Complete the blank fields with the insurance check number and the bank.

Some insurance companies send funds by electronic payment. These are accounted for the same way, but be sure to check Electronic Payment so you aren't looking for a check you don't have at the end of the day.

When your entries are complete and accurate. Hit OK/Post to complete the transaction. You can return to the ledger to check your work and to the family file to see how it changed the account balance.

By managing patient accounts and payments correctly, it is very easy to see at a glance if the balance is the patient's responsibility and if additional insurance payments are expected.

WALKOUT STATEMENTS

A walkout statement is an update for the patient regarding their account. It can be used as a receipt or a bill. Within any dental office the best way to receive payment for the treatment done is on the same day as the visit. This saves staff time and the cost of printing and mailing statements. It also eliminates possible collection problems at a later date. If patients' financial arrangements allow them to pay the fee after the appointment, or for some reason they are unable to pay at the time of appointment, a walkout statement is a good alternative. Some offices even give patients an envelope to send payment to encourage them to do so promptly.

For clarification: Bulk statements can be sent electronically, much like insurance claims, but there are fees associated with doing both of those things because they go through a clearinghouse. Fees are small but electronic doesn't mean free. A small number of statements could be sent as attachments to emails without additional cost, but this method would be too time consuming on a large scale.

Patient statements are started when treatment is completed. To examine how practice management software works, start by accessing a patient chart; any adult chart will work. Highlight Tooth #18 with your explorer in the clinical chart and choose MOD amalgam from your procedure short cuts. Because we are only interested in the statement part of treatment, go to Completed, which is shown as a check mark at the right of EO, Ex, Tx.

Now you have a completed procedure so you can create statements.

You will be doing bookkeeping functions from the ledger, but you will also be able to print a walkout statement.

Select *Print* from the line above the graphic icons, then *Walkout* from the options in the drop-down menu. You will see a dialog box like in Figure D-24.

You have several areas that allow you to customize the walkout statement, including a place to include a message. Try including your own message.

Enhanced Form or Plain Form is determined by the printer the office uses so once this is set, it does not need to be changed.

Family Walkout will include any charges pending for family members as well as the patient. Then DENTRIX® prints appointment reminders for upcoming appointments for each family member.

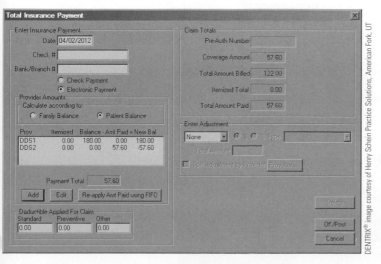

Figure D-23 Total Insurance Payment

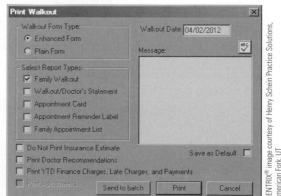

Figure D-24 Print Walkout

The Walkout/Doctor's Statement is used by offices that ask patients to do their own insurance billing. This form gives them the information needed.

You can also print an appointment card or an appointment label.

The additional fields are optional but could be added if it is your office protocol.

If you had a message you wanted to print on all your walkout statements, such as "Our office will be closed on Fridays beginning in June," you would save it as a default, When you are ready, you would either print it from the dialog box or send it to batch.

Helpful Hint: *When you send an item to batch, you will see it on the Office Manager's Desk. Doing that enables you to print everything at the end of the day or at a later date. From the Manager's Desk, you can view an item, print an item, or send it electronically. To view any of the items in the Batch Processor, highlight it and use the icon to the left of the printer that looks like a monitor screen.*

For practice: send your walkout statement to batch. Go to the Office Manager, highlight it, and then view it by using the monitor icon for print preview. Can you see your message?

QUICK CHECKOUT

Once you understand the checkout system and the individual steps in checking a patient out, you can graduate to the Quick Checkout. This will enable you to quickly post treatment and payments, and file insurance.

Choose a patient and go to the *Fast Checkout* icon, which looks like a little man going out the door.

If the patient you chose had no new treatment today, don't expect to see any; but if there had been something done, the insurance for that treatment would automatically go to the Batch Processor, so click OK to acknowledge that you understand. Enter any payment just for practice, and then go ahead and post it as cash.

Remember that anytime you handle cash payments, you will want to make sure you give the patient a walkout statement with the amount on it immediately.

You can check a patient out that quickly and you will use this method all time.

CORRESPONDENCE

Writing Quick Letters

As you work on writing letters, printing is an option but is not necessary. All exercises can be done without making a hard copy, so don't be concerned if you are not connected to a printer. If you do have access to a printer, it is fun to have some samples of your work.

After accessing the DENTRIX® program, go to *Family File* to begin exploring the basic letter-writing process. Select a Patient (you can use yourself for fun), and click on the icon with the envelope for quick letters. You should see a dialog box like the one in Figure D-25.

To view what each letter looks like before the actual patient information is added, highlight the letter name and open the template.

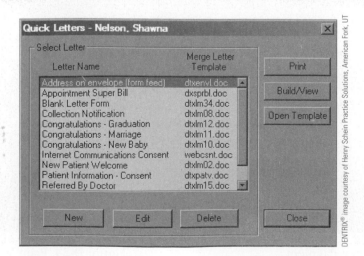

Figure D-25 Quick Letters

Please take the time to open each letter and see the variety of prewritten letters available. Now let's personalize the letter.

For this exercise choose the New Patient Welcome letter and highlight it.

To create the letter without looking at it, just click Print,

If you want to see how your letter looks before you print it, click on Build/View. Your letter will be merged with the patient's information and you can make any changes necessary.

Helpful Hint: *Unless you send this letter all the time, and even if you do, it is a good idea to view it before you waste letterhead on a letter that doesn't represent the professionalism of your office. For example: recently I received a "Thank you for visiting us" letter from a car dealer. Because of capitalization errors in the salutation, it was obvious that it was computer generated without taking time to double check it. Small things can make an impression; make sure your written communication makes an excellent impression.*

Use the Build/View button to see your letter. There are a couple of things you will want to correct before you print.

First, make sure the salutation is correct. For example: "Dear Cindy" or the more formal salutation of "Dear Ms. Lamkin," if appropriate.

Please note this can be set in *Patient Information* under *Salutation* to make writing letters even quicker. How you address patients will depend on office policy or the individual patient.

Second, in the body of the letter, in the third line is the term "reasonable prices," please change that to "reasonable fees.'

When you have made these changes, you are ready to print the letter. Go to File, Print, and your letter is ready to be sent.

A dialog box will ask if you want to save the changes to the letter. You could save it to a file to print later. Otherwise, once you have printed the letter, you can click No to saving it.

You also have an icon on your toolbar (next to the *Quick Letters* icon) that allows you to create a label.

Continue using yourself as the patient and open *Quick Labels* from the toolbar. You will see the dialog box shown in Figure D-26.

As you read through the list of possible labels, note how each would be used. If we were sending a letter to the person financially responsible for the account or the guarantor, you wouldn't want to click on *Quick Label* for the patient.

Once you have selected to whom the correspondence should be addressed, highlight the label and click on the Print key if you want to print it.

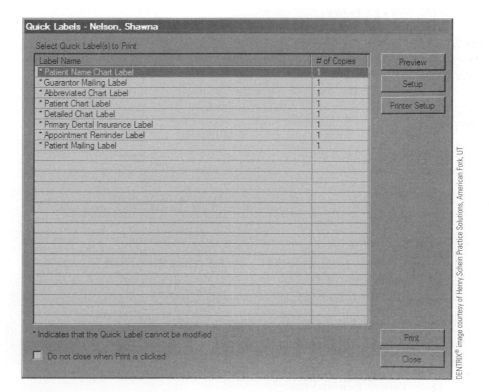

Figure D-26 Quick Labels

RECURRING CARE/RECALL

It is common for offices to send out postcards to patients who have appointments for routine cleaning and check-up appointments. Offices often use postcards to save on printing, paper cost, and also postage. To do this, we will be merging a list of patients with the postcard we want to send.

Go to *Office Manager* and from the toolbar (above the icons) choose *Letters* and click on it.

A dialog box should open with choices of several types of letters as seen in Figure D-27.

Choose *Continuing Care* by clicking on it and then clicking on *Cont, Care Cards–Appt,* and finally click on the *Edit* button so you can customize who these postcards should go to. That series of selections will bring up the dialog selection box with criteria for sending cards as seen in Figure D-28.

Helpful Hint: *Most offices have a regular protocol for making recurring care contacts. If you chose not to edit who you were sending postcards to, the system will send out cards to everyone. According to office protocol, you will want to be specific. If you send cards one month ahead, in December you set the system to send for January, etc.*

The *Patient Report View* dialog box will enable you to select the patients to receive cards. For this exercise, you should select patients who have appointments or the letter name *Cont. Care Cards–Appointment.*

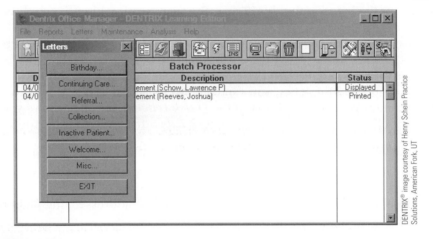

Figure D-27 Letters

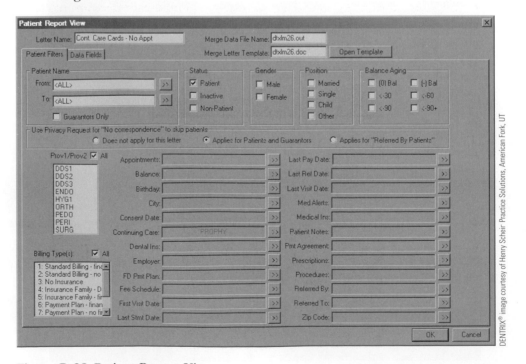

Figure D-28 Patient Report View

To the right of the letter name is the selection for Merge Letter Template. You would make this selection in an office based on the type of postcards you have purchased. Your User's Guide has specific information.

If you were sending out recurring care/recall postcards for January of 2012 to patients with appointments, use the arrows next to appointments in *Patient Report View* to select the dates shown in Figure D-29, *Select Appointment Range*. Under Search, choose existing patients with an appointment in date range.

After you have examined all your fields and determined these are the people to send cards out to, click the OK button.

You then return to the *Continuing Care Letters* dialog box (this happens after you click OK). Check to make sure the Cont. Care Cards–Appointment line is still highlighted.

If it is, click on the bottom left button for *Create/Merge*.

Under *Create/Merge* options select *Create Data File* and *Merge Letters* along with *Add to Journal*.

There are probably no patients in our tutorial database that fit these exact criteria so to practice, we'll repeat with different information.

Helpful Hint: *By covering the basics of what DENTRIX® is able to do with correspondence, you will be able to transfer your knowledge to a dental office. Just remember each office has its own procedures and they may be slightly different than what we have practiced. When you are confident with the basics, the transition will be effortless.*

Repeat the steps above with the exception of:
Use *Cont, Care Cards–No Appt*
Under *Select Appointment Range* "search" using Existing Patients with no appointments in the date range.
Use *Edit* to set your criteria
Use a date range of 1/1/2005 to 1/31/2008
Hit OK until you return to *Continuing Care Letters*, confirm that *Cont. Care Cards –No Appt.* is still selected, and then go to Create/Merge

There are several patients within this broader search range. You will see what would be printed on postcards to those patients. At this point you would print your postcards.

LETTERS

Sometimes you will want to send letters to a group of patients. While *Quick Letters* works great for single pieces of correspondence, it is not practical for larger mailings.

Follow the same basic steps for letters that we did for the continuing care postcard mailing.

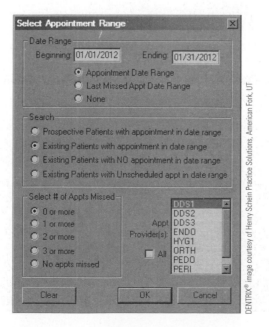

Figure D-29 Appointment Range

We will be sending out birthday letters using the Create/Merge function; go to the *Office Manager* (shown by the office chair icon or an icon on your desktop) and use the drop-down menu for letters from above the icon toolbar.

Look at the letter choices shown in Figure D-27 and choose Birthday at the top of the list. You will see a dialog box for Birthday Letters that shows you there are actually two versions of the letter: an adult letter and a child letter.

For this exercise choose the adult letter by highlighting it. You can complete your date range from this dialog box or go to Edit. We are sending out a January birthday letter to adults, so our date range is 01/01 to 01/31; then select the years to include as adults. Because we want to include any of the oldest patients in the practice, we'll choose a date well before the year anyone was born. Let's put 1900 as the beginning date and let's include anyone born up to 1996 as an adult.

Who you include as an adult may depend a lot on the wording of the letter and your practice, so adjust your dates accordingly. Don't offend the teens in your practice by sending a juvenile letter.

Instead of using the Fast Date selection box you could also use the edit function to add the dates included in this birthday mailing. The edit function allows you to make other choices such as: Do you send the letter just to patients? Or do family members that are nonpatients also get a birthday greeting? Do you want to send this to inactive patients as well as active patients?

When you are satisfied with your "birthday group," go to Create/Merge, create a data file, merge letters, and add to journal.

You will be able to see the letters in the group and you are ready to print.

Practice using the different letters and different criteria available until you feel comfortable.

CHANGING AN EXISTING LETTER

While DENTRIX® has carefully chosen the wording in the letters available, occasionally you may want to change a letter to make it reflect your practice. When you change the template you will be doing so for all future letters, so make sure you want to make the change and, if needed, that you have permission from the dentist/office manager.

To change letters, go to the *Office Manager* and open the letters from the drop-down menu.

Select *Anniversary in the Practice* from the *Welcome* group to change.

Select Edit to access the *Patient Report View* as previously seen. This time in the upper right corner, select *Open the Template*. The template is like the recipe for the letter, so you will want to be careful.

Find the line in the letter that reads "reasonable prices" and change it to "reasonable fees."

Close the letter from the upper right X, and when asked, say yes to save the change.

From now on this letter will include that change. For practice, repeat the steps and confirm the change, and then try making another one.

It is possible to create custom letters in DENTRIX® but doing so takes an excellent knowledge of word processing. Practice for now with the letters available in *Quick Letters* or from the drop-down menu under *Letters*. When you have mastered those you can refer to the User's Manual for step-by-step instruction on custom letters.

RUNNING REPORTS

If you have entered information completely and correctly, DENTRIX® can put it together for you in just about any report you would want to see. To run management reports, begin from *Office Manager*, go to *Report* from the top of your screen, and then *Management* and a list of possible reports will appear.

> **Helpful Hint:** *Some of these you can choose to run automatically with the Month End report, but let's look at running a couple manually. So if they print out automatically, why ever print them manually? Often doctors want specific information and they want it now, not at the end of the month. If your employer is having a meeting with colleagues, it is nice to have information about referrals that were sent to the office. Maybe there are financial decisions being made, such as large equipment purchases, and the doctor may want a practice analysis.*

To practice running reports begin by running a practice analysis. Choose *Analysis Summary* from the list displayed to get the dialog box with the specific information you would like to include in your report (Figure D-30).

If you are working in a multiple doctor office, you can choose to run your report for all of the providers or just one or a group; for example, just the information for the specialists in the practice.

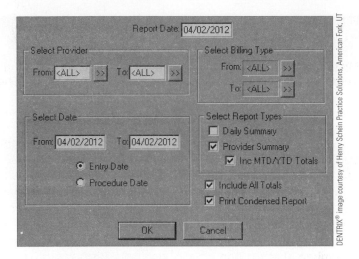

Figure D-30 Analysis Summary

Because the sample practice is small, you can select dates for an extended time to get more information. For an actual report, choose the dates that are important to your report.

On the right side of the dialog box, you can choose billing types; choose *Daily Summary, Provider Summary,* or both.

Helpful Hint: *If you are asked to run an analysis for your employer, ask what information is needed and be ready to give options. It will save you running a report that includes too much or not enough information.*

Once you are satisfied with your report criteria, click OK.

Where did it go? Look at the Batch Processor on the *Office Manager* screen. When you find it, highlight it and use the *Print Preview* icon from the toolbar to view it.

Try running other management reports on your own to see the information available. Give your reports a big date range because the database we are using is small.

Try running a Referred to Doctor report from 2005–2011.

View the report from the Batch Processor. It should look like Figure D-31.

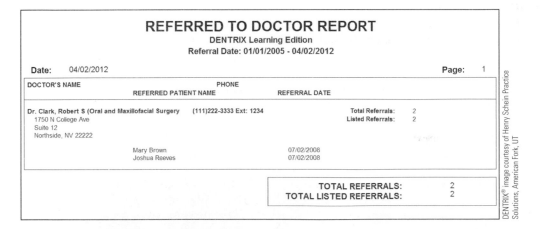

Figure D-31 Referral Report

PRACTICE GOALS ANALYSIS

Another type of report that is helpful when evaluating the production of a practice is the *Practice Goals Analysis*.

From the *Office Manager*, go to *Analysis* and begin with *Practice* or choose the icon on the toolbar. Because the end-of-month reports were not run for this practice last month, you will get a pop-up reminder; just click OK to Continue for now.

With the screen shown in Figure D-32, *Practice Goals Analysis,* each practitioner is able to set production goals and then evaluate their achievement.

Go to *Setup* and choose *Goals*; set up a goal to see this report.

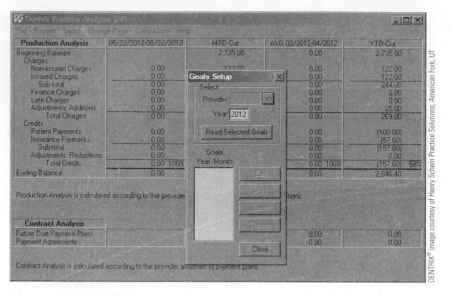

Figure D-32 Practice Analysis Goals

USING PRACTICE ASSISTANT

DENTRIX® Practice Assistant provides you with reports and graphs that are automatically scheduled to print or can be printed on demand. The Practice Assistant can also send these reports via email when set up to do so.

Find the icon for *Practice Assistant* and click on it or go to *Office Manager,* find *Analysis,* and choose *Practice Assistant* from the drop-down.

There are three tabs: *Reports, Scheduled Reports,* and an *Address Book* for storing e-mail addresses. Click on each tab and review.

View the list in the *Reports* tab. Highlight each report and use the view button to the right to see the type of report it generates (Figure D-33).

Highlighting and viewing *Adjustment Summary Report* should show you a report similar to Figure D-34.

To create a report, double click on the folder and fill in the desired criteria.

Reports in the *Practice Assistant* can be scheduled to print automatically by following the directions in your User's Guide.

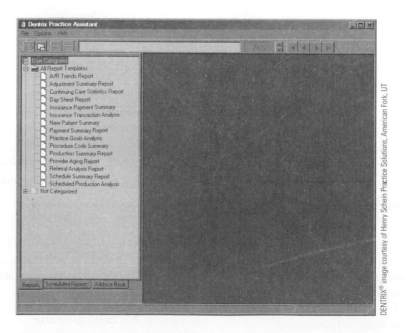

Figure D-33 Practice Assistant

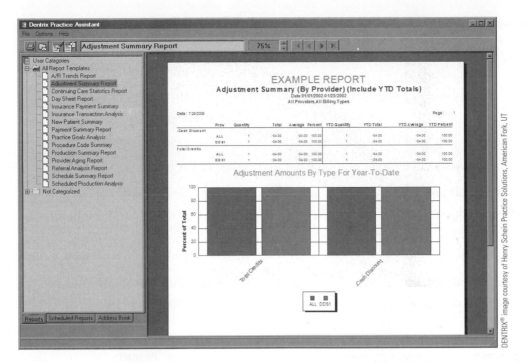

Figure D-34 Sample Report

SUPPLEMENTARY ONLINE INSTRUCTION

To view *On Demand Training* you will need Internet access; use the *Help* drop-down menu from any DENTRIX®
screen and select *On Demand Training*. From *On Demand Training* you will see a list of resources you can
view to help you in learning the Dentrix system.

MULTIPLE CHOICE

1. Corey Hansen has an outstanding balance of $377.00. How much of it is expected from the insurance company?

   a. Insurance should pay the entire amount.

   b. Insurance was not filed, no estimate on file.

   c. Insurance should pay $155.

   d. This patient does not have insurance.

2. What is the balance for Adria Johnson?

   a. $300

   b. $150

   c. $75

   d. No balance

3. What is the patient alert for Peggy Perkins?

   a. There is no alert.

   b. She has been sent to collections.

   c. She has a privacy request.

   d. Her alert is suspended.

4. Mary Brown has a balance on her account of $377.00. On which date were the fees posted?

   a. July 2, 2008

   b. April 5, 2005

   c. July 8, 2008

   d. July 2, 2009

5. Your patient, Harmon Davis, would like to know what percentage of endodontic treatment is covered by
   his dental insurance plan.

   a. 50%

   b. 70%

   c. No endo coverage

   d. 80%

6. What is the group number for Kimberly (Kim) Edward's insurance plan?

   a. VC

   b. 88442

   c. 442

   d. 1500

7. Which of the following is Michelle Keller's maximum annual insurance benefit?

   a. $1500

   b. $1000

   c. $2000

   d. $2500

8. Spencer Kenner would like to get braces. What percentage of his treatment would be covered?

   a. 50% up to $1000 per person or $3000 per family

   b. 60% up to $1500 per person

   c. 50% up to $2000 per person

   d. 50% with a $1500 lifetime max for orthodontics

9. Chad Little has dual insurance coverage. What is his annual maximum for the primary carrier?

   a. $1000 per individual

   b. $2000 per individual

   c. $1500 per family

   d. $2000 per family

10. Where are reports viewed before printing?

    a. The Ledger

    b. The Batch Processor

    c. View Reports

    d. Office Journal

11. The Appointment List includes which of the following?

    a. Balance Due

    b. Patient's Address

    c. Patient's Phone Number

    d. Health Status

12. To print a list of current insurance carriers, you would access it through:

    a. Ledger and Insurance Claims

    b. Reports and Reference

    c. Reports and Management

    d. Reference Insurance Maintenance

13. Which of these is not found in the Practice Assistant?

    a. E-Mail addresses

    b. Production Summary Report

    c. Archived Patient Summary

    d. Production Code Summary

14. Courtesy discounts should be taken off:

    a. Before posting

    b. After the insurance has paid

    c. After posting

    d. Done in secret

15. Incorrect clinical charting can affect:

    a. Insurance claims

    b. Amount of courtesy discount

    c. Patient statement

    d. All of the above

16. When a patient assigns benefits they go to the:

    a. Dentist/dental practice

    b. Employer repayment fund

    c. Patient/responsible party

    d. Subscriber

17. Electronic insurance claims and patient statements are:

    a. More expensive than paper statements

    b. Done at no cost online

    c. Not advisable due to HIPAA

    d. Handled through a clearinghouse for a small fee

18. Examples of Quick Letters include:

   a. New patient welcome

   b. Congratulations

   c. Consent

   d. All of the above

19. The salutation can be added to:

   a. Patient information

   b. Ledger

   c. Family File

   d. Letter only

20. Existing letters can be changed:

   a. But only with consent of dentist or office manager

   b. Changed for a single letter

   c. On a permanent basis

   d. All of the above

Critical Thinking

1. It is easy to create reports using practice management software. Explain the advantages of the entire dental team being able to access this information.

2. Letters are preprogrammed into the dental management software. Describe the steps that should be taken to send out high-quality correspondence that represents your practice well.

3. Because practice management software intertwines information, explain the potential errors that could result from incorrect chart management.

CASE STUDY 1

Dan stops by your office to discuss why he continues to get statements for procedures that he thought would be covered by his insurance. Do not assume blame; just figure out the problem.

1. Explain step by step how you could discover the discrepancy.

2. If the problem is yours, what could be done so this problem might be avoided in the future?

3. If the misunderstanding is the patient's, what could be done so this situation could be avoided in the future?

CASE STUDY 2

Susan comes to her appointment without her dental insurance card. She insists that she doesn't have a separate card for dental.

1. Using the information you do have, what can you find out about Susan's insurance.

2. What questions would you want to ask Susan about her coverage?

SKILLS ASSESSMENT

	Successful	Needs Assistance
Demonstrates entering a new employer.		
Demonstrates adding new insurance for patient.		
Demonstrates use of drop-down arrows to save time.		
Creates Quick Letter.		
Creates letter.		
Creates postcard mailing.		
Produces referral report.		
Produces production report.		
Explains how to view items prior to printing.		
Shows how to edit an existing letter.		
Accesses and navigates the patient ledger.		
Locates specific icons quickly.		
Produces patient walkout statement.		

IMPORTANT! READ CAREFULLY: This End User License Agreement ("Agreement") sets forth the conditions by which Cengage Learning will make electronic access to the Cengage Learning-owned licensed content and associated media, software, documentation, printed materials, and electronic documentation contained in this package and/or made available to you via this product (the "Licensed Content"), available to you (the "End User"). BY CLICKING THE "I ACCEPT" BUTTON AND/OR OPENING THIS PACKAGE, YOU ACKNOWLEDGE THAT YOU HAVE READ ALL OF THE TERMS AND CONDITIONS, AND THAT YOU AGREE TO BE BOUND BY ITS TERMS, CONDITIONS, AND ALL APPLICABLE LAWS AND REGULATIONS GOVERNING THE USE OF THE LICENSED CONTENT.

1.0 SCOPE OF LICENSE

1.1 <u>Licensed Content</u>. The Licensed Content may contain portions of modifiable content ("Modifiable Content") and content which may not be modified or otherwise altered by the End User ("Non-Modifiable Content"). For purposes of this Agreement, Modifiable Content and Non-Modifiable Content may be collectively referred to herein as the "Licensed Content." All Licensed Content shall be considered Non-Modifiable Content, unless such Licensed Content is presented to the End User in a modifiable format and it is clearly indicated that modification of the Licensed Content is permitted.

1.2 Subject to the End User's compliance with the terms and conditions of this Agreement, Cengage Learning hereby grants the End User, a nontransferable, nonexclusive, limited right to access and view a single copy of the Licensed Content on a single personal computer system for noncommercial, internal, personal use only. The End User shall not (i) reproduce, copy, modify (except in the case of Modifiable Content), distribute, display, transfer, sublicense, prepare derivative work(s) based on, sell, exchange, barter or transfer, rent, lease, loan, resell, or in any other manner exploit the Licensed Content; (ii) remove, obscure, or alter any notice of Cengage Learning's intellectual property rights present on or in the Licensed Content, including, but not limited to, copyright, trademark, and/or patent notices; or (iii) disassemble, decompile, translate, reverse engineer, or otherwise reduce the Licensed Content.

2.0 TERMINATION

2.1 Cengage Learning may at any time (without prejudice to its other rights or remedies) immediately terminate this Agreement and/or suspend access to some or all of the Licensed Content, in the event that the End User does not comply with any of the terms and conditions of this Agreement. In the event of such termination by Cengage Learning, the End User shall immediately return any and all copies of the Licensed Content to Cengage Learning.

3.0 PROPRIETARY RIGHTS

3.1 The End User acknowledges that Cengage Learning owns all rights, title and interest, including, but not limited to all copyright rights therein, in and to the Licensed Content, and that the End User shall not take any action inconsistent with such ownership. The Licensed Content is protected by U.S., Canadian and other applicable copyright laws and by international treaties, including the Berne Convention and the Universal Copyright Convention. Nothing contained in this Agreement shall be construed as granting the End User any ownership rights in or to the Licensed Content.

3.2 Cengage Learning reserves the right at any time to withdraw from the Licensed Content any item or part of an item for which it no longer retains the right to publish, or which it has reasonable grounds to believe infringes copyright or is defamatory, unlawful, or otherwise objectionable.

4.0 PROTECTION AND SECURITY

4.1 The End User shall use its best efforts and take all reasonable steps to safeguard its copy of the Licensed Content to ensure that no unauthorized reproduction, publication, disclosure, modification, or distribution of the Licensed Content, in whole or in part, is made. To the extent that the End User becomes aware of any such unauthorized use of the Licensed Content, the End User shall immediately notify Cengage Learning. Notification of such violations may be made by sending an e-mail to infringement@cengage.com.

5.0 MISUSE OF THE LICENSED PRODUCT

5.1 In the event that the End User uses the Licensed Content in violation of this Agreement, Cengage Learning shall have the option of electing liquidated damages, which shall include all profits generated by the End User's use of the Licensed Content plus interest computed at the maximum rate permitted by law and all legal fees and other expenses incurred by Cengage Learning in enforcing its rights, plus penalties.

6.0 FEDERAL GOVERNMENT CLIENTS

6.1 Except as expressly authorized by Cengage Learning, Federal Government clients obtain only the rights specified in this Agreement and no other rights. The Government acknowledges that (i) all software and related documentation incorporated in the Licensed Content is existing commercial computer software within the meaning of FAR 27.405(b)(2); and (2) all other data delivered in whatever form, is limited rights data within the meaning of FAR 27.401. The restrictions in this section are acceptable as consistent with the Government's need for software and other data under this Agreement.

7.0 DISCLAIMER OF WARRANTIES AND LIABILITIES

7.1 Although Cengage Learning believes the Licensed Content to be reliable, Cengage Learning does not guarantee or warrant (i) any information or materials contained in or produced by the Licensed Content, (ii) the accuracy, completeness or reliability of the Licensed Content, or (iii) that the Licensed Content is free from errors or other material defects. THE LICENSED PRODUCT IS PROVIDED "AS IS," WITHOUT ANY WARRANTY OF ANY KIND AND CENGAGE LEARNING DISCLAIMS ANY AND ALL WARRANTIES, EXPRESSED OR IMPLIED, INCLUDING, WITHOUT LIMITATION, WARRANTIES OF MERCHANTABILITY OR FITNESS FOR A PARTICULAR PURPOSE. IN NO EVENT SHALL CENGAGE LEARNING BE LIABLE FOR: INDIRECT, SPECIAL, PUNITIVE OR CONSEQUENTIAL DAMAGES INCLUDING FOR LOST PROFITS, LOST DATA, OR OTHERWISE. IN NO EVENT SHALL CENGAGE LEARNING'S AGGREGATE LIABILITY HEREUNDER, WHETHER ARISING IN CONTRACT, TORT, STRICT LIABILITY OR OTHERWISE, EXCEED THE AMOUNT OF FEES PAID BY THE END USER HEREUNDER FOR THE LICENSE OF THE LICENSED CONTENT.

8.0 GENERAL

8.1 Entire Agreement. This Agreement shall constitute the entire Agreement between the Parties and supercedes all prior Agreements and understandings oral or written relating to the subject matter hereof.

8.2 Enhancements/Modifications of Licensed Content. From time to time, and in Cengage Learning's sole discretion, Cengage Learning may advise the End User of updates, upgrades, enhancements and/or improvements to the Licensed Content, and may permit the End User to access and use, subject to the terms and conditions of this Agreement, such modifications, upon payment of prices as may be established by Cengage Learning.

8.3 No Export. The End User shall use the Licensed Content solely in the United States and shall not transfer or export, directly or indirectly, the Licensed Content outside the United States.

8.4 Severability. If any provision of this Agreement is invalid, illegal, or unenforceable under any applicable statute or rule of law, the provision shall be deemed omitted to the extent that it is invalid, illegal, or unenforceable. In such a case, the remainder of the Agreement shall be construed in a manner as to give greatest effect to the original intention of the parties hereto.

8.5 Waiver. The waiver of any right or failure of either party to exercise in any respect any right provided in this Agreement in any instance shall not be deemed to be a waiver of such right in the future or a waiver of any other right under this Agreement.

8.6 Choice of Law/Venue. This Agreement shall be interpreted, construed, and governed by and in accordance with the laws of the State of New York, applicable to contracts executed and to be wholly preformed therein, without regard to its principles governing conflicts of law. Each party agrees that any proceeding arising out of or relating to this Agreement or the breach or threatened breach of this Agreement may be commenced and prosecuted in a court in the State and County of New York. Each party consents and submits to the nonexclusive personal jurisdiction of any court in the State and County of New York in respect of any such proceeding.

8.7 Acknowledgment. By opening this package and/or by accessing the Licensed Content on this Web site, THE END USER ACKNOWLEDGES THAT IT HAS READ THIS AGREEMENT, UNDERSTANDS IT, AND AGREES TO BE BOUND BY ITS TERMS AND CONDITIONS. IF YOU DO NOT ACCEPT THESE TERMS AND CONDITIONS, YOU MUST NOT ACCESS THE LICENSED CONTENT AND RETURN THE LICENSED PRODUCT TO CENGAGE LEARNING (WITHIN 30 CALENDAR DAYS OF THE END USER'S PURCHASE) WITH PROOF OF PAYMENT ACCEPTABLE TO CENGAGE LEARNING, FOR A CREDIT OR A REFUND. Should the End User have any questions/comments regarding this Agreement, please contact Cengage Learning at Delmar.help@cengage.com.

MINIMUM SYSTEM REQUIREMENTS

Hardware:

Intel Pentium® IV 2.4 GHz
1 GB RAM
3 GB available disk space
DVD drive preferred. CD-ROM Drives are acceptable on workstations as long as there is a DVD drive on the network to be used to install Dentrix G4.
100 Mbps Ethernet card
Standard CRT/LCD monitor and video card capable of displaying 32-bit color and a resolution of at least 1024×768
USB chipset with two or more powered USB 2.0 ports
Additional PCI Express, AGP, PCI or USB 2.0 expansion slots may be required.

Supported 32-bit Operating Systems:

Windows® XP Professional
Windows® XP Tablet PC Edition
Windows® Vista Business
Windows® Vista Ultimate
Windows® 7 Professional
Windows® 7 Ultimate

Supported 64-bit Operating Systems:

Windows® XP Professional
Windows® Vista Business
Windows® Vista Ultimate
Windows® 7 Professional
Windows® 7 Ultimate

NOTES

NOTES

NOTES

NOTES

NOTES

NOTES

NOTES

NOTES